Occupational Therapy and Ergonomics

Applying Ergonomic Principles to Everyday
Occupation in the Home and at Work

'Gör det du tycker om,
och tyck om det du gör!'
('Do what you like,
and like what you do!')

Word: 'Anonymous'
Original painting on a postcard: Barbro Slotts, Borlänge, Sweden

Occupational Therapy and Ergonomics

Applying Ergonomic Principles to Everyday Occupation in the Home and at Work

Franklin Stein PhD, OTR, FAOTA
Ingrid Söderback Dr. Med. Sci, OT/L
Susan K. Cutler PhD
Barbara Larson MA, OTR/L, FAOTA

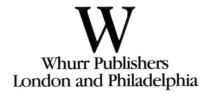

Whurr Publishers
London and Philadelphia

Other Wiley Editorial Offices

John Wiley & Sons Inc., 111 River Street, Hoboken, NJ 07030, USA

Jossey-Bass, 989 Market Street, San Francisco, CA 94103-1741, USA

Wiley-VCH Verlag GmbH, Boschstr. 12, D-69469 Weinheim, Germany

John Wiley & Sons Australia Ltd, 42 McDougall Street, Milton, Queensland 4064, Australia

John Wiley & Sons (Asia) Pte Ltd, 2 Clementi Loop #02-01, Jin Xing Distripark,
Singapore 129809

John Wiley & Sons Canada Ltd, 22 Worcester Road, Etobicoke, Ontario, Canada M9W 1L1

Wiley also publishes its books in a variety of electronic formats. Some content that
appears in print may not be available in electronic books.

British Library Cataloguing in Publication Data

A catalogue record for this book is available from the British Library

ISBN-13   978-1-86156-504-4
ISBN-10   1-86156-504-6

Typeset by SNP Best-set Typesetter Ltd., Hong Kong

Printed and bound in Great Britain by TJ International Ltd, Padstow, Cornwall

This book is printed on acid-free paper responsibly manufactured from sustainable forestry
in which at least two trees are planted for each one used for paper production.

Contents

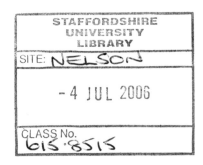

Preface

The field of ergonomics has broadened greatly since its development in the early part of the twentieth century. Occupational therapists have traditionally applied the principles of ergonomics in adapting the environments of individuals with disabilities so that they can be as functional as possible as well as teaching clients preventative techniques in the home and at work.

This book originated out of the clinical and teaching experiences of the authors. The first author, Franklin Stein, has taught a course in ergonomics at university level for over ten years and has taken a number of advanced courses in ergonomics, notably at the University of Michigan in Ann Arbor. Ingrid Söderback has used ergonomics in working with clients in their homes and in simulated kitchens in clinics. Susan Cutler, a professor of special education, has applied ergonomic principles as a consultant in the schools system. The fourth author, Barbara Larson, has applied ergonomics in her full-time work with corporations in developing healthy work environments.

As we work with our clients in a holistic manner, we incorporate ergonomic principles into interventions and preventative strategies in the home, work, leisure and school environments. The Occupational Therapy Practice Framework (American Occupational Therapy Association, 2002) includes the domains of ADL, IADL, education, work, play, leisure and social participation as the focus of the occupational therapist. We apply these guiding principles from the practice framework to the areas of the home and work environments while citing the importance of ergonomics in one's everyday life. The emphasis in the book is on ergonomic principles that are important in carrying out everyday occupation in the home or at work, such as lifting a heavy object without causing back pain, transferring successfully from a wheelchair to a bed, working on an assembly-line and preventing repetitive motion injuries, and using a computer while maintaining a neutral position. The concepts and principles derived from ergonomics are used to prevent musculoskeletal injuries, conserve energy and to use the body most efficiently when engaging in any activity or occupation. At first, ergonomic principles were applied primarily in work environments to prevent injuries on the job. In this book we have extended the concepts of ergonomics to other environments as well as in interventions and rehabilitation. We have also included psychosocial factors related to ergonomics, such as stress management, since this is a very important part of health and wellness and is an important risk factor in many diseases.

The principles of ergonomics are derived from the research of many professions including industrial engineering, human factors psychology, occupational medicine, nursing, vocational counselling as well as occupational therapy. Ergonomics is a multidisciplinary field. Each profession has a unique contribution to make in the application of ergonomics. Theory, research and practice are interrelated and cited throughout the book. We examine ergonomics from the unique perspectives of occupational therapy and special education.

The book is targeted at students taking courses in ergonomics and applying occupational therapy to work, home and school environments, occupational therapy and physical therapy practitioners who use a holistic approach in their treatment and incorporate ergonomic principles during intervention, special education teachers who apply ergonomics in the school environment and other healthcare professionals who are interested in the principles of ergonomics.

Reference

American Occupational Therapy Association (2002) Occupational Therapy Practice Framework: Domain and Process. American Journal of Occupational Therapy 56: 609–639.

Acknowledgements

Our heartfelt thanks are to:

- Students through the years who have asked questions and challenged us and by so doing have sharpened our thinking and helped us to apply evidence-based clinical practice and to use scientific results. We have organized the chapters in the book to foster critical thinking and to encourage students to apply an ergonomic approach as a model for interventions in occupational therapy. We especially acknowledge the occupational therapy graduate students at the University of South Dakota and at the Department of Public Health and Caring Sciences, Uppsala University who, through their assignments and discussions, taught us to appreciate how important teaching becomes as a learning tool for the professor.
- Occupational therapy colleagues who have contributed their expertise and clinical experience through their many publications and research, generating the content of this book. We acknowledge that the information and concepts in this book rest on the shoulders of many scholars and clinicians who have used ergonomics as a framework for occupational therapy.
- Occupational therapy researchers, clinicians, and rehabilitation and healthcare scholars who have contributed to this textbook through their publications that have been cited throughout the book.

Our special thanks are to:

- Karen Jacobs who helped us in the initial planning for this book and to the occupational therapy clinicians Birgit E. Hagsten, Åsa Gruwswed, Susanne Guidetti, Gunilla Hammarskiöld, Marina Härtull, Anita Lassfolk, Christina Nyström, Kerstin Sandberg and Marianne Söderström who supported us in our work.
- Our colleagues in Sweden: Professor Birgitta Bernspång, Umeå Professor Susanne Iwarsson, Lund; Doctor Maria Müllersdorf, Eskilstuna; Doctor Ulla Nordenskiöld, Göteborg; Doctor Marie-Louise

Schult, Danderyd-Stockholm; Associate Professor Inga-Britt Bränholm and Medicine Licenciate Gunvor Kratz, Stockholm.

Our deepest thanks for financial support are to:

- Principal Bo Sundqvist through The Principal's Foundation of Uppsala University, Uppsala.
- The Department of Public Health and Caring Sciences, Section of Caring Science, Uppsala University, Uppsala.

We also thank the University of South Dakota for granting a sabbatical to the first author in 1999 and travel expenses to Sweden in 2001 and 2005 and the University of Uppsala which generously supported our collaboration in writing this book.

We express much gratitude to our families, Jennie and Per and Sue's eight cats! We are thankful for the support in our many trips from Vermillion, South Dakota to Sioux City, Iowa, to Sweden and from Sweden to South Dakota and to Madison, Wisconsin in December 2002.

Finally, we acknowledge the value of e-mail and long-distance telephone calls in keeping us on track.

CHAPTER 1

Introduction: Purposes, theory and assumptions

Ergonomics is interdisciplinary: it bases its theories on physiology, psychology, anthropometry, and various aspects of engineering.

E. Grandjean, 1982, p. ix

Universal Design is defined as the design of products and environments to be useable by all people, to the greatest extent possible, without adaptation of specialized design.

Jon Christophersen, 2002, p. 13

Learning objectives

By the end of this chapter the learner will:

1 Be introduced to the content of the book.
2 Understand definitions of ergonomics that encompass a broad concept that includes adaptation, coping and environmental modification.
3 Understand the assumptions of the book.
4 Understand basic concepts underlying ergonomic principles.
5 Recognize those individuals with disabilities, according to the International Classification of Functioning, Disability and Health (ICF), who can potentially benefit from ergonomic interventions. The definitions of disabilities used in this chapter are, for the most part, based on the *International Classification of Functioning, Disability and Health (ICF)*, formerly entitled ICIDH-2 (World Health Organization, 2001).
6 Understand the relationship between ergonomics and occupational therapy.
7 Understand the differences between interdisciplinary roles in ergonomics.
8 Understand how to formulate a client-centred intervention plan using ergonomic principles.
9 Understand the importance of client compliance.

10 Gain knowledge about educational curriculum for ergonomics.
11 Gain knowledge about research evidence supporting the application of ergonomics.
12 Gain knowledge about ethical treatments in ergonomics.

Introduction

What is ergonomics and how can occupational therapists incorporate ergonomic principles into their everyday practice? Ergonomics is an interdisciplinary field that has evolved during the past century to create environments, tools, work methods and conditions to enable an individual to function efficiently in a safe environment. Universal design, ergonomics and client participation are the current integrative models for creating functional environments while increasing quality of life and client independence (Demirbilek and Demirkan, 2004).

Ergonomics first applied in work environments showed positive effects for both employers and employees. It is a win-win situation for the employer and employee if production is efficient and accidents on the job are reduced. The basic principles that underlie ergonomics are also key elements in occupational therapy practice, such as in modifying and adapting environments and in homemaking tasks to meet the needs of the client. The major premise of ergonomics is that machines are designed to fit the biological and psychological capacities of the individual rather than fitting the individual to the machine. This concept is very important in facilitating maximum production and in preventing injuries that could result from workers placed in vulnerable positions that cause undue stresses on nerves, joints, ligaments, tendons and muscles. By creating a healthy environment, the ergonomic concept reduces work-related injuries and, in the long run, increases industrial production. Ergonomic principles have been used to introduce such changes in the work environment as:

- altering the position of machines such as automobile assembly (Joseph, 2003)
- adjusting the pace of industrial work (Chee et al., 2004)
- incorporating rest breaks and warm-up exercises (Balci and Aghazadeh, 2003)
- changing and designing tools (Duke et al., 2004)
- improving environmental conditions, such as lighting, temperature, humidity and noise (Niemela et al., 2002).

At the same time, workers have been educated about healthy biomechanical practices, ergonomic principles and stress management.

Ergonomics is a dynamic field that is continually developing and expanding its range of practice. The history of ergonomics starts with the introduction of occupational medicine where physicians became aware of the relationship between work and disease (e.g. mining and black lung disease, or lead-based ceramics and brain damage). Currently, ergonomics incorporates research findings from a wide range of fields including occupational medicine, anatomy and physiology, biomechanics, industrial engineering and human factors psychology. Knowledge of ergonomics is applied to practice by professionals in various disciplines, including the industrial engineer, occupational physician, nurse hygienist, physical therapist, industrial psychologist and occupational therapist. Each professional discipline examines ergonomics from a unique perspective. The occupational therapist, as an essential member of a multidisciplinary team, works alongside the industrial engineer, human factors psychologist, industrial nurse, physical therapist, occupational physician, special educator and architect in creating a safe environment for the worker, home-maker or student.

Table 1.1 describes the major professions that are related to ergonomic practice in the work environment. It shows the overlap in the role functions between each profession; for example, the occupational therapist and physical therapist both provide services that restore and promote function and facilitate reasonable accommodation. The ergonomist and occupational therapist both do onsite job analyses.

Table 1.1 Interdisciplinary approach in ergonomics

Profession	Education	Job description	Typical work activities
Environmental Health Officer	Degrees in environmental health sciences, including courses in physics, chemistry, biology, earth science and ecology	Environmental Health Officers are responsible for interpreting and monitoring governmental rules and regulations regarding environmental and public health standards	• Inspecting commercial and industrial environments for factors and incidents related to environmental health • Recommending legal action • Educating the public and private sectors on environmental health practices • Using statistical analysis to measure air, water and chemical pollution • Writing reports on environmental health • Co-operating with other agencies • Keeping abreast of legislation related to environmental and public health standards

Table 1.1 Interdisciplinary approach in ergonomics (continued)

Profession	Education	Job description	Typical work activities
Ergonomist	Postgraduate education, with professional credentials. Unless the first degree is relevant, a one-year MA in Ergonomics or Human Factors is recommended. Relevant fields include: • Computer Science/Software Engineer • Engineering • Mathematics • Medicine • Occupational Therapy • Operational Research Scientist • Physical Therapy • Physics • Physiology • Psychology • Sports Science	Investigates the relationship between individuals and their work environments and then uses the findings to design safe and healthy workstations, systems, tools and equipment without compromising productivity	• Assessing the physical and psychological capacities of the individual in the work environment • Completing a job analysis, including how equipment, tools and machinery are used • Analysing the work environment for noise, lighting, toxic fumes, hazards, obstacles and any other environmental components • Generating possible solutions based on the findings • Selecting the best solutions based on a cost-effective analysis • Making recommendations for an implementation plan that considers cost, time, safety and productivity
Health and Safety Officer	Relevant experience with responsibility for health and safety in an industrial plant and a degree in a scientific, engineering or technical field	Health and Safety Officers provide advice to their employers to ensure that the workplace is complying with current and forthcoming legislation on health and safety (e.g. OSHA and NIOSH). A major role is the prevention of job-related accidents	• Advising management on safety policy and environmental factors • Educating employees regarding safety requirements and promoting safe practices with machinery or equipment • Assessing the hazards of dangerous materials or toxic fumes • Investigating job-related accidents • Maintaining statistics regarding job-related accidents

Table 1.1 Interdisciplinary approach in ergonomics (continued)

Profession	Education	Job description	Typical work activities
Health Promotion Specialist	Degrees in health-related, social or behavioural science preferred. Postgraduate studies in health education or health promotion	Health Promotion Specialists develop, implement and evaluate programmes to promote health within an industrial and governmental environment	• Working with organizations and local communities to assess health needs and promote health education • Researching and evaluating health prevention projects
Human Factors Psychologist or Industrial/ Organizational (I/O) psychologists	University courses offer MA, MSc or PhD degrees in psychology that specialize in Human Factors Psychology or Industrial-Organizational Psychology	Applies psychological principles and research methods to the workplace in order to improve productivity and to increase human comfort and safety. They conduct research on management and marketing problems, applicant screening, training and development, counselling, stress-management, and organizational development and analysis	• Developing governmental campaigns for health promotion • Supporting health education professionals by offering information, training and research • Selecting and placing new employees, and developing criteria for promotion • Setting up training programmes to improve worker skills • Facilitating organizational change • Measuring organizational work performance • Increasing quality of work environment and job satisfaction • Assessing and developing consumer demand • Designing safe work environments
Industrial Engineer	A BA in industrial or mechanical engineering is generally required for entry-level engineering jobs	Industrial Engineers carry out systems analysis by interfacing with management goals and operational performance. They examine the most effective ways for an organization to employ the	• Analysing the product and its requirements and applying mathematical methods to meet product requirements and design manufacturing and information systems • Developing organizational systems for cost analysis, design production and physical distribution of goods and services

Table 1.1 Interdisciplinary approach in ergonomics (continued)

Profession	Education	Job description	Typical work activities
Industrial Engineer (contd)		essential factors of production: people, machines, materials, information and environment	• Examining optimal plant locations with regard to availability of raw materials, transportation and overall costs
Industrial or Occupational Health Nurse	Occupational and environmental health nurses are registered nurses (RN). A BSN is preferred for an industrial nurse.	Occupational and environmental health nursing is the specialty practice that provides for and delivers healthcare services to workers at the work site. They work towards providing a safe and healthy work environment. They work in a variety of roles including nurse practitioner, case manager, educator, consultant and corporate director. They often work with the other members of an occupational health and safety team	• Providing nursing care to those with minor injuries and illnesses • Providing emergency care, preparing accident reports, and referring to physicians for further care if necessary • Offering health counselling • Assisting with health examinations and inoculations • Assessing work environments to identify potential health or safety problems
Occupational and Environmental Medicine Physician	Entry into postgraduate specialist medical training in Occupational and Environmental Medicine follows the same pattern as other clinical fields. On completion of a medical degree, the physician specializes in occupational medicine through a residency or fellowship programme	Occupational and environmental medicine physicians provide health advice to organizations to ensure worker safety. They work to reduce injuries and disease related to work, increase the flexibility of work options for injured or ill workers and assist other health professionals to ensure an early return to work.	• Treating individuals with work-related injuries and job-related diseases • Referring individuals to other medical specialists • Instituting rehabilitation methods with interdisciplinary teams • Evaluating the ability of individuals with work-related injuries to return to work • Recognizing workplace hazards and designing injury prevention programmes

Table 1.1 Interdisciplinary approach in ergonomics (continued)

Profession	Education	Job description	Typical work activities
Occupational Therapist	A BA or MA degree from an WFOT (or similar) approved programme is the minimum requirement for entry into this field. A course or clinical experience in work hardening, job analysis and ergonomics is preferred	Occupational therapists prevent, treat and restore function. Under ADA guidelines, they modify work environments for individuals with disabilities to function maximally on the job and recommend reasonable accommodations. Their main goal is to enable the individual to be independent, productive, and increase their quality of life. In the workplace they work with an interdisciplinary team in preventing work injuries. They may also act as case manager to individuals	• Using assessments such as Functional Capacity Evaluations (FCE) for screening and intervention planning • Interviewing clients to obtain work and medical history, vocational, leisure interests • Conducting a job analysis • Implementing services such as job modifications, psychoeducation, splinting, assistive devices, job simulation, stress and pain management • Documenting evaluation findings, intervention plan, progress and discharge planning • Supervising OT assistants • Engaging in consultative services and educational presentations
Physical Therapist	A BA or MA degree from an approved educational programme and passing scores on a licensure exam is the minimum requirement for entry into this field. A course or clinical experience in work hardening, work conditioning, and ergonomics is preferred.	Physical therapists provide services that help restore function, improve mobility, relieve pain and prevent or limit permanent physical disabilities of individuals sustaining injuries or disease. They restore, maintain and promote overall fitness and health. Under ADA, physical therapists collaborate with employers on issues regarding accessibility and	• Examining workers' medical and work histories, and making referrals to other agencies and medical professionals • Administering FCE and/or evaluation of strength, range of motion, respiration and neuromuscular function • Implementing work hardening, work conditioning, back schools, pain management and on-site work modification

Table 1.1 Interdisciplinary approach in ergonomics (continued)

Profession	Education	Job description	Typical work activities
Physical Therapist (contd)		reasonable accommodations. They may serve as case managers	• Documenting evaluation findings, progress, discharge planning and fitness to return to work • Supervising PT assistants
Rehabilitation Counsellor or Vocational Rehabilitation Consultant	Any of the following: • MA in vocational rehabilitation, rehabilitation counselling or vocationally-related field • professional member of rehabilitation counselling association • certification by Commission on Rehabilition Counselling or Work Adjustment and Vocational Evaluation Experience in industrial rehabilitation programme is preferred	Rehabilitation counsellors help people deal with the personal, social and vocational effects of disabilities. They evaluate the strengths and limitations of individuals, provide personal and vocational counselling, arrange for medical care, vocational training and job placement. They may serve as case managers	• Screening individuals for appropriateness of services • Interviewing individuals with disabilities and their families, in areas of education, training, work history, interests and personal traits • Arranging for and administering aptitude and achievement tests • Conferring and planning with other health professionals to determine the capabilities and skills of the individual • Conferring with client to develop a rehabilitation programme that includes training in job skills • Documenting evaluation findings, case management reports, rehabilitation plans, discharge plans and on-going consultative plans • Working with individuals to develop job search skills • Job coaching
Systems Analyst	Graduate study in industrial technology recommended with	Systems analysts use problem-solving methods in a business and technical context to	• Translating management requirements into highly specified strategic plans

Table 1.1 Interdisciplinary approach in ergonomics (continued)

Profession	Education	Job description	Typical work activities
Systems Analyst (contd)	undergraduate degree in psychology, business, engineering or health-related field	evaluate the production requirements of an organizational system. They are active in the design, testing and implementation phases of a project. They usually work with a team in close coordination with management and the workforce	• Identifying logical and innovative options for potential solutions and assessing them for both technical and business suitability • Ensuring technical compatibility and user satisfaction with recommended decision • Planning and working in flexible manner to meet deadline • Preparing detailed reports in a timely manner

Note: Adapted from *Careers in Occupational and Environmental Medicine* by the American College of Occupational and Environmental Medicine, *Careers in Occupational Medicine: Specialist Training in Occupational Medicine*, Society of Occupational Medicine, *Careers in Occupational Medicine: What is Occupational Medicine?*, Society of Occupational Medicine, *Certification*, American Board for Occupational Health Nurses, *Occupational Outlook Handbook: 2004–2005*, Bureau of Labor Statistics, 2004–2005; *Environmental Health Officer in Close-up*, Graduate Prospects Ltd, 2004; *Ergonomist in Close-up*, Graduate Prospects Ltd, 2003; *Health Promotion Specialist*, Graduate Prospects Ltd, 2004; *Inspectors in Public and Environmental Health and Occupational Health and Safety*, Human Resources Development Canada; *Systems Analyst in Close-up*, Graduate Prospects Ltd, 2003; *What Is an Occupational Physician?*, Chiropractic and Osteopathic College of Australasia, 1998; *Occupational and Environmental Health Nursing Profession Fact Sheet*, American Board for Occupational Health Nurses, *What Are Industrial-Organizational Psychologists?*, Society for Industrial and Organizational Psychology.

Ergonomics and occupational therapy

The application of ergonomic principles is a key dimension to holistic occupational therapy practice. What are the primary roles of occupational therapists? Occupational therapists traditionally have three primary roles: healer, teacher/facilitator and environmental adapter using ergonomic principles. As a healer, the occupational therapist uses purposeful and meaningful activities during intervention. For example, the occupational therapist may use relaxation therapy as an activity to reduce the symptoms of depression (Stein and Cutler, 2002). The Range of Motion Dance (ROM; Valentine-Garzon et al., 1992) could be used with clients with osteoarthritis to reduce pain. In this role, the occupational therapist uses activities as a healing mechanism to restore health to the individual. This is the traditional role of the occupational therapist. The selection of the specific occupation or activity depends on the purpose, which is the therapeutic goal and the meaningfulness of the activity to the client. Activities are applied in a client-centred approach which serves to reduce the symptoms of a disability and to increase the health of the client.

The second role of the occupational therapist is to serve as a teacher/facilitator to the client. In this role, the occupational therapist teaches or facilitates the client's knowledge of health and wellness strategies, steps in independent living and biomechanical principles. For example, the occupational therapist may teach energy conservation methods to a patient with multiple sclerosis (Mathiowetz et al., 2001). In another example, the occupational therapist teaches proper biomechanics in lifting objects for a client who has back pain (Randolf, 1984). This approach is referred to as psychoeducational practice. Psychoeducational techniques are also used with clients with psychosocial problems, such as depression and schizophrenia. Lectures, discussion and hands-on techniques are explored in teaching the client relaxation techniques, prescriptive exercises, nutrition, biofeedback, creative arts, poetry and anger management (Stein and Cutler, 2002).

In the third role, the occupational therapist applies ergonomic principles in preventing injuries and disabilities (Rhomberg et al., 1995), and adapts and accommodates the environment for an individual with a disability by improving function in the areas of self-care, work and leisure. This third role of the occupational therapist in applying the principles of ergonomics in practice (Drake and Ferraro, 1997) is the primary focus of this book. A brief history of ergonomics is included as the last chapter (see Chapter 9) to give the reader an understanding of the interdisciplinary nature of ergonomics. The Socratic Case Study Method was selected as a teaching model in this book to engage the reader in active learning, clinical reasoning and problem-solving while applying the principles of ergonomics.

Ergonomics began as a method to improve production and to prevent injuries in industrial workers (Melhorn et al., 1999). The methods used were to fit the machines and tools to the biomechanical and physiological characteristics of the worker. In contemporary practice, occupational therapists use ergonomic principles not only in work environments, but also in the home (Iwarsson and Isacsson, 1996), at school (Stonefelt and Stein, 1998) and in leisure settings (Kratz et al., 1997). Occupational therapists adapt and modify the environment to meet the needs of the individual (Matthews and Tipton-Burton, 2001) while the individual is developing independent living skills. The individual with a disability learns to be as functional as possible in work, self-care and leisure through assistive technology and the modification of the environment.

During the twenty-first century, universal design is a model for modern living in the areas of home, school, work and leisure. In universal design (Christophersen, 2002), the environment is modified to enable all people with or without disabilities to access buildings and function independently in the home and work environments. For example, pavements are modified so that wheelchair users can have independent mobility. Christophersen (2002) proposes seven principles that form the basis for the application of universal designs.

1 Equitable use: The design is useful for all people with diverse abilities, such as lowering curbs in streets for individuals in wheelchairs and children on bicycles.
2 Flexibility in use: The design can be modified to accommodate a wide range of preferences and abilities, such as tools that can be used by left- and right-handed individuals.
3 Simple and easy to understand: Individuals with all levels of cognitive functioning, literacy or language skills can understand the design. Feedback is provided to the individual during and after task completion.
4 Perceptual information: The design can be used by individuals with sensory loss (visual, auditory, tactile). For example, sub-titles are used in television programmes for individuals with hearing disabilities.
5 Tolerance for error: The design prevents serious accident or injury by having fail-safe features. Fail-safe environments are provided to eliminate hazards or accidental errors.
6 Low physical effort: The design allows individuals to be in a neutral body position and use minimal effort.
7 Size and space for approach and use: The design accommodates for individual differences in body size, posture and mobility.

The concept of universal design is futuristic and its implementation is based on the resources of a nation. In developed countries throughout the world universal design is perceived as a right of the individual, while in developing countries universal design is not a priority issue when compared with universal healthcare, elimination of poverty and economic development. However, the concept of universal design is an underlying principle of modern living and should serve as a model for adapting and modifying work and home environments.

Purposes of the book

The major purpose for this book is to integrate theory and research from the ergonomic literature and to apply it to clinical practice. The primary principles used to (a) prevent injuries in the worker and homemaker and (b) increase function in the individual with a disability are introduced. A pragmatic approach to intervention is used.

Specifically, the main aims of the book are to:

1 Define ergonomics within the broad concepts of environmental adaptations in work and home environments

2 Explain or clarify how environments can be adapted to:
   a) prevent injury
   b) facilitate occupation at work and in the home for individuals with disabilities

3 Utilize the language of International Classification of Functioning, Disability and Health (ICF, World Health Organization, 2001)

4 Apply ergonomics to the fields of:
   a) prevention
   b) intervention
   c) habilitation
   d) rehabilitation

5 Help students to understand the history of occupational medicine and human factors psychology in its relationship with ergonomics

6 Provide means for occupational therapists to help individuals and corporations comply with recommendations to ergonomic adaptations such as Occupational Safety and Health Association (OSHA) regulations and ergonomic standards

7 Incorporate a psychosocial and person-centred approach to ergonomics by recognizing the importance of:
   a) job satisfaction
   b) reduction of occupational stress
   c) job competence
   d) realistic goal-setting
   e) social skills
   f) self-esteem and efficacy
   g) development of client responsibility and compliance
   h) family interactions

8 Help the learner to:
   a) assess and evaluate the needs of the client in the home and at work
   b) identify assessments for developing an ergonomic intervention programme

9 Incorporate ergonomics into the broad areas of:
   a) orthotics
   b) adaptive devices
   c) prosthetic devices
   d) self-care
   e) accessibility designs

10 Develop intervention protocols that are consistent with the Americans with Disabilities Act of 1990 and adapted to the individual needs of the client

11 Examine interventions and outcomes in case study designs

12 Use the Socratic case-based learning method to apply the principles of ergonomics in various case studies.

13 Incorporate research findings and scientific principles into applying ergonomics.

Theory and assumptions underlining this book

The major theories underlying the application of ergonomics include cybernetics and person-centred ergonomics. In general, a theory presents an explanation of events or phenomena that can be tested and confirmed. How can a theory guide ergonomic principles that are applied in the home or in the work environment? A theory can generate principles guiding interventions and assumptions that can be applied in practice. For example, ergonomics starts with the theory that the work environment should be adapted or designed to meet the needs and physical and mental characteristics of the individual. In other words, fitting the environment to the individual rather than fitting the individual to the environment is a basic principle in ergonomics. This theoretical concept assumes that the environment should be altered to fit the individual. This concept, which is accepted as a truism in the industrial world, was not always practised as evidenced in the history of occupational medicine where there are numerous examples in the nineteenth century of children working in mines suffering extreme temperatures and unhealthy conditions, or chemical workers being exposed to toxic substances without concern for their health and welfare.

The practice of ergonomics is a twentieth-century idea. It is based on awareness of occupational diseases; respect for the individual; knowledge regarding the relationship between trauma to the joints, nerves and muscles of the body and musculoskeletal diseases; the interrelationship between the mind and the body and the effects of stress on health; understanding of anthropometry (the measurement of human physical characteristics) and work capacity; and the application of engineering to design efficient and healthy work environments and tools to prevent occupational injuries and diseases.

Cybernetics

The theory of cybernetics as first proposed by Norbert Wiener (1948) generated a scientific revolution in computers, industrial manufacturing and robotic devices. Wiener invented the term 'cybernetics', from the Greek word meaning governance, to generate a new field of enquiry into the understanding of human and machine systems through interdisciplinary efforts. He conceived that scientists from established fields such as engineering, physics, chemistry, mathematics, neurophysiology and psychology could work together in a creative way to understand how systems work. Cybernetics led to the development of the computer, artificial intelligence, robotics in industry, biofeedback and indirectly to ergonomics. What is the relation between cybernetics and ergonomics? Both fields are interdisciplinary and incorporate knowledge from engineering and psychology. Cybernetics relies on feedback to gain an understanding of how systems function. For example, in a cybernetics approach to memory, the mathematician von Neumann (1958) made an analogy between computers and the human nervous system:

> The observation I wish to make is this: processes which go through the nervous system may, as I pointed out before, change their character from digital to analog, and back to digital, etc., repeatedly. Nerve pulses, i.e., the digital part of the mechanism, may control a particular stage of such a process, e.g. the contraction of a specific muscle or the secretion of a specific chemical. (pp. 68–69)

In ergonomics, engineering knowledge is used to modify work environments and, in addition, research from psychology is used to help decrease stress in the worker. Both cybernetics and ergonomics apply feedback to understand and modify how systems work. For example, cybernetics researchers use biofeedback to understand how an individual can control blood flow. In the case of ergonomics occupational therapists use feedback in understanding how modifying work positions can reduce musculoskeletal injuries. Feedback is an important concept that is derived from the initial work of Wiener and von Neumann. Wiener (1950), in his influential book on cybernetics and society, analysed the industrial age and the implications for the future. He stated:

> Let us consider what for example the automobile factory of the future will be like; and in particular the assembly line, which is the part of the automobile factory that employs the most labor. In the first place, the sequence of operations will be controlled by something like a modern high-speed computing machine. (p. 209)

Wiener's view in 1950 had proved true by 2006. The revolutionary ideas of Wiener have generated creative thinking in the manufacturing area that indirectly led to the design of machines and equipment that are efficient, cost-effective and fit the human anatomy and psychological characteristics.

Person-centred ergonomics

Person-centred ergonomics began in the 1950s shortly after ergonomics developed in the late 1940s. In a way, person-centred ergonomics fits into the model of cybernetics in that the ergonomist in this approach considers the man–machine system as 'dynamic and constantly responding to the inputs of the human operator' (Osborne et al., 1993, p. 9). Paul Branton, a psychologist, is considered to be the founder of person-centred ergonomics (Osborne et al., 1993). Person-centred ergonomics focuses on the complete needs of the worker within the work system. The worker's values, perceptions, motivations and even philosophy of life are considered when designing and altering work environments. Ergonomic solutions will vary depending on the worker's psychology, education, personality and values. In addition to these variables, the ergonomist in this approach considers the psychophysiology of the worker, including worker physical and psychological characteristics that can affect the work tasks. For example, the ergonomist in this approach would focus on the worker's ability to handle stress, the worker's interests, factors that create boredom in the worker, the skills necessary in performing the work tasks, physical comfort of the worker in performing the work tasks and the amount of decision-making, responsibility and authority that is part of the job. All of these factors would be considered as well as the traditional engineering approach that examines the tools, machines and work processes. The person-centred approach is humanistic and considers the importance of the individual's needs and characteristics in designing ergonomic workstations. It is the opposite of a Procrustean bed where the engineer designs a workstation based only on average physical characteristics that are required to perform a work task without considering the whole individual and the psychological factors that are required to do a job effectively.

> Altogether the Brantonian View represents a major shift in emphasis in ergonomics thinking towards what Paul Branton described as a 'Design from the Man Out' approach. In this view, the human being is at the center of the working situation, and we must understand the abilities, responsibilities and requirements which people bring to the situation, not just the foibles, in order to be able to deal adequately with the system. (Osborne et al., 1993, p. 15)

Cybernetics and person-centred ergonomics provide the theory base applying ergonomic principles in occupational therapy. These theories are congruent with occupational therapy's philosophy of humanism, scientific reasoning, beneficence and client-centred treatment.

Assumptions of an ergonomic model in occupational therapy

Ergonomics is an integrative concept that ties together the interplay between the human being and the environment. It is a basic concept in occupational therapy because the environment is used as an intervention, such as when the home environment is adapted for an individual with a residual disability from a brain injury. The environment used as an intervention media is translated as a mediator between the occupational therapist and the client. Case studies and clinical reasoning are used to facilitate learning. Research has shown that students incorporate what they learn into practice more efficiently if they can apply problem-solving methods to actual cases (Keller et al., 2001). In this context, occupational therapy students learn how to apply results obtained from assessment instruments by using a holistic approach to evaluate the client's disability status in a simulated environment.

The client's unique solutions in coping with his or her disability should be respected. For example, the therapist should respect the wishes of the client if he or she decides not to use a prosthetic device, but seems to cope well by using unimpaired parts of the body to compensate for the loss of a limb. The client should also be supported when requesting an assistive device, even though the client has a progressive disease and may or may not benefit from the appliance.

The knowledge derived from ergonomics is directly related to how occupational therapists adapt and modify environments to increase client independence. It fits into our use of occupation, it is humanistic, increases the choices of clients, encourages clinical reasoning and provides a tangible way to explain the purposes of occupational therapy to clients and health colleagues.

Evidence-based practice is substantiated by research. Ergonomic practices that are applied are based on research. In general, research from the fields of industrial engineering, architecture, occupational medicine and human factors psychology has generated knowledge that occupational therapists can apply in clinical settings. In this book research evidence is cited to support the principles of ergonomics used in occupational therapy.

Fitting in with a humanistic philosophy, we ally ourselves with patient groups that advocate the integration of individuals with disabilities in society. We maintain a holistic view of treatment and a compassionate approach to the client by using people-first language and client-centred interventions. Alternative or complementary interventions offer clients a choice. By advocating a preventative approach we can reduce the overall medical expenses of clients and create healthy environments. We realize that client motivation and compliance are essential if interventions are to be successful. In general, we must consider occupational therapy as an ergonomic means to intervention.

Basic concepts and terms related to ergonomics

A common terminology is needed when communicating with the client, family members and colleagues regarding findings from evaluations, progress notes and discharge summaries. Occupational therapy as an interdisciplinary profession needs to use the same terminology in assessment and intervention shared by the ergonomic team. For example, the terms job analysis, accommodation, work hardening, work conditioning, accessibility and job coach should be used uniformly (see Glossary). The terms defined in the following paragraphs include variables related to personal, environmental, occupation and activity factors. The definitions described are adapted from the MESH terms in the National Library of Medicine database (http://www.pubmed.org) and the ICF (World Health Organization, 2001).

Personal factors

These relate to the psychological variables that affect an individual's ability to cope with a disability while adapting to home and work environments.

- Clients are those individuals who seek ergonomic counselling and interventions from the occupational therapist. Caregivers are also included as clients when necessary.
- Individuals with disabilities are usually limited in their ability to perform *activities of daily living* (ADL). ADL is divided into two areas:
  1 Personal activities of daily living (PADL) are those used in self-care or self-maintenance. These include activities requiring basic cognitive and motor planning, such as eating, toileting, dressing and undressing, grooming, ambulating and communicating.
  2 Instrumental activities of daily living (IADL) include high-level executive functioning and decision-making, such as shopping (Söderback, 1988), completing school assignments, commuting to work or school, and engaging in a leisure activity. Stress management is also considered an IADL (Stein and Cutler, 2002) because the client plans and incorporates relaxation activities into his or her everyday schedule.
- *Human factors* are intrinsic to the individual and include the personality characteristics, attitudes, beliefs, values, roles and habits of the client and the family members, caregivers and friends who interact with the client. These psychological factors are considered when the occupational therapist plans with the client an intervention programme. When a person has a disability, attention must be paid to the client's attitudes towards independence as well as functional limitations and capacities (World Health Organization, 2001). For example, an elderly woman who has broken her hip in a fall may choose to live at home after leaving hospital rather than moving to a residential home for the elderly, even though her bedroom at home is on the second floor. A staircase elevator could be considered critical to maintain her independence. Another solution is to relocate the bedroom to the ground floor if feasible. The three choices are carefully evaluated by the occupational therapist considering the financial implications of installing the lift, the client's ability to live at home with a disability and the input from family. Another consideration is to have a visiting nurse and occupational therapist home team to monitor the individual's self-care abilities. This is a common example of how human factors can affect the client's decision to remain in his or her home or apartment rather than living in a nursing home.
- *Functioning* denotes the individual's ability to engage in activities of daily living, work, leisure and social interactions.
- *Disability* is an 'umbrella term which covers impairments, activity limitations and participation restrictions' (World Health Organization, 2001, p. 6). Disability is any limitation to perform activities in daily life and/or restrictions to participate in life situations in the home and at work. Disabilities comprise (a) cognitive and social issues, such as learning new information, applying knowledge to everyday situations or communicating with others; (b) mobility problems in everyday

settings, such as using public or private transportation; (c) a psychoso-cial illness, such as depression, which may result in an inability to cope at work or school and to perform daily occupations; (d) learned help-lessness that causes dependence on others and a passivity in decision-making; or (e) negative attitudes or stigmas towards the client with a disability that limits the individual's opportunities. A disability can be mild, moderate and severe in its impact on functioning. Often, the severity of the disability is in proportion to the individual's capacity to function. For example, an individual diagnosed with a moderate trau-matic brain injury (TBI) may have a disability that restricts his ability to dress independently, work a full eight-hour shift, and participate in bowling activities. Other individuals with a diagnosis of mild TBI may have no restriction in activity or participation.

• *Impairments* are abnormalities of a body structure or function that cause a significant deviation or loss, and may result in functional limi-tations or restrict participation in social activities. The following impairments are those relevant to clients seeking occupational therapy interventions in a home or work environment:

1 *Mental impairments* include low cognitive function, or mild to severe brain damage caused by a trauma, infection or deterioration of brain function.

2 *Sensory, voice and speech impairments* include blindness or low vision, deafness or hearing loss, and speech impediments.

3 *Neuromusculoskeletal and movement-related impairments* include muscle and reflex dysfunction, joint restrictions, and movement and mobility limitations. Examples of neuromuscu-loskeletal disease include (a) stroke or traumatic brain injury resulting in pareses or hemiplegia, (b) spinal cord injuries (para-plegia, quadriplegia or tetraplegia), (c) post-polio syndrome and (d) progressive degenerative disease (e.g. multiple sclerosis, Parkinson's disease). Musculoskeletal diseases are characterized by symptoms of pain, stiffness, restricted range of joint motion and muscle weakness. They include (a) rheumatoid arthritis, (b) anky-losing spondylitis, (c) muscular dystrophy, (d) osteoarthritis and (e) herniated disk resulting in low back pain. Individuals with amputations (e.g. removal of pelvis, parts of the legs or parts of the arms) are considered examples of neuromusculoskeletal and movement-related impairments.

4 *Impairments of skin and related structures* include pressure or ulcer sores. People who sit more than 75 per cent of the day or who lie in bed most of the time are at risk of developing these impair-ments.

5 *Psychosocial limitations* include individuals with severe mental ill-ness such as schizophrenia, depression, bipolar mental disorders or other psychiatric diagnoses that interfere with everyday functioning.

Environmental factors

Environment is defined as 'the external elements and conditions which surround, influence, and affect the life and development of an organism or population' (World Health Organization, 2001, p. 14). The environment is composed of concentric layers that are comprised of objects, tasks, social groups and culture.

'Environmental factors are extrinsic to the individual' (World Health Organization, 2001, p. 16) and include the person's immediate setting (e.g. home, furniture, appliances) and social interactions within the environment (e.g. family members, relatives, acquaintances, peers, caregivers). The physical settings include the architectural characteristics that may be influenced by the legal system. For example, Federal laws (e.g. Americans with Disabilities Act [ADA, 1990]) require public buildings and public transportation to be accessible to persons with disabilities (Kornblau et al., 2000; Lathrop, 1997). Additionally, in some of the European countries, individuals with a disability may receive a grant to adapt or modify the home. Ergonomically designed equipment, utensils and furniture make the environment more accessible to individuals with disabilities. However, just the availability of these objects is not enough; the occupational therapist, with knowledge of biomechanics and the functional limitations of the client, can determine which of the ergonomically designed equipment are most appropriate (Mace, 1998).

Occupation and activity factors

Occupation refers to the purposeful and meaningful activities in which individuals engage in the home, school, work and leisure environments. These activities range widely, depending on the environment, and may include such occupations as working in the garden, handwriting, cooking and biking. The occupational therapist uses occupation in working with clients to improve their everyday functioning by embedding goals, such as increasing upper extremity range of motion and muscle strength by prescribing a horticulture activity.

• *Purposeful activities* fulfil individual needs in everyday living. For example, a purposeful activity such as cooking fulfils the individual's everyday need for basic nutrition. Another example is walking, where the activity fulfils the individual's need for physical exercise. Therapeutic activities refer to goal-directed activities when they are used with individuals with disabilities. For example, a computer activity could be helpful for an individual who has had a stroke in improving cognitive and perceptual abilities. In another example, ceramics can be used as a purposeful activity for an individual with depression in helping the individual to express inner feelings.

- *Meaningful activities* are directly related to the individual's unique interests. A meaningful activity does not necessarily have to be purposeful, although it can be. These activities arise from the individual's interests and personal characteristics. For example, a meaningful activity for a ten-year-old child may be taking apart an appliance (e.g. old television, computer, etc.), while a 50-year-old man may enjoy gambling. In both cases, the activity is meaningful to the individual, but not necessarily purposeful or therapeutic. The goal of the occupational therapist is to select an activity that is purposeful and therapeutic as well as meaningful to the client.

Definitions of ergonomics

- Ergonomics is the study of those human abilities and characteristics that affect the design of equipment, systems and jobs. The terms ergonomics and human factors can be used interchangeably (Cornell Univeristy, nd, para 1).
- 'The American Industrial Hygiene Association (AIHA) defines ergonomics as a multidisciplinary science that applies design principles based on the physical and psychological capabilities of people to the design of jobs, equipment, products, and workplaces' (American Industrial Hygiene Association, 1994, p. 1).
- 'Ergonomics includes both the physical and psychological aspects of adaptation. When there is a mismatch between the physical requirements of the job and the physical capacity of the worker, work-related musculoskeletal disorders (WMSDs) can result. Workers who must repeat the same motion throughout their workday, who must do their work in an awkward position, who must use a great deal of force to perform their jobs, who must repeatedly lift heavy objects or who face a combination of these risk factors are most likely to develop WMSDs' (Occupational Safety and Health Administration (OSHA), US Department of Labor, 2001, p. 1).
- In the psychological aspects of ergonomics the emphasis is on placing the worker in the most favourable position by matching the workers' psychological and cognitive capacities to the requirements of the job. The goal in psychological ergonomics is to help the worker to achieve maximum job satisfaction. In the cognitive aspect of ergonomics the workload is considered as a potential factor in creating stress and job burnout (Folts et al., 1995).

The term ergonomics is also equated with the term *Human Engineering*, which is defined as the 'science of designing or equipping mechanical devices or artificial environments to the physiological, or psychological requirements of the people who will use them' (National Library of Medicine, 2002–2005).

In general, ergonomics is referred to as the study of work and working conditions in order to improve efficiency. This term constitutes the base for the occupational therapist in adapting and modifying the home and work environments to prevent work-related injuries and to facilitate independent function in the individual with a disability.

Using these definitions and concepts, the definition of ergonomics may be expanded to:

> Ergonomics is the modification of the environment, design of tools and application of biopsychosocial strategies to prevent injuries to the worker, student, and homemaker, and to increase functional independence for individuals with disabilities.

In this definition, the environment is conceptualized as the setting in which the individual engages in purposeful and meaningful occupations. The study of ergonomics, then, allows the occupational therapist to create a healthy environment, design tools and use psychosocial methods to prevent injuries and enable the person with a disability to function independently.

Relationship between ergonomics and occupational therapy

In this expanded definition of ergonomics, occupational therapists deal with adapting the environment so that individuals with a disability can function maximally (see Table 1.2, pp. 22–3). The environment is fitted to the individual. For example, in an individual with a stroke, the environment is modified to meet the needs of the individual to be independent in activities of daily living (Pedersen et al., 1997). The school environment (e.g. the desk, chair, computer, lights, psychosocial factors, etc.) is adapted to enable the student with a disability to learn. Ergonomic principles have been used by occupational therapists in many ways, such as adapting the position of equipment such as looms (Maughan, 1962), or adapting writing utensils for individuals with a spinal cord injury (Cooperman and Vendetti, 2000). In the course of practice, occupational therapists routinely integrate ergonomic principles with occupational therapy to enhance function and to solve problems related to a person's interaction with the environment. Ergonomic principles as they are utilized by occupational therapists optimize the individual's occupational performance in the areas of self-care, productivity/work and leisure (see Figure 1.1).

Intrinsic to the occupational therapist's role is a holistic understanding of the functional impact of injury or disease and of the multiple factors linking the person and his or her environment (whether physical, social, psychological, cultural or spiritual) affecting performance (Canadian Association of Occupational Therapists, 1997).

INTERVENTIONS IN THE ENVIRONMENT

GOALS	
Prevent injuries and disabilities	Improve the client's performance in self-care, productivity and leisure activities

TYPE OF INTERVENTIONS		
Adapt the environment	Use of assistive technology in the home and workplace	Teaching-learning-process

THE PERSON WITH A DISABILITY

THE OCCUPATIONAL THERAPIST

DESIRED OUTCOME				
Independence in self-care activities	Improve quality of life	Improve well-being	Improve satisfaction with assistive technology	Improve client's follow-through to recommended and agreed upon interventions

Figure 1.1 Interventions in the environment. The model is an interactive system between the occupational therapist and an individual with a disability. Goals, interventions and outcome are an integral part of this ergonomic model.

Table 1.2 Relationship between ergonomics and occupational therapy

	Ergonomics	Occupational therapy
Definition	Ergonomics is the modification of the environment, design of tools and the application of biopsychosocial strategies to prevent injuries to the worker, student and homemaker, and to increase functional independence for individuals with disabilities	Occupational therapy, based on a holistic biopsychosocial scientific model, assists individuals with and without disabilities to perform occupations at their maximum functional level in work, self-care, leisure and interpersonal relationships
Purposes	To prevent injury and enhance safety and performance based on fitting machines and the environment to individual capacities while maintaining production standards	To develop and restore functional skills and prevent injuries by employing purposeful and meaningful occupation
Methods	• human–machine interactions • problem-solving approach • interdisciplinary • evolving theory and applied research to discover best methods to fit machines to humans • design of machines and tools to accommodate maximum work capacity	• human–occupation interactions • problem-solving approach • single discipline • evolving theory and applied research to discover best methods to restore functions and design environments to enable individuals with and without disabilities to master independent living

Table 1.2 Relationship between ergonomics and occupational therapy (continued)

	Ergonomics	Occupational therapy
Assessment procedures	Assess the job requirements and environment to ensure adequate functioning, safety and injury prevention through:	Assess the ability to master the environment and prevent injuries in home, school, leisure and work through:
	• job analysis (including cognitive workload, stress and psychosocial issues) • work-site analysis • anthropometry • biomechanics • environmental considerations • psychometrics	• task analysis • clinical observation • behavioural evaluation • individual assessment (including self-care, leisure, cognition) • functional capacity evaluation

Ethical considerations in ergonomics

Ethical principles guide the practice of ergonomics in the relationship between the therapist and client. The values and cultural differences in the client are recognized and respected. The American Occupational Therapy Association's Code of Ethics (American Occupational Therapy Association, 2000) is a guide for clinicians in working with clients and colleagues in a just and fair manner. The Code includes six principles of ethical behaviour. These include:

1 avoiding harm to clients
2 respecting the rights of clients to privacy and request for accurate information
3 providing competent treatment
4 abiding by the laws governing the profession
5 being truthful in communicating with clients, other professionals and the public
6 interacting with colleagues in a fair manner without prejudice or deceit.

These ethical principles are important in the occupational therapist's everyday practice. It is especially important in the ergonomics arena where the therapist works in the community interacting with clients in their homes, and work, school and leisure environments. Therapists are placed in a position of responsibility and trust with clients who may be vulnerable to abuse and harmful practice. The personal values and attitudes of the therapist are also important in communicating to the client a sense of trust and security. The client should feel secure that the therapist is concerned for his or her well-being, treats the client with respect regardless of creed, religion or nationality, allows the client freedom in making decisions throughout the intervention process, expresses empathy and respect for the client, is honest and direct in interacting with the client and uses good judgement and clinical reasoning in working with the client. Ethical behaviour reflects the honesty of the therapist in interacting with clients and their families, co-workers and the public.

Formulating an intervention plan using ergonomic principles

Table 1.3 provides a guide for designing an intervention plan using ergonomic principles. In the ergonomic model, an intervention plan is devised by the therapist and the client working together. The programme is based on an initial evaluation, goal-setting, implementation of interventions, measurement of outcome and redesign of a new intervention plan as needed. 'Evaluation is an analysis of an individual's behavior, characteristics, aptitudes, and present functioning gained through specific tests, clinical observations, and procedures that can be used for treatment planning or discharge recommendations' (Stein and Roose, 2000, p. 102).

In the ergonomic model, the term intervention is used rather then treatment since the therapist works towards preventing injury and disease as well as restoring function. The evaluation process is used to identify factors in the home, school, work and leisure environments that impact on the client's ability to be independent. For example, in the work environment the occupational therapist evaluates the job tasks, tools used, risk factors and facilities. In the home, the occupational therapist evaluates the client's ability to cook, clean and perform other home-making tasks. The therapist also assesses the accessibility of the entrance, risk factors for falling, and other factors related to living independently in the home. In the school environment, the occupational therapist would evaluate the student's academic tasks, classroom furniture, writing utensils, environmental lighting, noise, distractions and other factors affecting the ability to learn. In the leisure environment, the occupational therapist evaluates the client's ability to engage in meaningful leisure activities. The factors related include a task analysis of the activity, the tools and implements involved in the activity and the environment in which the activities take place.

Another aspect of the evaluation process is the assessment of the client's functional performance. Normative tables can be used to establish standards of performance. The results of the evaluation process, using both the environmental factors and functional performance, help determine the direction and strategies used in the intervention.

In organizing the intervention strategies, the occupational therapist works in alliance with the client. Short- and long-term goals are planned that are both relevant and meaningful to the client, and understandable, so that the client can see the purpose of the interventions. The outcomes of intervention should be measurable by using standardized instruments, physiological measures and self-evaluations. Short-term goals are usually related to performance components of sensorimotor, cognitive or psychosocial factors. Long-term goals are related to the performance areas of work, school, self-care and leisure. Other factors in planning intervention strategies involve preventing injury such as cumulative trauma injuries on the job, falls in the home, or learning difficulties in school. Other goals involve supporting the client's functional independence in the home, such as helping the client with a disability to maintain his or her cooking skills by rearranging the placement of kitchen appliances. Another goal is to promote functional independence by using assistive devices, orthoses, cue cards, language boards and assistive technology.

The implementation of the intervention plan will depend on the resources available to the therapist in the environments where the intervention takes place. For example, in the work environment, the goal may be to prevent carpal tunnel syndrome in an individual working on a computer for six hours a day. The therapist can recommend use of an ergonomically appropriate computer keyboard, chair or mouse and placement of the computer, and consider the use of copyholders or a footrest. The therapist would do an onsite job analysis in the evaluation phase and then set up goals with the client and a time schedule for implementation. Behavioural interventions at the job site could include rest breaks, stretching one's hands or wrists and standing up at the workstation.

The next step in the intervention plan is to evaluate the outcomes related to the established goals. The assessments used in the initial evaluation are re-administered by the therapist and compared with the initial evaluation results. In this phase of the intervention plan the therapist discusses with the client his or her compliance with the suggested recommendations and the ability to self-regulate behaviour. Outcome also includes the client's quality of life and functional independence. This can help the client to understand where his or her functional level is compared with clients of similar disabilities, age or job title.

Based on the outcome results the therapist and client might redesign an intervention plan. In general, the intervention plan is dynamic and should be changed or adapted to the needs and wishes of the client. It is truly client-centred and democratic in that decisions are the joint responsibility of the client, family and treatment team.

Table 1.3 Guide for designing intervention plan using ergonomic principles

Initial evaluation	Set intervention plan and generate goals	Select modalities as part of the intervention plan	Implement the intervention plan	Evaluate outcome	Redesign intervention plan
Evaluate the home, work, school or leisure environment considering accessibility, workstation, classroom and recreation facility	Set goals using RUMBA: Relevant, Understandable, Measurable, Behavioural, Achievable	Intervention media or modalities including assistive devices, orthoses, cue cards, language boards, assistive technology	Consider the architectural accessibility; the ergonomical designed furniture, assistive devices, orthoses and psychosocial strategies	Clients' compliance to intervention plan	New intervention plan based on outcome results
Client identifies problems interfering with functional independence	Short-term goals are tied to performance components: • sensory-motor • cognitive • psychological	Strategies to teach the client methods to perform activities such as self-care activities, energy conservation, joint protection, proper positioning and biomechanics	Consider cognitive aptitudes, personality traits, physical capacity, vocational and avocational interests, and personal values	Level of functional independence	Change interventions based on outcome results
Therapist does a task analysis of activities related to the homemaker, worker, student and targeted leisure occupation	Prevent injury or disease	Rearrange placement of furniture and other objects. Recommend, ergonomically designed furniture, chairs and cushions	Redesign environment so that client is as independent as possible in self-care, work and leisure	Increased quality of life, health and wellness, and independence	Redesign tools and environment based on outcome results

Table 1.3 Guide for designing intervention plan using ergonomic principles (continued)

Initial evaluation	Set intervention plan and generate goals	Select modalities as part of the intervention plan	Implement the intervention plan	Evaluate outcome	Redesign intervention plan
Assess psychosocial factors that impact on the client's ability to carry out the task	Support the client's independence and growth in motivation	Plan intervention based on establishing rapport and therapeutic alliance, and increasing client motivation	Consider therapeutic strategies to help client to be motivated and goal-directed	Increased client motivation to improve function	Reconsider therapeutic strategies in gaining cooperation of the client toward reaching personal goals
Assess the impact of the disability on the client's performance	Compensate for client's disability and functional independence	Adapt the environment and design tools to increase independence	Psychoeducational instruction regarding environmental control	Increased independence and performance	Revise implementation plan to foster maximum performance

Importance of client compliance

The client's motivation to change and to comply with recommended ergonomic solutions is an important part of the intervention process. How can occupational therapists help clients to incorporate ergonomic adaptations, good biomechanical principles and stress management strategies into their everyday lives? Compliance to prescribed interventions for clients is a significant problem for all healthcare workers. Clients who are prescribed therapeutic diets, medications, exercise programmes, relaxation protocols and bladder management, for example, need assistance in compliance with the regime. Behavioural management techniques to improve a client's compliance have been studied extensively and they are an important focus of current researchers in healthcare. For example, in one study of factors associated with compliance to therapeutic diets Thomas et al. (2001) found that favourable attitudes towards compliance, a supportive environment and the clients' knowledge about their diets all contributed to increased compliance. Another study of clients with osteoporosis (Silverman and Schein, 2001) indicated that communication between the health professional and client was a key factor in compliance. The quality of the client–provider relationship was a factor recognized as important in compliance in a study of adherence to treatment recommendations in clients with diabetes (Ciechanowski et al., 2001).

Other factors identified in the literature to increase client compliance included goal-setting, informant support and self-care monitoring (Ocampo-Balabagno, 1999), readiness of the client to change his or her behaviour (Reust et al., 1999), consideration of the client's lifestyle (Yavuzer et al., 2000), and mutual communication and decision-making between the health provider and client (Silverman and Schein, 2001).

On the other hand, factors associated with non-compliance include time conflicts, lack of client effort and poor health status (Sabati et al., 2001). Incorrect interpretation of treatment recommendations (Gago et al., 2000), not recognizing individual differences between clients (Lahdenpera and Kyngas, 2001), complications or side effects of treatment (Alvarez, 2001), poor client–provider communication (Ciechanowski et al., 2001), and financial, transportation, barriers and increased stress (Reust et al., 1999) were also identified as interfering factors with client compliance.

In general, client compliance will increase if the occupational therapist considers the following principles:

1 Inform the client why he or she should follow the prescribed recommendations.
2 Establish rapport with the client that ensures client trust.
3 Involve the client in decision-making by asking for input into the intervention process.
4 Provide opportunities for the client to report any side effects or contraindications of interventions or use of assistive devices.

5 Decrease barriers to communication especially with speakers using a second language.
6 Establish behavioural contracts where clients are given written instructions on how to perform an activity or treatment procedure.
7 Have the client keep a daily log of activities to monitor compliance.
8 Use diagrams and pictorial representations to demonstrate prescribed activities to client.
9 Have the client use videos, DVDs, CDs and audio tapes explaining procedures in steps and providing feedback to client to change behaviour.
10 Be aware of cultural differences in clients.
11 Do follow-up with the client to evaluate the client's compliance and progress.

Types of principles of ergonomics

What are the types of principles, supported by research evidence, that can be applied by an occupational therapist to all clients, whether working in a school, work, home or leisure environments? The following paragraphs describe two types of principle: (a) those that prevent physical injuries in promoting function, and (b) those that foster psychological health in these environments.

Physical principles

• Always try to place joints in a neutral position when doing repetitive motions such as typing, lifting objects, working on an assembly-line, engaging in a sport or doing housework. The neutral position while sitting is the position where the feet are on the floor; ankle, knee and hip joints are in approximately 90 degree angles; the back is straight; and the elbow joints are at approximately 90 degrees. The wrist should be in a neutral position when performing tasks, meaning that the wrists are not in ulnar or radial deviation. In this position the individual can be efficient in a work task without putting undue pressure on any of the joints of the body (Richards et al., 1996; Timm et al., 1993). While standing and performing an activity, the individual should be able to use his or her arms close to the body, with the elbows in approximately 90 degrees angles (Iwakiri et al., 2002).
• Face the work directly without twisting the body, back, neck or hips when completing a task (Torén, 2001).
• Take short rest breaks (micro-pauses) when working intensively at a task (Henning et al., 1997).
• Bend at the knees when picking up items from the floor. This movement takes the load off the back and prevents injury (Yip, 2001).
• Use warm-up stretching exercises before engaging in prolonged tasks. This prevents tears in tendons, ligaments or muscles that are tight and prone to injury (Safran et al., 1989).

- After doing prolonged movements do the opposite movement. For example, if an individual is doing an activity which involves flexion of the wrist take a short break and exercise the wrist in extension (Nathan et al., 2001).
- In the morning do warm-up exercises that gently stretch muscles and joints through each range of motion slowly and rhythmically such as a T'ai-Chi-type exercise (Kirsteins et al., 1991).
- Condition back muscles through Williams flexion exercises (Blackburn and Portney, 1981) and McKenzie extension exercises (Al-Obaidi et al., 2001).

Psychological principles

Psychological factors can affect an individual's performance at work, school, in the home or at leisure. These factors, such as job satisfaction, competency, security, freedom of expression, tolerance towards one's diversity, respect from others and self-actualization, will influence self-perception. This, in turn, can lead to increased productivity, motivation and commitment to change. Ergonomics as a model does not exist in a vacuum. The environment can be effectively adapted and changed, the workstation can be improved and yet the individual may feel alienated and ineffective. The occupational therapist working in a holistic framework looks at the individual as well as the environment. The following factors should be considered in this model:

- Involve the client in all decisions while changes are being made. For example, if a computer workstation involves changes in the position of the monitor and mouse or the selection of an ergonomic chair, then the client should feel free to express his or her opinion during the process and enter into the decision process (Sumsion, 1993).
- Recognize that the individual's attitude towards the job, school, work, home tasks and leisure activities will affect success in the activity (Dehlin et al., 1981). If an individual has low job satisfaction it will definitely negatively interfere with the ergonomic adaptations (Iverson and Deery, 2001).
- Stress can be a negative factor to the individual and affect the person's performance (Reed, 1984).
- Self-esteem will affect the individual's motivation, efforts and efficacy (Sharma and Mavi, 2001).
- The client's relationship with the family (Alexy et al., 2001; Clark, 2001) will affect the success of the ergonomic intervention.
- Social skills can affect the client's ability to work (Tsang, 2001), be successful in school (Gonzalez and Sellers, 2002), engage in leisure activities and relate to the family in the home (Greco and Morris, 2001).
- Consistency between the client's aptitude and potentials and goal-setting in the work, school, home and leisure environments (Jenkins, 2002).

Summary

In this introductory chapter, ergonomics is defined, as applied by the occupational therapist, as fitting the environment to meet the needs of the worker, student and homemaker. The occupational therapist in this role adapts and accommodates the environment to prevent injuries and disabilities, and to maximally increase the function and independence of individuals with disabilities. The occupational therapist works with an interdisciplinary team of professionals to accomplish these goals. Universal design principles are advocated as a method to design products, tools and environments that can be used by all individuals. In achieving these goals the occupational therapist works in conjunction with architects and engineers to design homes, offices, parks and communities that can be used by all individuals whether they are in a wheelchair, use a walker or have cognitive impairments. The general principles of ergonomics are applied to create these user-friendly environments. Ethical considerations and client compliance are important factors in the success of an ergonomic intervention plan.

Review questions

1 What role does the occupational therapist play in the field of ergonomics?
2 How does the occupational therapist differentiate his or her role from other professionals in the field of ergonomics?
3 What is the origin of ergonomics?
4 How is ergonomics defined?
5 What is universal design and what are the seven principles of universal design?
6 What are the underlying concepts in the ergonomic model?
7 What is the relationship between ergonomics and occupational therapy?
8 What are the differential roles of the various disciplines in ergonomics?
9 What are the ethical standards for the occupational therapist?
10 What are the steps involved in setting up a client-centred intervention plan.

References

Alexy, B., Benjamin-Coleman, R. and Brown, S. (2001). Home healthcare and client outcomes. Home Healthcare Nurse, 19, 233–239.
Al-Obaidi, S., Anthony, J., Dean, E. and Al-Shuwai, N. (2001). Cardiovascular responses to repetitive McKenzie lumbar spine exercises. Physical Therapy, 81, 1524–1533.

Alvarez, C.A. (2001). Noncompliance or human nature? Clinical Nurse Specialist, 15, 51.

American Board for Occupational Health Nurses (nd, a). Certification. Retrieved 23 December 2004, http://www.abohn.org/certif.htm and http://stats.bls.gov/ocohome.htm

American Board for Occupational Health Nurses (nd, b). Occupational and Environmental Health Nursing Profession Fact Sheet. Retrieved 23 December 2004 from http://www.aaohn.org/press_room/fact_sheets/profession.cfm

American College of Occupational and Environmental Medicine (nd). Careers in Occupational and Environmental Medicine. Retrieved 23 December 2004 from http://www.acoem.org/guidelines/article.asp?ID=29

American Industrial Hygiene Association (1994). An Ergonomics Guide to VDT Workstations. Fairfax, VA: AIHA.

American Occupational Therapy Association (2000). Occupational therapy code of ethics. American Journal of Occupational Therapy, 64, 614–616.

Americans with Disabilities Act of 1990, Pub. L. No. 101-336, 2, 104 Stat. 328 (1991).

Balci, R. and Aghazadeh, F. (2003). The effect of work-rest schedules and type of task on the discomfort and performance of VDT users. Ergonomics, 46, 455–465.

Blackburn, S.E. and Portney, L.G. (1981). Electromyographic activity of back musculature during Williams flexion exercises. Physical Therapy, 51, 878–885.

Bureau of Labor Statistics, US Department of Labor (2004–2005). Occupational Outlook Handbook. Retrieved 23 December 2004 from http://www.bls.gov/oco

Canadian Association of Occupational Therapists. (1997). Position statement on occupational therapy and ergonomics. The Canadian Journal of Occupational Therapy, 64, 229.

Chee, H.L., Rampal, K.G. and Chandrasakaran, A. (2004). Ergonomic risk factors of work processes in the semi-conductor industry in Peninsular Malaysia. Industrial Health, 42, 373–381.

Chiropractic and Osteopathic College of Australasia (1998). What is an Occupational Physician? Retrieved 23 December 2004 from http://www.coca.com.au/newsletter/1999/SEP9906a.htm

Christophersen, J. (Ed.) (2002). Universal Design: 17 Ways of Thinking and Teaching. Oslo: Husbanken.

Ciechanowski, P.S., Katon, W.J., Russo, J.E. and Walker, E.A. (2001). The patient–provider relationship: Attachment theory and adherence to treatment in diabetes. American Journal of Psychiatry, 158, 29–35.

Clark, R.E. (2001). Family support and substance use outcomes for persons with mental illness and substance use disorders. Schizophrenic Bulletin, 27, 93–101.

Cooperman, M.S. and Vendetti, T. (2000). Outcomes of tendon transfers on school-related activities for children with tetraplegia. Topics in Spinal Cord Injury Rehabilitation, 6(Suppl), 233.

Cornell University (nd). DEA 651 class notes; Ergonomics origin and overview. Retrieved 23 December 2004 from http://ergo.human.cornell.edu/student-downloads/dea325notes/ergorigin.html

Dehlin, O., Berg, S., Andersson, G.B. and Grimby, G. (1981). Effect of physical training and ergonomic counseling on the psychological perception of work and on the subjective assessment of low-back insufficiency. Scandinavian Journal of Rehabilitation Medicine 13, 1–9.

Demirbilek O. and Demirkan, H. (2004). Universal product design involving eld-erly users: A participatory design model. Applied Ergonomics 35, 361–370.

Drake, M.R. and Ferraro, M.C. (1997). VDT ergonomics: Upper extremity assess-ment requires a holistic approach. Work: A Journal of Prevention, Assessment and Rehabilitation, 8, 15–28.

Duke, K., Mirka G.A. and Sommerich, C.M. (2004). Productivity and ergonomic investigation of bent-handle pliers. Human Factors, 46, 234–243.

Folts, D.J., Giannini, A.J. and Otonicar, B. (1995). Cognitive workload. In K. Jacobs (Ed.), Ergonomics for Therapists (pp. 43–54). Newton, MA: Butterworth-Heinemann.

Gago, C., Gruss, E., Gonzalez, S., Marco, B., Fernandez, J., Jarriz, J., Martinez, S., Gonzalez, A., Galvez, C., Andrea, C., Hernando, P. and Hernandez, J. (2000). Compliance of haemodialysis patients with prescribed medication. EDTNAER-CA [European Dialysis and Transplant Nurses Association, European Renal Care Association] Journal, 26, 4–6.

Gonzalez, L.O. and Sellers, E.W. (2002). The effects of a stress-management pro-gram on self-concept, locus of control, and the acquisition of coping skills in school-age children diagnosed with attention deficit hyperactivity disorder. Journal of Child and Adolescent Psychiatric Nursing, 15, 5–15.

Graduate Prospects Ltd (2003a). Ergonomist in Close-up. Retrieved 23 December 2004, http://www.prospects.ac.uk/cms/ShowPage/Home_page/Explore_types_of_jobs/Types_of_Job/p!eipaL?state=showoccandidno=444andpageno=1

Graduate Prospects Ltd (2003b). Systems Analyst in Close-up. Retrieved 23 December 2004, http://www.prospects.ac.uk/cms/ShowPage/Home_page/Explore_types_of_jobs/Types_of_Job/p!eipaL?state=showoccandidno=481and pageno=1

Graduate Prospects Ltd (2004a). Environmental Health Officer in Close-up. Retrieved 23 December 2004, http://www.prospects.ac.uk/cms/ShowPage/Home_page/Explore_types_of_jobs/Types_of_Job/p!eipaL?state=showoccan-didno=210andpageno=1

Graduate Prospects Ltd (2004b). Health Promotion Specialist in Close-up. Retrieved 23 December 2004, http://www.prospects.ac.uk/cms/ShowPage/Home_page/Explore_types_of_jobs/Types_of_Job/p!eipaL?state=showoccan-didno=176andpageno=1

Grandjean, E. (1982). Fitting the Task to the Man: An Ergonomic Approach. London: Taylor & Francis.

Greco, L.A. and Morris, T.L. (2001). Treating childhood shyness and related behaviour: Empirically evaluated approaches to promote positive social inter-actions. Clinical Child and Family Psychology Review, 4, 299–318.

Henning, R.A., Jacques, P., Kissel, G.V., Sullivan, A.B. and Alteras-Webb, S.M. (1997). Frequent short rest breaks from computer work: effects on productiv-ity and well-being at two field sites. Ergonomics, 40, 78–91.

Human Resources Development Canada (2004). Inspectors in Public and Environmental Health and Occupational Health and Safety. Retrieved 23 December 2004 from http://www23.hrdc-drhc.gc.ca/2001/e/groups/2263.shtml

Iverson, R.D. and Deery, S.J. (2001). Understanding the 'personological' basis of employee withdrawal: The influence of affective disposition on employee tar-diness, early departure, and absenteeism. Journal of Applied Psychology, 86, 856–866.

Iwakiri, K., Yamauchi, S. and Yasukouchi, A. (2002). Effects of a standing aid on loads on low back and legs during dishwashing. Industrial Health, 40, 198–206.

Iwarsson, S. and Isacsson, Å. (1996). Development of a novel instrument for occupational therapy of assessment of the physical environment in the home – a methodologic study on 'The Enabler'. Occupational Therapy Journal of Research, 16, 227–244.

Jenkins, R. (2002). Value of employment to people with learning disabilities. British Journal of Nursing, 11, 38–45.

Joseph, B.S. (2003). Corporate ergonomics program at Ford Motor Company. Applied Ergonomics, 34, 23–28.

Keller, T.E., Whittaker, J.K. and Burke, T.K. (2001). Student debates in policy courses: Promoting policy practice skills and knowledge through active learning. Journal of Social Work Education, 37, 343–355.

Kirsteins, A.E., Dietz, F. and Hwang, S.M. (1991). Evaluating the safety and potential use of a weight-bearing exercise, Tai-Chi Chuan, for rheumatoid arthritis patients. American Journal of Physical Medicine and Rehabilitation, 70, 136–141.

Kornblau, B.L., Shamberg, S. and Klein, R. (2000). Occupational therapy and the Americans with Disabilities Act (ADA). American Journal of Occupational Therapy, 54, 622–625.

Kratz, G., Söderback, I., Guidetti, S., Hultling, C., Rykatkin, T. and Söderström, M. (1997). Wheelchair users' experience of non-adapted and adapted handicap clothes during sailing, guard rugby, or wheel-working. International Disability Studies, 19, 26–34.

Lahdenpera, T.S. and Kyngas, H.A. (2001). Levels of compliance shown by hypertensive patients and their attitude toward their illness. Journal of Advanced Nursing, 34, 189–195.

Lathrop, D. (1997). Home sweet home. . . How to make client's home accessible. Rehabilitation Management: The Interdisciplinary Journal of Rehabilitation, 10, 40–44.

Mace, R.L. (1998). Universal design in housing. Assistive Technology, 10, 21–28.

Mathiowetz, V., Matuska, K. and Murphy, M. (2001). Efficacy of energy conservation course for persons with multiple sclerosis. Archives of Physical Medicine and Rehabilitation, 82, 449–456.

Matthews, M.M. and Tipton-Burton, M. (2001). Treatment Contexts (5th edn). St. Louis: Mosby.

Maughan, I.V. (1962). Graduated supination-pronation: Attachments for table and floor looms. American Journal of Occupational Therapy, 16, 285–286.

Melhorn, J.M., Wilkinson, L., Gardner, P., Horst, W.D. and Silkey, B. (1999). An outcomes study of an occupational medicine intervention program for the reduction of musculoskeletal disorders and cumulative trauma disorders in the workplace. Journal of Occupational Medicine, 41, 833–846.

Nathan, P.A., Wilcox, A., Emerick, P.S., Meadows, K.D. and McCormack, A.L. (2001). Effects of an aerobic exercise program on median nerve conduction and symptoms associated with carpal tunnel syndrome. Journal of Occupational Environmental Medicine, 43, 840–843.

National Library of Medicine (2002–2005). MeSH subject headers. Available at http://www.nlm.org/cgi/mesh/2005/MB_cgi

Niemela, R., Rautio, S., Hannula, M. and Reijula, K. (2002). Work environment effects on labor productivity: An intervention study in a storage building. American Journal of Industrial Medicine, 42, 328–335.

Ocampo-Balabagno, A.V. (1999). Functional health performance outcomes of compliance to home instruction program after myocardial infarction. Philippine Journal of Nursing, 69(3-4), 20–29.

Occupational Safety and Health Administration (OSHA0, US Department of Labor (2001). Proposal for an Ergonomics Program Standard. Retrieved 4 July 2002 from http://www.osha.gov/ergonomics-standard/PROPOSED/ergo-faq.html

Osborne, D.J., Branton, R., Leal, F., Shipley, P. and Stewart, T. (Eds) (1993). Person-centred Ergonomics: A Brantonian View of Human Factors. London: Taylor & Francis.

Pedersen, P.M., Jorgensen, H.S., Nakayama, H., Raaschou, H.O. and Olsen, T.S. (1997). Comprehensive assessment of activities of daily living in stroke. The Copenhagen Stroke Study. Archives of Physical Medicine and Rehabilitation, 78, 161–165.

Randolf, J. (1984). The role of occupational therapy in back school. Occupational Therapy in Health Care, 1, 93–102.

Reed, J.C. (1984). Excessive stress affects worker health, productivity. Occupational Health Safety, 53, 33–35, 38.

Reust, C.E., Thomlinson, R.P. and Lattie, D. (1999). Keeping or missing the initial behavioural health appointment: A qualitative study of referrals in a primary care setting. Families Systems and Health, 17, 399–411.

Rhomberg, S., Wolf, L. and Evanoff, B. (1995). An integrated program for the prevention and management of musculosketal work injuries. Work: A Journal of Prevention, Assessment and Rehabilitation, 5, 115–122.

Richards, L.G., Olson, B. and Palmiter-Thomas, P. (1996). How forearm position affects grip strength. American Journal of Occupational Therapy, 50, 133–138.

Sabati, N., Snyder, M., Edin-Stibbe, C., Lingren, B. and Finkelstein, S. (2001). Facilitators and barriers to adherence with home monitoring using electronic spirometry. AACN [American Association of Critical Care Nurses] Clinical Issues: Advanced Practice in Acute and Critical Care, 12, 178–185.

Safran, M.R., Seaber, A.V. and Garrett, W.E. (1989). Warm-up and muscular injury prevention. An update. Sports Medicine, 8, 239–249.

Sharma, V. and Mavi, J. (2001). Self-esteem and performance on word tasks. Journal of Social Psychology, 141, 723–729.

Silverman, S. and Schein, J.R. (2001). Physician–patient decision making in osteoporosis management: The outcome of treatment is only as good as patient compliance. Journal of Musculosketal Medicine, 18, 124–128, 130.

Society for Industrial and Organizational Psychology (nd). What are Industrial-organizational Psychologists? Retrieved 23 December 2004 from: http://www.siop.org/Media/What.htm

Society of Occupational Medicine (nd,a). Careers in Occupational Medicine: Specialist Training in Occupational Medicine. Retrieved 23 December 2004 from http://som-old.foxsoft.net/carinom/car4_stio.html

Society of Occupational Medicine (nd,b). Careers in Occupational Medicine: What is Occupational Medicine? Retrieved 23 December 2004 from http://som-old.foxsoft.net/carinom/car1_wiom.html

Stein, F. and Cutler, S.K. (2002). Psychosocial Occupational Therapy: A Holistic Approach (2nd edn). Albany: Delmar.

Stein, F. and Roose, B. (2000). Pocket Guide to Treatment in Occupational Therapy. San Diego: Singular.

Stonefelt, L.L. and Stein, F. (1998). Sensory integrative techniques applied to children with learning disabilities: An outcome study. Occupational Therapy International, 5, 252–272.

Sumsion, T. (1993). Client-centered practice: the true impact. Canadian Journal of Occupational Therapy, 60, 6–8.

Thomas, L.K., Sargent, R.G., Michels, P.C., Richeter, D.L., Valois, R.F. and Moore, C.G. (2001). Identification of the factors associated with compliance to therapeutic diets in older adults with end stage renal disease. Journal of Renal Nutrition, 11, 80–89.

Timm, W.N., O'Driscoll, S.W., Johnson, M.E. and An, K.N. (1993). Functional comparison of pronation and supination strengths. Journal of Hand Therapy, 6, 190–193.

Torén, A. (2001). Muscle activity and range of motion during active trunk rotation in a sitting posture. Applied Ergonomics, 32, 583–591.

Tsang, H.W. (2001). Applying social skills training in the context of vocational rehabilitation for people with schizophrenia. Journal of Nervous Mental Disease, 189, 90–98.

Valentine-Garzon, M.A., Maynard, M. and Selznick, S.Z. (1992). ROM dance program: Effects on frail elderly women in an adult daycare center. Physical and Occupational Therapy in Geriatrics, 11, 63–83.

von Neumann, J. (1958). The Computer and the Brain. New Haven: Yale University Press.

Wiener, N. (1948). Cybernetics, or Control and Communication in the Animal and the Machine. Cambridge, Massachusetts: The Technology Press.

Wiener, N. (1950). The Human Use of Human Beings: Cybernetics and Society. New York: Avon.

World Health Organization (2001). International Classification of Functioning, Disability and Health [ICF]. Geneva, Switzerland: WHO.

Yavuzer, G., Gok, H., Tuncer, S., Soygur, T., Arikan, N. and Arasil, T. (2000). Compliance with bladder management in spinal cord injury patients. Spinal-Cord, 38, 762–765.

Yip, Y. (2001). A study of work stress, patient handling activities and the risk of low back pain among nurses in Hong Kong. Journal of Advanced Nursing, 36, 794–804.

CHAPTER 2

Applying ergonomic principles in the home environment

Human factors methodologies have been used to successfully analyze the (progressive) problems encountered by (older) persons (with a disability) as they. . . [are] performing specific tasks of daily living. This approach characterizes person–environment transactions as a quantification of the . . . demands associated with a specific task such as meal preparation, lifting an object or driving. Intervention strategies may include the development (and prescription) of an assistive technology or/and the modification of a characteristic of the person.

Laura N. Gitlin, 1998a, p. 146

The home environment protects you, gives you meaning and comfort, if it is designed to suit your personality, interests and your ability to perform activities in the home.

Ingrid Söderback, 16 June 2002

Learning objectives

By the end of this chapter the learner will:

1 Understand how ergonomic principles are applied in the home through the process of initial evaluation, goal-setting, intervention plan, evaluation of outcome and the redesign of the intervention plan if necessary.
2 Demonstrate understanding of the terms used for interventions regarding the individual, home environment and activities.
3 Recognize those individuals with disabilities, according to the International Classification of Functioning, Disability and Health (ICF) (World Health Organization, 2001a, 2001b) who potentially can benefit from ergonomic home interventions. The definitions of disabilities used in this chapter are, for the most part, based on this classification.
4 Identify ergonomic methods to (a) prevent injuries in the home; (b) encourage independence in self-care and home-making; and (c) compensate for impairments and disabilities.

5 Develop specific interventions related to self-care and home-making that
   (a) protect joints and prevent injuries; (b) reduce home hazards; (c)
   eliminate architectural barriers in the home and garden; (d) modify the
   home environment and use ergonomically (universally) designed furniture, chairs and cushions; (e) adapt tools and utensils making them more
   functional; and (f) prescribe assistive technology and orthoses.
6 Identify principles for teaching biomechanical and ergonomic principles and functional strategies when performing self-care and
   home-making tasks.

Principles and concepts used in the home environment

Housing and shelter comprise apartments, flats, houses, independent living
arrangements and nursing homes. The home environment incorporates the
immediate surroundings, including the entrances, lifts, garages, cellars, gardens, porches and backyards, as well as the layout of the buildings and
arrangement of the furniture and appliances. An application of ergonomic
principles to the home consists of adapting and modifying the home
environment to (a) promote safety in the living spaces; (b) facilitate independent living by providing useful products and devices; (c) increase
accessibility within the home and surrounding environment by removing
barriers; (d) place objects and tools within the client's reach; and (e) increase
ease of living through ergonomic utensils and furniture.

Interventions

Ergonomic interventions within the home primarily focus on commonly
available objects and on those occupations, activities or tasks performed
within this context. Common objects include furniture, kitchen and laundry appliances, stairs, telephones, bathrooms and household utensils.
Tasks may include use of any of these objects in performing personal
activities of daily living (PADL; e.g. showering) and instrumental activities
of daily living (IADL; e.g. using a telephone). Social and cultural considerations include the attitudes and dispositions of the client and how these
impact on home activities. The role of each individual in the home may
influence activities that are performed. For example, a husband who is
unaccustomed to doing household activities may need outside help when
his spouse is injured or unable to carry out typical activities. Likewise, cultural expectations affect patterns of cooking, cleaning and daily routines.

Preventive interventions

Preventive interventions are employed to prevent further deterioration in
the person's function. Preventive interventions take place at three levels:

primary prevention, secondary prevention and tertiary prevention. At the level of *primary prevention*, occupational therapy interventions are implemented before the critical incident has occurred. In the home, primary prevention may focus on teaching caregivers ergonomic principles to protect them from sustaining back injuries when they are caring for clients with mobility impairments or who are bedridden. For example, the caregivers may be taught ergonomic principles for lifting a person from the bed to a wheelchair by using a transportable lift (Edlund et al., 1998a; Edlund et al., 1998b). Primary prevention may also be used to reduce barriers in the home setting so that individuals have an opportunity to perform desired meaningful activities (Harlowe, 2001). For example, use of primary prevention interventions may reduce accidents such as tripping on electrical wires, slipping on scatter rugs, falling from unstable ladders or receiving burns while cooking. Steultjens et al. (2004) state that primary prevention using home hazard assessments has been implicated in decreasing the incidence of falls in elderly people and increasing their functional ability, social participation and quality of life.

Secondary prevention refers to preventing the recurrence of an injury or disability. For example, in the home the client may experience frequent falls. How can the occupational therapist prevent the recurrence of falls in the home to a client who is vulnerable? This question is presented as a clinical question in Chapter 4.

Tertiary prevention relates to secondary effects from the primary disability. For example, clients with a progressive neurological disease such as amyotrophic lateral sclerosis (ALS) or multiple sclerosis (MS) are often at risk of developing musculoskeletal disorders. The occupational therapist focuses on preventing joint stiffness or joint contractures by recommending conservative or passive exercises to maintain function.

Accessibility

Accessibility, in general, refers to the freedom or ability of an individual to make full use of a product or environment. Independence in ADL is compromised in people older than 75 years (Fänge and Iwarsson, 2003). A product or environment is accessible to individuals with disabilities only if they are able to use it to carry out everyday functions in the same way as individuals with similar skills and training who do not have disabilities (Americans with Disabilities Act of 1990, 1991; Cooper et al., 1991). For example, a doorknob may not be negotiable for an individual with quadriplegia if the individual does not have the muscle strength to use it. However, the doorknob can be redesigned so that an individual with an upper extremity disability can use it independently or the door can be controlled with an electrical switch. Barrier-free entrances refer to buildings, houses and gardens that are free from physical obstacles. Accessibility within the home considers the interior layout, furniture and ventilation.

The principles for making the home accessible for persons with disabilities consider (a) construction or redesign of the home to eliminate architectural barriers, such as constructing outdoor ramps; (b) rearrangement of furniture, utensils and objects to make them more functional; (c) use of ergonomically designed furniture and tools; and (d) prescription of assistive technology. Owens et al. (1996) have suggested that accessibility requires the application of ergonomic principles to issues of safety and reasonable accommodations. Similarly, Eberhardt (1998) has described how modification of homes for people with spinal cord injures might promote their function in daily life. If the environment is accessible the client will strive to become independent in daily and personal activities. The principles used for implementing architectural home accessibility are identified in Table 2.1.

Table 2.1 Examples of home environmental interventions according to the accessibility guidelines of the Americans with Disabilities Act

Principle	Examples
Make homes assessible	Use ramps and lifts (see specific recommendations from ADA: http://www.cs.wright.edu/bhe/rehabengr/ramps/adaramp.htm)
Remove barriers	Electric flexes on the floor, thresholds, loose carpets, furniture obstacles
Rearrange objects	Place items used daily so that they are easily accessible
Use of modern technology	Microwave oven, micro-switches, computer-operated appliances, electric utensils
Use ergonomically designed furniture, devices and tools	Chairs, household equipment, utensils with neutral position on the grip or handle, devices and tools with built-up handles
Facilitate independent living and cooking	Consider the nutritional value, time, energy and convenience of pre-manufactured foods or TV dinners
Consider safety and security in the home	Security alarm, help-bars in bathroom, shower chair, safety caps on medication
Structure comfort in the home	Aesthetics of colour and form in furniture and everyday household objects
Choose functional practicality	Consider the adage 'form follows function'. Objects in the home are designed with functional purposes, so the activities of daily living can be performed efficiently while conserving energy

Adapted from 'ADA Accessibility Guidelines for Buildings and Facilities', Federal Register, 1991.

Environmental or architectural *barriers* are factors in the home that restrict independent living and interfere with family life and social activities (World Health Organization, 2001a). For example, a person with paraplegia or tetraplegia is less likely to engage in social activities outside of his or her immediate surroundings when there are several steps between the apartment and the pavement outside. Other barriers include narrow hallways, carpeting that prevents wheelchairs from rolling smoothly, objects and utensils placed in inaccessible locations, or environmental conditions affecting sensory impairments or allergies (World Health Organization, 2000). Barriers preventing environmental accessibility can lead to disengagement from activities and depression (Söderback et al., 1993).

Environmental *facilitators*, on the other hand, are factors in the environment that enable the client to perform occupations and activities of daily living and to participate in family life as independently as possible (World Health Organization, 2001a). For example, the presence of a lift is a facilitator that enables an individual in a wheelchair to use a building.

Adaptation

Adaptation is the adjustment or modification of an environment (Stein and Roose, 2000) to achieve a good fit between the person and his or her environment. Adaptations are made so that the client can reach his or her optimal level of competence in performing activities of daily living (Law et al., 1994; Law et al., 1997). In the home, adaptation refers to changing or adapting the design of the house or apartment and the objects (e.g. tools, utensils, furnishings) belonging in the home. For example, adaptation of computers (e.g. input and output devices, input processing) to fit the needs of the individuals assist people with disabilities in becoming more productive (Brodwin et al., 2004). Adaptation may also refer to modifying the ways that the individual performs daily tasks. Purposeful environmental adaptations can meet the needs of all people, regardless of disability, and support independent living in the home (Gignac and Cott, 1998).

The *Consumer's Guide to Home Adaptation* (Adaptive Environments Center, 1996) is a practical workbook designed to help the consumer to make intelligent decisions regarding adaptation of homes, including constructing outdoor ramps; modifying doorways, kitchen counters or bedroom closets; or mounting bathroom grab bars. Adaptations are based on the consumer's evaluation of need, using questions such as the following, to guide the consumer:

1 Do you prefer to hold on to something when you are walking around the house?
2 Do you prefer any particular lighting?
3 Do you prefer to sit while cooking and grooming?
4 Is it easier to store things at higher or lower levels?
5 Do you find any kind of doorknob or tap easier to operate?
6 Is there a need for handrails in the hallways?
7 Is the sink at the best height for you?

8 Is there good lighting in your work areas and where you read?
9 Is the bath easy to get into and out of?
10 Do you need grab bars by the toilet or shower?

Adaptations are based on the responses, as well as consideration of cost, practicality and appearance.

Adaptations are (a) important determinants that enable the client to function in the home environment (Gitlin, 1998b); (b) applied to ergonomic strategies; and (c) individually designed by the occupational therapist in cooperation with the client. The occupational therapist's role is to identify and implement acceptable adaptive solutions based on the person's individual needs and lifestyle (Gitlin, 1998b; Gitlin and Burgh, 1995; Gitlin et al., 1999; Jackson et al., 1998; Levine and Gitlin, 1990; Levine and Gitlin, 1993; Pedretti and Early, 2001). For example, utensils used in the home may be adapted to meet the client's special needs and to accommodate his or her residual abilities. Some of these kitchen utensils include rocker knives, built-up handles on spoons and forks, cutting boards with suction cups, easy-grip mugs, plate surrounds, one-handed cutlery 'sporks', easy-use jar openers, easy-grip vegetable peelers, stable trays and tap turners. Objects are functional if they enable the client to perform daily self-care and home activities (Breines, 2001). The success of the adaptations depends on the client's willingness to accept and use them. The occupational therapist can support compliance by explaining the purpose and meaning of the adaptation to the client.

- *Physiological adaptation* is the adjustment of a person's biological responses to environmental stimuli, measured by, for example, body temperature, heart rate, blood pressure and biomechanical load. In some situations, these conditions are relevant for measuring outcomes, especially when determining how suitable and comfortable the adaptations of the home environment will be for individuals with disabilities.
- *Psychosocial adaptations* are the outcomes that describe a person's psychological and or social adaptations to altered health or life circumstances. The term is related to terms such as attitude, behaviour, coping, motivation, personality and psychological adjustment (Breines, 2001).

Assistive technology

An assistive technology device is defined as 'any item, piece of equipment, or product system, whether acquired commercially, off the shelf, modified or customized, that is used to increase or improve functional capabilities of individuals with disabilities' (Assistive Technology Act of 1998, 2001a Section 3(2)) by compensating for motor, sensory and cognitive impairments. Stein and Roose (2000) state, 'assistive technology includes any adaptation or creation of a device to assist a person with self-care' (p. 24). Assistive devices, tools for living, equipment or aids are interchangeable concepts and include orthotic and prosthetic devices (Foti, 2001; Gitlin, 1998a). When the device involves the use of technology, it is referred to as assistive technology (AT).

The use of assistive devices increases significantly with age because an individual's muscle strength and joint range of motion decrease with age, causing difficulties in mobility. Gitlin et al. (1999) found that 22 per cent of elderly people aged between 65 and 74 years used a mobility aid (e.g. crutches or canes), while 43 per cent of individuals older than 75 used an aid.

Although assistive devices are designed for individuals with disabilities, individuals without disabilities also use them. Many assistive devices prescribed by therapists are available on the commercial market in local pharmacies and department stores. For example, ergonomically designed eating utensils or tools and night lights or light lines are considered assistive devices, but are found in many homes, even when there is no one with a disability. Another example is an ergonomically designed knife where the handle is at a right angle to the knife blade (Nordenskiöld, 1997), thereby allowing the individual to grip the knife handle in a neutral position. This protects the wrist joint while using less muscle strength. These objects facilitate occupational performance for everyone, not just for those with disabilities (Christenson, 1999).

- *Protective devices* are 'designed to provide personal protection against injury to individuals exposed to hazards in industry, sports, aviation, or daily activities' (National Library of Medicine, 2005). Examples of protective devices are goggles to prevent eye injuries, special gloves to protect against vibration, anti-fatigue mats, elasticated belts to support back activities and ear muffs to protect ear drums.
- *Orthotic devices* are used 'to support, align, prevent, or correct deformities or to improve the functions of movable parts of the body' (Mann et al., 1995, p. 811). Common orthotic devices include crutches, splints, braces, slings, traction and foot and shoe adaptations. For example, wrist orthoses (splints) are prescribed for joint protection and prevention of pain in people with rheumatoid arthritis when performing housework (Callinan and Mathiowetz, 1996; Nordenskiöld, 1997). Michlovitz et al. (2004) found that continuous, low-level heat warp therapy for three days with two days' follow-up was effective in reducing moderate wrist pain and disability.
- *Prosthetic devices* are the replacement of a missing part by using a man-made material. Prostheses include artificial arms, legs or eyes, which may be cosmetic or functional. As a functional device, prosthetic devices are used to enhance performance.
- *Universal (ergonomic) design* is the application of sound biomechanical principles to the manufacture of utensils and tools used for self-care and housework in order to make them useful for all people including individuals with disabilities (Ahmadi, 1997; Christophersen, 2002; Mace, 1998; Trachtman et al., 1999).

Therapeutic strategies

Therapeutic interventions help the client to develop strategies to compensate for impairments (Söderback, 1988b). The occupational therapist uses a problem-solving process in a creative and ingenious manner in this process (Breines, 2001). The end result of the process enables the client to perform self-care and housework tasks independently or with less pain.

In the teaching–learning process, the occupational therapist teaches the client to substitute previously learned behaviours for a new strategy. As the client uses the new strategy, it becomes habitual. For example, the occupational therapist might teach a homemaker to turn his or her entire body when loading a washing machine, rather than twisting the back to pick up the clothes. The client remains in a neutral position and the joints and the spine are protected.

Occupational performance factors

Occupational performance or task performance involves both ability and capability. *Ability* refers to the individual's competence to perform a task. The abilities may or may not be realized, depending on the individual's motivation and determination to succeed. *Capability* refers to an individual's capacity to use his or her ability to complete a task. The individual's ability to perform a task is dependent on (a) the time of day when the task occurs; (b) how frequently the task occurs during this period; and (c) how long the task takes (Söderback, 1999). These factors often restrict a person's capability to perform an occupation independently because of the time the task takes, or the fact that the task is not a priority in the person's daily schedule (Guidetti and Söderback, 2001). For example, an elderly individual who is recovering from a stroke may find that cooking a meal from basic ingredients takes too long (e.g. $1\frac{1}{2}$ hours compared with $\frac{1}{2}$ hour before the stroke occurred), and so may fail to cook three meals a day. If, however, the individual uses prepared meals, the time required to cook is lessened, thus increasing the likelihood of cooking and the ability of the individual to cook for oneself. Occupational performance areas are related to the dynamic interaction between the client, environment, interventions and social/cultural norms.

The dynamic integrative process of ergonomic interventions

Several theorists have described the interface between the person, the task performance and the environment as a dynamic interacting process that constantly influences the individual's functioning, or disability, and his or her capability to perform daily occupations in the home (Bronfenbrenner, 1977; Calkins and Namazi, 1991; Fougeyrollas, 1995;

Law et al., 1994; Marks, 1997; World Health Organization, 2001a). This interface is depicted in Figure 2.1.

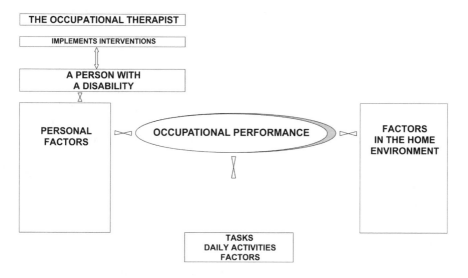

Figure 2.1 The interface of the dynamic interaction of components in the home environment using ergonomic principles. Thus, personal factors and factors in the home affect the occupational performance of the individual with disabilities.

According to these theorists, the dynamic interaction occurs between (a) an individual's internal psychological state, including one's belief about competency and the desire to seek meaning for oneself; (b) the physical environment; and (c) the environmental and task demands (Law et al., 1994). Within the home environment individuals with or without diseases or disorders interact dynamically in social situations. Interactions between family members affect the independence of other family members. When individuals are encouraged to be independent, they can participate as fully as possible in activities of daily living (Söderback et al., 1993).

Related to the dynamic interaction is the 'ecology of human development' framed by Bronfenbrenner (1977). This theory is defined as 'the progressive, mutual, accommodations throughout the life span, between a growing human organism and the changing immediate environment' (p. 514). The four major concepts of the ecology of human development consist of:

1 the reciprocal interaction between a person's developing skills in the changing immediate environment and the environmental changes caused by that person's action
2 the microsystem, restricted to the people, animals and things that belong to the immediate environment and in which the actors (members of the household) engage in activities of daily life and participate in various roles

3 ecological validity, which refers to the congruence between environmental expectation and reality
4 the outcome of the interaction viewed by how well the person adapts (adjusts) to the changes, or takes control of and influences the ecological system in a personally rewarding way. This ecological theory contributes to the understanding of the process of the person–environmental interaction (Bronfenbrenner, 1977; Law et al., 1994).

Partly based on the theory of the ecology of human development (Bronfenbrenner, 1977), Fougeyrollas (1995) conceptualized a holistic model where environmental factors have a determining effect on the role of the person with disabilities and on one's ability to complete activities of daily life. Fougeyrollas's model is comparable to the conceptualization of the International Classification of Functioning, Disability and Health (ICF) (World Health Organization, 2001a, 2001b). The ICF model views aspects of the person's health domains and well-being from a biological, psychosocial and social perspective. It can be used as a therapeutic approach by combining environmental adaptations, rearrangements and designs in creative ways (Marks, 1997; World Health Organization, 2001a), and as a needs assessment by providing a classification system (World Health Organization, 2001b) for individuals needing interventions in their home environment and for which adaptations are appropriate and available (Calkins and Namazi, 1991).

Ideally, every person desires to gain a sense of well-being by obtaining a good life and by being healthy (World Health Organization, 2001a). Success in obtaining a sense of well-being is dependent on integrating the components of a person's functioning and the way in which the context of the environment influences this functioning. Modification of the environment in a way that increases comfort, security and safety may influence one's sense of well-being (Calkins and Namazi, 1991).

Home environmental factors, such as the layout of furniture and the availability of functional utensils, can contribute to a person's success or failure to perform activities of daily living and household tasks. In applying ergonomics, the environmental factors are prioritized when developing home interventions. The person's resources, subjective perceptions, attitudes and coping strategies influence how the home interventions are carried out (Gignac and Cott, 1998). Appropriate clinical decisions, therefore, require an understanding of the way in which personal and environmental factors influence task performance.

As stated previously, a disability is any limitation to perform activities in daily life and/or restriction to participate in life situations in the home, work, school or leisure settings. There are a number of reasons why individuals with disabilities cannot perform functional activities: (a) an inability to perform because of an impairment; (b) over-protectiveness by the caregiver; (c) the caregiver's desire to have an activity performed in a certain way; (d) the caregiver's need to care for the individual, thereby refusing to allow the client to perform the activity; (e) the caregiver's intolerance in waiting for the client to perform the activity (i.e. time intolerance); and (f) barriers in the home environment. Decreased capabilities may also occur because of infirmity, old age or the interactions between people in the home environment that may limit the individual's functional independence. Söderback et al. (1993) have described the ways in which interactions between family members affect the independence of other family members. In one case, a man with hemiplegia was not allowed to use his teeth on the sleeve when taking off a jacket because his mother thought this would destroy the new jacket. Therefore, she took off his jacket, rather than allowing him to be independent. This led to his developing a 'learned helplessness' attitude in which he allowed others to do things for him that he had the ability to do. In another example, a woman who used a wheelchair at all times had not been outdoors because she was not able to open the door to the lift.

Applying ergonomic principles to home interventions

A clinical decision-making process is used to develop ergonomic interventions for clients in the home environment. The components of this process are shown in Figure 2.2. Clinical reasoning is usually described as a linear process (Rogers, 1983); however, the different components may occur simultaneously (Söderback et al., 1994). It is best to complete the decision-making process during home visits rather than in a clinic, because the therapist and client can problem solve together and discuss the best solutions acceptable to the client. The occupational therapist considers the client's and family's social environment, culture, beliefs, values, attitudes, roles and habits during the process of formulating a client-centred intervention plan. The occupational therapist begins with an initial evaluation, which includes an analysis of the tasks which the client performs in the home environment. Individual goals are set with the client based on the purposes for the intervention. Finally, the intervention is evaluated in terms of the outcome expectations. The individual with the disability is included in all aspects of the clinical decision-making process, as his or her compliance with the interventions is essential.

The clinical decision-making process is illustrated in the following example. A woman, who lives alone, had no difficulty with independent living in her home environment until she sustained a femur fracture causing a disability. The use of a functional status assessment during the initial evaluation showed that the client had decreased ability to (a) ambulate safely around the living areas; (b) sit and get up from the toilet; (c) pick up objects off the floor; and (d) put on or take off her shoes and stockings. The short-term goal was to help the client compensate for the

THE OCCUPATIONAL THERAPIST

○   **Initial evaluation of the client's functional status**
(ADL, work, leisure) and occupational performance factors

○   **Task analysis of the home environment**
(Tasks client performs in the home environment)

○   **Identifying purposes for occupational**
therapy interventions

○   **Setting individual goals using**
client-centred approach

○   **Implementing relevant interventions**
(Accessibility, adaptation, assistive technology and
therapeutic strategies)

○   **Outcome evaluation**
(Evaluating effectiveness of interventions)

A PERSON WITH A DISABILITY
(Compliance with the interventions)

Figure 2.2 Steps involved in the clinical decision-making process when developing interventions using ergonomic principles. The occupational therapist begins with an initial evaluation which includes an analysis of the tasks which the client performs in the home environment. Individual goals are set with the client based on the purposes for the intervention using relevant interventions finally, the intervention is evaluated in terms of the outcome expectations. The individual with the disability is included in all aspects of the clinical decision-making process, as his or her compliance with the interventions is essential.

musculoskeletal impairments related to movement (ICF classification s770) (World Health Organization, 2001b). The long-term goal was to help the client to become as independent as possible in the home in self-care activities, perhaps to the same level as before the accident occurred. Possible interventions included the prescription of assistive devices to allow her to be independent in bathing, dressing, toileting and ambulating in the house. Rearrangement of the home might include (a) moving the bed nearer to the bathroom; and/or (b) designing the bed to be more ergonomically appropriate by lowering it so that it is easier for the client to get in and out of the bed. An ergonomically designed chair at the appropriate height in which she can sit down and get up easily might also be recommended. Another solution, although more expensive, is to recommend a hydraulic chair that lifts the client to a standing position. The therapist needs to be aware that the client's fear of fracturing her hip again could prevent her from trying to walk. Evaluation of the client's ability to walk should be done before the operation, two to three days after the operation, and two weeks and three months respectively during the home visits (Hagsten and Söderback, 1994).

Purposes of the home interventions

The overall purpose of an intervention is to maintain function and increase independence in activities of daily living. Interventions applying ergonomic principles are accomplished by (a) preventing negative outcomes; (b) therapeutically supporting the client's efforts to be independent; (c) therapeutically promoting the client's independence through adaptations in the home; (d) compensating for impairments by reducing disability; and (e) facilitating care by working cooperatively with the client's family or caregiver. The integration of these purposes into the clinical decision-making process is depicted in Figure 2.3. The client and the occupational therapist work together in selecting realistic and suitable purpose(s) before the goal(s) are set or the interventions are implemented (Müllersdorf and Söderback, 2002; Northen et al., 1995).

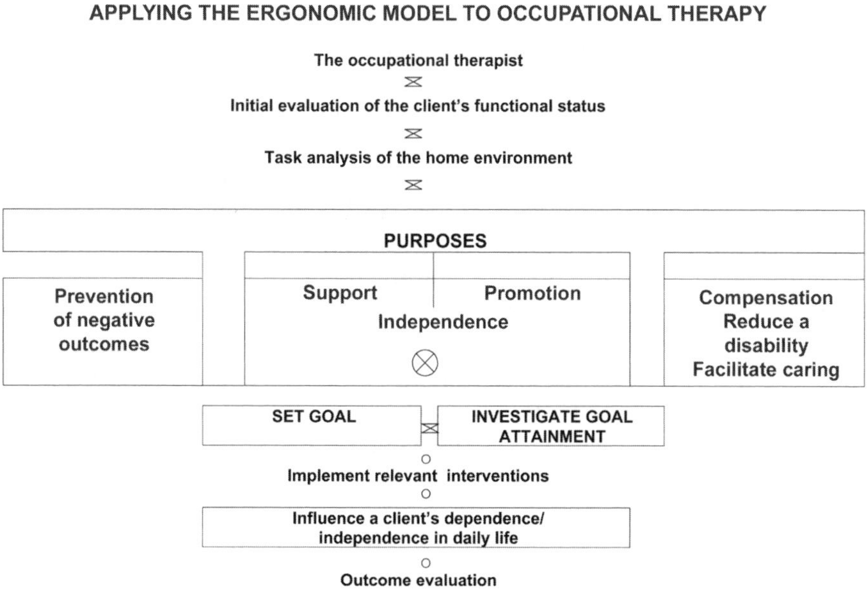

APPLYING THE ERGONOMIC MODEL TO OCCUPATIONAL THERAPY

The occupational therapist

⧖

Initial evaluation of the client's functional status

⧖

Task analysis of the home environment

⧖

PURPOSES		
Prevention of negative outcomes	Support Promotion Independence ⊗	Compensation Reduce a disability Facilitate caring

SET GOAL	⧖	INVESTIGATE GOAL ATTAINMENT

○

Implement relevant interventions

○

Influence a client's dependence/ independence in daily life

○

Outcome evaluation

Figure 2.3 Purposes (prevention, support, promotion and compensation) for applying ergonomic principles to interventions in the home environment.

Prevention of a negative outcome

Prevention includes strategies in the home environment to (a) stop an initial injury from occurring; (b) deter further deterioration of the client's present functional or activity status (Harlowe, 2001); or (c) maintain the present functional status by avoiding the occurrence of a negative condition because of the impairment or disability (Jacobs, 2000). For example, an accidental fall might cause a hip fracture resulting in an inability to ambulate in the home. This negative condition might be prevented by arranging furniture appropriately, using night lights or light lines, or removing loose floor carpets and eliminating obstructive door thresholds. In another example, asthma may restrict an individual's social participation and employment. Asthmatic attacks might be avoided by teaching the client about house cleaning and the importance of daily airing of bedding (Frisk et al., 2002). Likewise a decubitus (pressure sore) might be avoided by prescribing an appropriate wheelchair cushion. Ergonomic environmental interventions are employed to prevent further deterioration in the person's function.

Supporting independence in daily life

A second purpose for implementing interventions is to support independence. Support involves three types of intervention. First, support is given in order to maintain or increase the independence of an individual with disabilities to perform activities in daily life in an appropriate ergonomic way. This occurs by making sure that the environment, including the objects used in the environment, is comfortable, or by prescribing assistive devices. For example, prescribing soft or hard resting hand splints for a client with rheumatoid arthritis may be prescribed to maintain present hand functioning (Callinan and Mathiowetz, 1996). Second, spouses, family members and caregivers support the individual in the performance of functional activities (Olsen et al., 1999). Using universal design in a home enables clients with disabilities to perform tasks more readily, thereby increasing independence and reducing dependence. Third, the therapist provides support to family members and caretakers. For example, they might be taught ergonomic principles for lifting a person from the bed to a wheelchair by using a transportable lift (Edlund et al., 1998a; Edlund et al., 1998b). Once the client perceives that the home environment (utensils and equipment) is accessible, comfortable and acceptable, and he or she can perform meaningful and purposeful occupations in the home, support will be accomplished.

Promotion of independence in daily life

A third purpose for intervening in the home is to enable the client to live at home (Forrest and Gombas, 1995) or an older person living in a nursing home to have access to his or her home environment (Liebig, 1999). Owens et al. (1996) have suggested that accessibility requires application of ergonomic principles to issues of safety and reasonable accommodations. Similarly, Eberhardt (1998) has described how modification of homes for people with spinal cord injures might promote their function in daily life. If the environment is accessible, the client will strive to become independent in daily and personal activities.

Compensation to reduce disability and facilitate caring

Compensation relates to interventions in order to reduce the effects of the disability. This process may involve substituting an intact muscle function for a paralysed or weakened muscle, or using an assistive device to perform a task that could not be performed in the typical manner because of a disability. Use of a prefabricated tenodesis splint that allows pinch and grasp movements may help a person with quadriplegia to perform tasks such as writing. Likewise a person with arthritic hands might use an electric can opener to compensate for limited joint movement. Compensation should have positive effects, but the therapist should also be cognizant of negative outcomes that may occur. Thus, an electric wheelchair may be helpful in some situations, but its use may cause joint contractures if the prescribed exercises are not followed (Harlowe, 2001). Table 2.2 lists some of the ways that interventions can compensate for specific disabilities by using assistive devices.

Table 2.2 Compensatory ergonomic interventions using assistive devices

Disability	Performances	Main assistive devices
Neuromusculo-skeletal movement impairments (Chen et al., 1998; Chung et al., 1997; Clemson and Martin, 1996; Cooper and Stewart, 1997; Gitlin, 1999; Nordenskiöld, 1997; Tuleja and DeMoss, 1999)	• Supporting 25 per cent of one's body weight • Balancing in an upright position • Ambulating • Walking up and down stairs or long hallways	• Canes • Banisters
	• Standing up and sitting down	• Lavatory raising chair • Shower stool • Bath stool • Supporting handrails • Power chairs • Elbow rests
	• Reaching for objects	• Reachers • Light-weight, one-handed clutching-tongs with adjustable length • Lock system for the grip and forearm support
	• Putting on shoes	• Adjustable long shoehorn • Supporting rails, available
	• Transferring from bed to chair, or from chair to toilet or shower	• Ergonomically designed bath chair allows the client to transfer into the bath safely by sitting on the edge of the chair first, and then swinging legs into the bath
	• Facilitate carrying of children	• Baby-care assistive reins

Table 2.2 Compensatory ergonomic interventions using assistive devices (continued)

Disability	Performances	Main assistive devices
Neuromusculo-skeletal movement impairments (contd)	• Supporting muscle strength by increasing tone or immobilizing joints when opening lids	• Various kinds of orthoses • Equipment with some kind of lever which decreases the need for muscle strength
Impairment of the joints and bones (Davis et al., 1999; Herrman et al., 1999; Prangrant et al., 2000; Saxena et al., 1995; Yuen and D'Amico, 1998)	• Grasping objects with paretic hands • Feeding • Eating • Swallowing • Dressing	• Electrical or pneumatic gripping systems • Assistive feeding devices • Cups with two handles help clients with weak muscles to lift the cup to mouth • Dressing stick to facilitate pulling up garments
Neuromusculo-skeletal movement and cognitive impairments Hemiparesis	• Various housework	• Suction pumps or other braking material to hold kitchen equipment • Nonslip mats
Cognitive impairments memory (Lindberg et al., 1999)	• Daily living activities	• Electronic or other memory equipment
Sensory impairments and pain Hearing impairments or deafness (Mann et al., 1993; Woodcock, 1997)	• Communicate	• Hearing aids • Increase speech and sound volume • Communication devices
Visual impairments or blindness	• Identifying objects	• Glasses • Magnification instruments • Braille system • Talking systems • Visual readers
Reducing pain	• Daily living activities	• Wrist orthoses

Occupational therapy interventions in the home environment

Using the home environment as an intervention mediator is a complex process that involves the occupational therapist, in cooperation with the client, caregivers and relatives, other rehabilitation team members, and other professionals (e.g. engineers, architects, technicians, ergonomic designers, healthcare providers and representatives of companies selling ergonomically designed adapted equipment and wheelchairs).

For example, for an elderly woman who has difficulty walking and moving (ICF classification, d450) (World Health Organization, 2001b), the purpose of the intervention is to prevent repeated accidental falls. With the help of the other team members, the client and the caregiver and relatives, the occupational therapist uses strategies to modify the environment. The furniture may be rearranged, barriers may be removed, or an assistive device may be prescribed to aid in walking.

The relationship of interventions in the home environment to the clinical decision-making process is depicted in Figure 2.4. The interventions used in an ergonomic model include (a) preventive interventions; (b) adaptive interventions, including accessibility; (c) prescription of assistive technology; and (d) strategies in the teaching learning process.

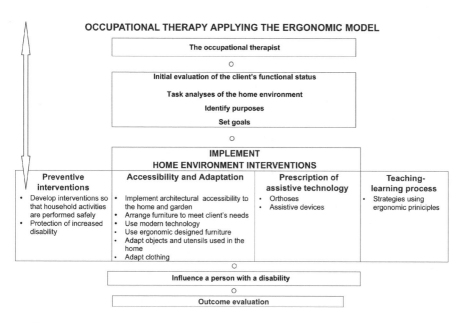

Figure 2.4 The relationship of implementing interventions in the home environment to the clinical decision-making process.

Preventive interventions

Interventions using ergonomic principles are designed to prevent injuries and avoid home hazards. The goal of the intervention is two-fold: (a) to protect the client from further deterioration of a neuromuscular and movement-related disorder in order to maintain one's present activity level in activities of daily life; and (b) to provide support to the client so that household activities can be performed safely. There are a number of interventions that may be used.

- *Joint protection*. Ergonomic intervention prevents increased pain or stiffness that may be due to inflammed or damaged joints, abnormal or irregular positioning and contractures. Ergonomically designed grips (e.g. angled or cane handles, built-up grips) or assistive devices (e.g. cheese-slicer, potato peeler, scissors) may be prescribed, as may a wrist splint (Brus et al., 1997; Chung et al., 1997; Nordenskiöld, 1997).
- *Lumbar (low back) and joint protection*. An ergonomically functional position in the wheelchair with major joints at a 90-degree angle can prevent low back pain, joint contractures or stiffness and increased spasticity (Dunn, 1996, 1997; Leonard, 1997; Patterson and Michael, 1991; Rader et al., 2000; Wong and Wade, 1995).
- *Skin protection*. The purpose of intervention is to protect protruding body parts, such as the hips and shoulders in the prone position and the buttocks in the sitting position, from pressure sores. Interventions focus on using various types of cushions in the wheelchairs and mattresses in the beds, which are designed to bring about pressure relief of the skin on the exposed body parts (Burns and Betz, 1999; Edlich, 1995; Hastings, 2000; Williams, 2000).
- *Prevention of home hazards*. Ergonomic intervention is designed to prevent injury by removing obstacles in the path where one walks, avoiding unsafe floor surfaces, and rearranging furniture and other equipment in the home environment, especially in the bathroom and the bedroom. These rearrangements include, but are not limited to, placement of the bed, removal of thresholds and carpets, and placement of night lights. Each of these rearrangements serves to avoid falls (Lange, 1996; Mahoney, 1998; Tibbitts, 1996).
- *Avoiding meaningless and restless wandering among people living with dementia-related syndromes*. Interventions include using visual and other subjective barriers. Examples of these subjective barriers are patterns on the floor or door, coloured tape on the door or doorknob, grids and stripes of tape, and coloured lines to show the directions for entrances and exits (Price et al., 2001).
- *Increasing safety*. Clients with memory and motor impairments may use various control devices to increase personal and environmental safety. For example, some devices may alert the client to scheduled events such as when to take medicine. Other devices may alert the client to safety issues, such as unlocked doors or windows, or stoves and ovens that have not been turned off (Cowan and Turner-Smith, 1999; Lindberg et al., 1999; Watzke, 1997).
- *Supporting weak muscles*. Ergonomically designed handles or chairs, bath stools and bath bars may support clients who have weak muscles or difficulties with balance resulting in difficulty in standing, sitting and walking (Aminzadeh et al., 1999; Clemson et al., 1999; Sweeney and Clarke, 1992).
- *Supporting postural balance*. Cushions designed to fit the body contour may support trunk posture and balance for people with cerebral

palsy, severe traumatic brain injury, amputated pelvis, or for the elderly sitting in a wheelchair (Kanyer, 1992; Patterson and Michael, 1991).

Accessibility and adaptations in the home environment

All people, but especially those with disabilities, can benefit from attractive, comfortable, ergonomically designed homes and furnishings (Benktzon, 1993). While universal design and accessibility benefit everyone, it is important to design the home to be accessible and barrier-free when there are individuals with disabilities (Branson, 1991a, 1991b). Adaptation of homes using ergonomic principles includes (a) implementing architectural changes to the home and garden to make it more accessible, (b) arranging furniture and objects in the home, and (c) adapting furniture, objects, tools and clothing. The following paragraphs describe some ways in which the home environment can become more accessible. These examples can serve as guides for occupational therapists in designing home interventions.

Architectural accessibility in the home

Architectural accessibility is a major intervention strategy used in the home environment that mediates how adaptation or rearrangements are used. For example, removing scatter rugs or other objects that might cause stumbling, or using night lights in the hallways, can prevent a hip fracture among the frail elderly. Likewise, using an electronic air cleaner, vacuuming frequently or changing furnace filters frequently can reduce the symptoms of asthmatic attacks. Table 2.3 outlines strategies used to modify and adapt the home environment, thereby making it more accessible and barrier-free.

Facile system

One of the most innovative uses of the home environment for facilitating independent living is the 'Support Tools for Home and Management, Integrated with Telematic Systems and Services, Devoted to Disabled and Elderly People' referred to as the FACILE System (Lindberg et al., 1999). The system is available at two rehabilitation-training flats: one in Sweden and one in Italy. The FACILE prototype was designed and developed by a cooperating frontier research European Union project, and its effectiveness has been demonstrated through clinical research.

This system is designed to give support in daily living activities to people with cognitive and/or motor disabilities. It is connected to a rehabilitation centre and hence the rehabilitation team can use the system to design goals and monitor progress for individuals in the rehabilitation programme.

Table 2.3 Using ergonomic principles in interventions in the home environment

	Examples of barriers	Examples of interventions	
		Assistive devices	*Architectural easements*
General Location			• Location should be close to public services, such as buses, shopping centres or main roads
Exterior surround-ings	• Steep incline to the home • Decks don't match indoor and outdoor floor levels • Outside steps prevent movement in and out of the house • Slippery ground • Garden paths too narrow to allow wheelchairs to pass • No access to garden		• Install wheelchair ramps • Terrace the landscape • Install lift • Change ground cover • Reconstruct garden area • Arrange garden in small raised beds
Stairs	• Unable to get to different parts of the home		• Install a stairlift • Build a wheelchair ramp • Mount handrails on both sides of the stairs
Doorways (e.g. exterior, interior and garage)	• Too narrow to allow wheelchairs to get through • Inability to open the door due to heavy door or inaccessible doorknobs • Thresholds prevent entrance	• Adapt door knobs with large handles • Install voice-activated or electric switches to automatically open doors	• Widen doors through reconstruction • Rebuild thresholds, or lower thresholds
Windows	• Difficult to open • Difficulties regulating incoming light	• Install auto-matic control to open the windows and adjust the Venetian blinds	
Interior rooms	• Not enough floor space • Inaccessible light switch		• Remodel to make room large enough for wheel-chair users • Lower light switches to waist high

Table 2.3 Ergonomic principles in interventions in the home environment (contd)

	Examples of barriers	Examples of interventions	
		Assistive devices	*Architectural easements*
Bathroom	• Inability to regulate temperature of water, possibly causing burns • Problems turning water tap • Electrical wires hanging freely • Inaccessible washbasin • Difficulty getting on or off toilet • Motor impairment prevents client from wiping oneself • Inaccessible shower or bathtub • No place to sit while bathing • No access to mirrors and medicine cabinet	• Enlarge the tap handle • Use appropriate assistive device • Provide manual and electrical hoists • Provide benches in the bath or shower	• Install a thermostat on taps to regulate temperature • Install ergonomically designed grips • Install safety devices for electrical wires • Remount washbasin higher • Use a bracket-supported countertop sink • Install special toilet that automatically wipes the client • Mount handrails on the wall beside the toilet, bath or shower • Place mirrors and medicine cabinets in accessible place at eye-level • Install mirrors so that client can inspect their back for pressure sores
Floors	• Too slippery, causing falls • Wheels on wheelchairs move sluggishly	• Change rubber material on wheelchair wheels	• Install non-slipping floor material
Kitchen	• Inaccessible countertops • Difficulty opening cabinet doors • Inability to reach the edge of counter, sink, or dishwasher		• Change the placement of counters, stove, oven and micro wave to meet individual needs • Allow for adjustable heights on countertops • Install automatic door opener activated by a voice-activated or electric switch for kitchen cabinets • Remove cabinet front and skirting on countertops, especially under sink

Table 2.3 Ergonomic principles in interventions in the home environment (contd)

	Examples of barriers	Examples of interventions	
		Assistive devices	*Architectural easements*
Cognitive disabilities or impairment	• Difficulty performing daily routines, including complicated tasks, because of specific mental impairments such as memory problems	• Computer-assisted or individualized computer programs that aid in memory (e.g. taking medicine) • Provide memory aids that cue the steps in house-keeping activities • Install automatic alarms to turn off appliances	
Physical impairments	• Difficulty carrying or moving household utensils or food • Difficulty in performing complicated tasks • Inability to reaching objects in high places		• Provide service cart specifically designed for people on crutches • Place kitchen utensils and cooking equipment, groceries, clothes and other personal articles in accessible places • Provide ways to obtain utensils or equipment in an energy-conservation manner
Epilepsy	• Increased epileptic seizures		• Remove shining and glittering surfaces on counters, fluorescent lights, or other objects that might trigger a seizure
Visual impairments			• Use highly contrasted colour schemes • Install dimmer switches

Adapted from 'Testing home modification interventions: issues of theory, measurement, design, and implementation', L.N. Gitlin (1998b).

*Assistive devices are adaptive equipment or software to help an individual to accomplish a task (Cook and Hussey, 2002).

**Architectural easements are permanent or fixed changes to entrances, buildings, rooms or gardens to remove barriers.

The FACILE system prototype includes a number of components:

- The Telematic Overview System (TOS) alerts the client at specific times according to an individually selected schedule. For example, the system can be programmed to (a) let the client know when to take medication; (b) show the daily schedule, including identifying which visitors are arriving and what time they can be expected; (c) list daily chores; (d) show when the client has free time; (e) keep track of health parameters (e.g. blood pressure, pulse rate, epileptic seizures); or (f) provide immediate connection to the ward.
- The Environmental Instrumental Button (EIB) system provides a convenient way to ensure security and safety. The remote control panel allows the client to control aspects of his or her environment, including opening and closing the windows, cutrains, and doors; turning lights on and off; or raising and lowering the bed both horizontally and vertically. Another control button can be used to make sure that everything is turned off and doors are securely locked.

The FACILE system can be preset in several different ways. For example, the system can be preset so that (a) components that might cause fire (e.g. cooker, iron) or overflow of water (e.g. taps) are automatically turned off. Alarms can alert the client to burning cigarettes or open refrigerator doors. Caregivers or rehabilitation personnel can be alerted when the client is having a seizure. Windows, blinds or curtains can be opened or shut at a specific time.

The physical environment of the FACILE system uses ergonomic principles and universal design. The furniture and utensils emphasize ergonomic functionality and convenience while providing comfort and harmonious beauty to the client. The apartments can be adapted for individuals with various disabilities, including hemiplegia, who have the use of only one hand; tetraplegia, who must use wheelchairs; individuals using crutches; and people with visual impairments. In summary, the training flat is designed to enable individuals with disabilities who are in a rehabilitation setting to develop independent skills in a safe, private environment. They can strive for maximum independence when performing activities of daily living (PADL and IADL). They can have guests, take part in social activities, and go out in the fresh air into an inspiring garden. The ultimate goal for these clients is eventually to return home having gained as much independence as possible. In some cases the home environment to which they return has been adapted or rearranged in the same manner as the training flat.

When designing an accessible house that allows people with cognitive disabilities (e.g. Alzheimer's disease, stroke) to live at home, the environment should assist the caregiver while providing protection and orientation for the client. The house should be built on one level, with adequate open floor space provided so that individuals can manoeuvre their wheelchairs. The floor plan should be easily understood. Objects and utensils used daily should be within reach and the location clearly labelled. Symbols may need to be used rather than words, especially if the client has lost his or her ability to read.

Safety is an issue in planning the home environment for individuals with dementia. Barriers may need to be provided to protect the individual. For example, double locks may need to be put on doors to prevent the client from wandering away (Olsen et al., 1999). Safety handles may need to be put on the stove and oven to prevent the client from turning on the appliances. Hot water taps may need to be disabled to prevent scalding. Automatic alarms, including fire and smoke alarms, can alert caregivers to possible danger.

Two examples of universally designed homes are the Lifetime Adaptable Home, designed with technology to make it accessible to all ages and to individuals with disabilities (Nielsen and Ambrose, 1999), and the Next Generation Universal Home, designed to be especially accessible for persons with impaired mobility and cognition, vision impairments or hearing impairments (Trachtman et al., 1999).

Architectural accessibility in the garden

Gardens, which include one's private garden, woods, city parks and children's playgrounds, are serene environments where people can enjoy leisure time. Horticulture and gardens can provide exercise, cognitive stimulation, and, in general, promote health and well-being (Barris, 1982; Barris et al., 1986). The meaning of growing plants, watching birds and butterflies, the intensity and quality of listening to the sounds in the garden, and responding to aromas and colours are therapeutic. It is well known that people who regularly visit gardens experience a healing effect and have fewer days of illness, develop increased immunity from physical illness and, through their positive attitudes, increase their well-being (Sandberg et al., 2000). Occupational therapists have had a long history of using horticulture and gardening for therapeutic purposes (Barris et. al., 1986; Sandberg et al., 2000). In this role, the occupational therapist designs a barrier-free garden, prescribes ergonomically designed garden tools and organizes gardening for individuals with differing needs (Söderback et al., 2004).

When gardening is used for therapeutic purposes, the following principles should be applied:

- *Increase accessibility or eliminate barriers.* Accessibility makes the garden available for people with disabilities, such as wheelchair users. Adaptations include very gradual inclines on the walks, use of railings to give support, and use of material that has minimal friction on the footpath surfaces (e.g. smooth concrete). Benches should be placed at frequent intervals to give the client and caregivers the opportunity to rest (Sandberg et al., 2000). City parks and gardens, when made accessible, provide individuals with disabilities an opportunity to retreat to a calm place for meditation and relaxation.

An example of an accessible forest park is in Järvsö, the county of Hälsingland, Sweden. Here, a 3000 metre-long wooden walkway is built above the ground on poles making it is accessible to everyone. The walkway passes through large enclosures where moose, bears, wolves and birds of prey live naturally. Because it is accessible, individuals with disabilities are able to view the wildlife.

When planning a new house for an individual in a wheelchair, it is important to plan for an accessible garden. Garden beds should be raised and built on a platform. Individuals in wheelchairs should be able to reach all the plants in the garden beds. Occupational therapists in conjunction with the landscape architect can be helpful in drawing up the plans (Sandberg et al., 2000).

- *Provide maximum stimulation.* This is especially helpful for people with dementia and visual impairments. For example, a garden with a 'scent grove' made up of flowers or bushes growing close together so that visitors can smell and touch the leaves encourages sensory stimulation.
- *Consider using the garden for socializing.* The garden can be used for entertainment, instruction and social interaction. Social meetings can be held in the garden while the produce taken from the garden can be used for cooking groups.
- *Remember that gardens can provide a symbolic link to a person's life experiences.* In a hospice, the garden can provide a link between present illness and past life. In some cases, patients are allowed to bring flowers and plants from their home, thus creating the symbolic link.
- *Provide physical and cognitive exercise.* While gardening, the individual is moving his or her body and giving gentle stimulation to muscles and joints. The individual is also making decisions regarding planting, weeding and arranging flowers. Thus, working in the garden and cultivating plants provide valuable experiences for an individual with a disability.
- *Use garden tools that are ergonomically designed.* The tools should (a) be of light-weight construction; (b) require as little muscle strength as possible to handle; (c) be constructed with a 90 degree angle between the tool and its handle, reachers or grippers based on biomechanical principles; (d) be covered with material to reduce friction on the grip; and (e) be able to be used with one hand (Söderback et al., 2004).

Arranging and adapting furniture, objects and utensils

For an individual with a disability, articles used daily (e.g. hair brush, personal care items or kitchen utensils) may be placed so that an individual with a restricted range of motion or muscle weakness can reach them without help. Tools using universal design are often commonly available on the open market. One example is an ergonomically designed knife where the handle is at a right angle to the knife blade (Nordenskiöld, 1997), thereby allowing the individual to grip the knife handle in a neutral position. This protects the wrist joint while using less muscle strength.

The following are examples of rearrangement, replacement, removal and adaptation of objects and furnishing:

• Arrange furniture to allow freedom of movement for individuals using wheelchairs or crutches, or to provide easy access for transporting lifts. For example, tables should be high enough so that the wheelchair can go under the table.
• Place the bed at a height and in a location that provides optimal ease for caregiving. The caregiver should be able to work in a biomechanically neutral position, without straining or bending, and should be able to move around the bed easily.
• Place the bed near a toilet and bathroom. This will make the bathroom more accessible to those who are bedridden, incontinent or who have difficulty walking.
• Use a night light to prevent injuries from falls during the night.
• The adage 'a place for everything and everything in its place' is applicable, especially for those individuals with memory difficulties. By making sure objects and utensils are always in the same place, items can be located quickly.
• Objects and utensils should be placed so that the client can reach them without a stool. This is especially important for kitchen utensils and toilet articles that are used daily.
• If the client is prone to seizures, remove objects that would prevent free passage or could cause injury. For example, polished surfaces in the kitchen may be slippery, while chairs or tables placed in hallways may prevent the client from moving quickly.
• Adapt canes for specific individuals by modifying the height of the cane, the type of handle grip, the angle of the grip and the tip.
• Use lever handles rather than knobs on doors and drawers, because they are easier for individuals with weak muscle grip.
• Adapt bath stools by raising or lowering the legs or changing the position in the shower or bath. This is especially useful for individuals with a pelvisectomy or for those with reduced balance or stamina.
• Add inserts to the toilet seat to raise it, or side railings beside the toilet to provide support for the individual to hold on to.
• Modify kitchen and eating utensils for those with restricted range of motion and/or weak muscles by using universal design (Aminzadeh et al., 1999; Breines, 2001; Clemson et al., 1999). Examples include building up the utensil handles to make them easier to hold, changing the angle of the utensil so that it can be grasped in neutral position, or combine a fork and spoon into one instrument (spork).

When recommending modifications and adaptations, the occupational therapist will apply his or her knowledge of biomechanics and ergonomics to determine the most appropriate design for specific clients (Mace, 1998). 'The physical and psychological characteristics of the individual are considered in devising an environment where the occupational therapist tries to place the homemaker in an anatomically neutral position as well as reducing the stressors' (Stein and Roose, 2000, p. 101). Instruction for use and monitoring of compliance are the responsibility of the occupational therapist or physical therapist.

Ergonomic design of furniture

Furniture, such as chairs, wheelchairs and cushions, bed and mattresses, mechanical lifts (hoists) and tables are prescribed by the occupational therapist in consultation with the client. Furniture should be adapted so that it is comfortable and appropriate for the client's disability. A well-designed piece of furniture correlates strongly with ease of use (Fricke and Worrell, 1991) and should take into account biomechanics, kinematics, muscle activity and functional perspectives (Kerr et al., 1991).

Optimal ergonomic designs of the parts of a chair include the seat height, seat depth, seat tilt, backrest, the armrests and the padding. When choosing chairs for persons with disabilities, especially those with amputations, ankylosing spondylitis, rheumatoid arthritis, osteoarthritis of the hips or generalized low back pain, ease of rising from the sitting position has been noted to be the most important feature (Sweeney and Clarke, 1992). When getting out of a chair, the ability to go from sitting to standing is dependent on the design of the chair, the distance between the seat and the arms, the muscle force generated in the joints and muscles of the lower extremities, and the joint angle motion positions (Kerr et al., 1991).

Special consideration should be given to the distance between the floor and the seat of chairs and sofas. The height of the seat on sofas and chairs should be comparable to the length of the person's calves or somewhat higher so that the feet can be flat on the floor. When the distance is appropriate, it is easier to sit down and get up. Special equipment, such as the Excelsior ejector chairs, is effectively used for assisting people in rising and standing from a seated position (Bashford et al., 1998).

Other examples of appropriate ergonomic designs in chairs affect the upper body. The distance from the shoulder to the armchair or the table surface should allow a 90-degree angle or more between the upper arm and lower arm when the shoulder is relaxed. This allows the shoulder and neck muscles to stay relaxed. A chair should have a lumbar back support. The chair's support and stability will assist people with arthritis and back pain to be comfortable (Sweeney and Clarke, 1992). Figure 2.5 shows the details for designing a chair ergonomically, while Table 2.4 provides a checklist useful for prescribing an individually adapted chair.

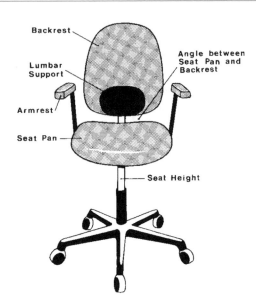

Figure 2.5 Description of parts of an ergonomic chair. Reprinted with permission from Jacobs, K. and Bettencourt, C.M. (1995). Ergonomics for Therapists (1st edn, p. 146). Boston: Butterworth-Heinemann, Elsevier Ltd.

Table 2.4 Checklist for designing an ergonomic chair

Identification of problem	Yes/No

Anthropometric fit
Does the individual's size and physical characteristics match the
   adjustment of the chair?
Does the seat height allow feet to rest on the floor?
Does the seat support the thighs to just behind the back of the knee?

Adjustments
Does the seat pan tilt forwards and backwards easily while seated?
Can the back be moved forwards and backwards easily while seated?
Can adjustments be made easily without the individual assuming an
   awkward position?
Can the height of the back be moved up and down while seated?
Has the individual been instructed in how to adjust the chair to fit
properly?
Are the seat and back contoured and do they adjust easily to the
individual's movements and body shape?

Back support
Does the chair support the individual's back?
Does the backrest provide firm support to the lower part of the back?
Does the seat configuration and material protect the person from
pressure sores?

Table 2.4 Checklist for designing an ergonomic chair (continued)

Identification of problem	Yes/No

If arms are present
Are the armrests adjustable in height and distance?
Can the armrests be removed easily without affecting the appearance
   of the chair?
Will the armrests allow the individual to move close to the desk?
Do the armrests allow the elbows and shoulders to remain in neutral
   position?

Other considerations
Does the individual experience a shock when touching the chair in
   cold weather?
Does the seat and back dissipate body heat?
Does the individual feel supported and comfortable in this chair?
If not, state why.
Does this chair come in a variety of models and sizes?
Does the individual like the overall appearance of the chair?

Adapted from Hermenau, 1995.

Wheelchairs

Wheelchairs are a major compensatory aid for people with reduced or lost ambulation due to conditions or diseases such as arthritis, decreased muscle force in the lower extremities, paralysis of the legs or old age. Electrically (battery) powered or manually driven wheelchairs are easily manoeuvred indoors, while the Permobil© (Permobil, 2000) was developed to be efficient in and out of doors.

In many cases the wheelchair is adapted to the specific need of the client. For example, wheelchairs for the elderly may need to address issues of stability, low energy and protection from falling (Redford, 1993). The design of a wheelchair is based on the factors of (a) biomechanical analysis of anthropometric measurements and (b) physical functioning. By taking these factors into account, the wheelchair will provide easier handling, more comfort and increased independence in carrying out daily activities (Cooper et al., 1997; Murata et al., 2001).

Guidelines for prescribing wheelchairs, partly based on biomechanical analysis involved in seating (Collins and Shipperley, 1999), are found in several articles (Burke, 1999; Cutter and Blake, 1997; Garber and Dyerly, 1991; Hastings, 2000; Hermenau, 1995; Minkel, 2000). (See also Chapter 3.) Determining the best wheelchair involves examining the fit between (a) the client's body contours, range of motion and orientation in space; (b) the environment where it will be used; (c) the activities in which the wheelchair is included; and (d) the design of the seating systems. The parts of the wheelchair must also be considered: (a) an ergonomically designed seating position; (b) the seat surface; (c) the backrest and contour; (d) the driving position to prevent injuries of the shoulder, wrists and hands; (e) the quality of the wheels; and (f) the safety properties. Other factors to be considered when prescribing a wheelchair include the cultural values and psychological attitudes of the user. A wheelchair should be individually adapted, and the therapist should consider the psychological impact on the client (Rader et al., 2000).

The wheelchair seat
The wheelchair seat is given the most attention in the literature. The cushion is designed to prevent (a) pressure sores by reducing perpendicular and parallel pressures of shearing of skin and (b) contractors on the iliotibinal band of the hips. Ergonomic principles used to bring about pressure relief involve the interaction between (a) the position of the sore(s); (b) adjustment of the body position; (c) the pressure between the body and the cushion; and (d) the material and design of the cushion (Pellow, 1999). Researchers have examined ways to decrease the pressure relief at the buttocks areas by (a) using a pneumatic system to tilt individuals forward with spinal cord injury above C7 (Hefzy et al., 1996) or (b) drilling small holes in the polyurethane foam cushion (Kang and Mak, 1997). The cushion should be designed to fit the body contour (see Figure 3.2) and provide postural support to balance the body. Balance is especially important with individuals with an amputated pelvis, ataxic cerebral palsy, severe traumatic brain injury or poor posture due to age (Kanyer, 1992; Patterson and Michael, 1991; Stinnett, 1997). A well-designed cushion can make bladder and bowel care easier.

The bed

People spend more than one-third of their time in bed. For people with long-term diseases or disability who receive rehabilitation or hospice home-care, the bed may become their primary living space. The bed position, that is the height from the floor to the edge of the mattress, should be adjusted based on whether the individual with a disability is wheelchair-bound or uses a walker. Higher beds are better for individuals using a walker because they can stand up or sit down more easily. For individuals in a wheelchair, the mattress should be at the same height as the wheelchair seat so that transfer can be made more easily. If the mattress is below the seat, transfer to the bed is made less difficult; however, the mattress needs to be raised electrically before transferring back to the wheelchair. The placement of the bed in the bedroom is dependent on the need for extra space around the bed. Extra space may be needed for the wheelchair, care-giving or to prevent the individual from falling out of bed.

An electrically adjusted bed may be prescribed by the occupational therapist (Söderback and Lassfolk, 1993). The client or the caregiver can adjust the height of the bed by using a control panel with a toggle switch adapted for a grip function. Raising the head of the bed, or raising or lowering the foot of the bed may increase comfort and enable the client to engage in independent activities. Caregiving can be facilitated and 'improve the caregivers' working posture and work environment' (Söderback and Lassfolk, 1993, p. 573). Neck or back injuries in the caregiver can be prevented when assisting in personal activities such as washing, dressing or making the bed. A bed hoist and a leg hoist should be available. The bed hoist assists in raising the individual's torso, while the leg hoist is used mainly to facilitate the heart–lung function. Other pieces of equipment associated with the bed include a sit-up support, bed bars and mattress. By using the sit-up support, the individual can raise him- or herself to a sitting position, thereby increasing independence and mobility.

Söderback and Lassfolk (1993) examined the usefulness and function of electrically adjustable beds for individuals with disabilities. Participants were asked to rank pictures of ten bed activities in order of importance (see Figure 2.6). The patients and the caregivers valued the ten bed activities in three ranked groups. The first-order bed activities were: getting into and out of bed without help, changing position in bed and getting out of bed. The second-order activities were: independent ability to change position in bed, a good sleep and a good rest. The third-order activities were: recreation in bed and being with other people (Söderback and Lassfolk, 1993, p. 577).

Ranking cards is a useful method of gaining important information from the client before making clinical decisions. The client's views can be sought regarding the design and placement of the bed in one's bedroom as well as the type and placement of other furnishings.

Mattresses and mattress covers

When individuals spend a large part of their day in bed, the type of mattress must be considered, especially in the prevention and treatment of pressure sores. Factors that cause pressure sores include keeping an individual bed-bound without changing his or her position. Specialized mattresses are available, and often recommended; however, Gunningberg et al. (2000) did not find that the use of a 7 cm viscoelastic foam plus 3 cm 35 kg/m^3 foam was more effective than the 'commonly used' mattress in preventing or treating pressure sores among elderly patients with hip fractures in an orthopaedic ward.

Another product associated with the bed is a special mattress cover, frequently prescribed to prevent asthmatic or allergic symptoms. The cover should be made of dense material that will prevent dust from getting through it.

Hoists

Although the hoist is relatively expensive and not affordable by most people, it is a valuable device for assisting non-ambulatory individuals to

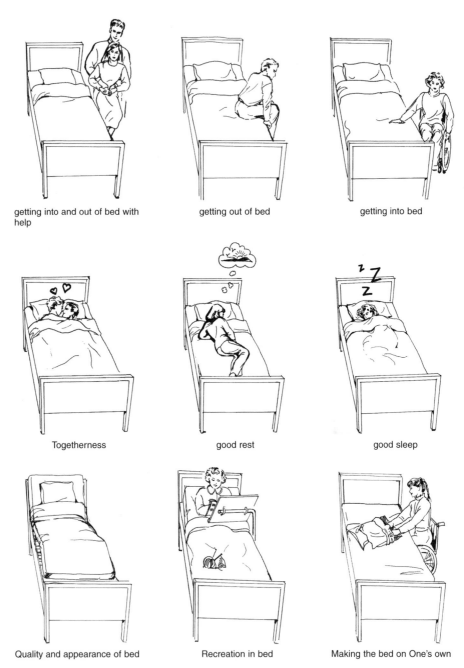

Figure 2.6 Illustration of bed functions. Reprinted with permission from Söderback, I. and Lassfolk, A. (1993). The usefulness of four methods of assessing the benefits of electrically adjustable beds in relation to their costs. The International Journal of Technology Assessment in Health Care, 9, 574–576.

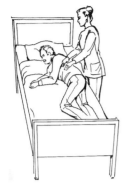

Changing position, relieving pain   **Figure 2.6**   continued.

transfer between bed and wheelchair, wheelchair and shower, or wheelchair and toilet, since it can help to prevent back and neck injures among caregivers. Two kinds of hoists are available: a manual hoist that remains on the floor and has wheels, and an electrical hoist that moves in a ceiling rail. Both types use a sling for the individual to sit in, and a spreader bar to determine the amount of room in the sling. The latter hoist should be more extensively promoted than the former (Edlund et al., 1998b). The biomechanical function of different types of manual hoists, hoist spreader bars and slings influences the comfort of the individual with disabilities during the lifting and transportation (Edlund et al., 1998a).

Adapting clothing and garments

Although not well documented, adapting clothing (overalls, capes, jackets, coats, trousers, skirts, dresses, shirts/blouses, waistcoats and aprons) is an effective ergonomic intervention, as it leads to increased functioning for individuals with disabilities such as musclar dystrophy, arthritis, body deformities such as scoliosis and spinal cord injuries (Kratz and Söderback, 1990; Kratz et al., 1997). This intervention requires (a) knowledge of construction of clothing patterns; (b) recognition of the best materials to use in making clothing; and (c) awareness of specialized clothing companies. The role of an occupational therapist is to design solutions that fit the client's specific clothing needs while increasing independence or facilitating caregiving.

Figure 2.7 provides examples of the ways that blouses, jackets and trousers have been adapted for specific individuals (Kratz and Söderback, 1990). Adaptations should be made based on the following considerations:

• Fit the garment according to individual anthropometric structure to allow for ease in movement. Increasing the shoulder span and sleeves may be more comfortable as the individual moves.

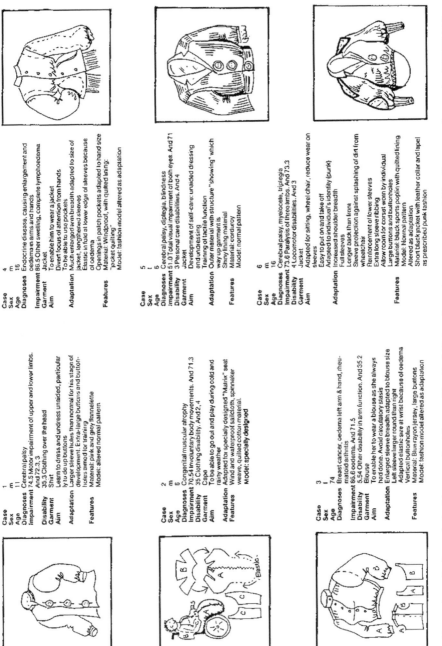

Figure 2.7 Examples of adapted clothing used with specific disabilities. Impairment and disability figures refer to the ICIDH II International Classification of Impairments, Disabilities and Handicaps II (WHO 1980). Reprinted with permission from Kratz, G. and Söderback, I. (1990). Individualised adaptation of clothes for impaired persons. Scandinavian Journal of Rehabilitation Medicine, 22, 166–168.

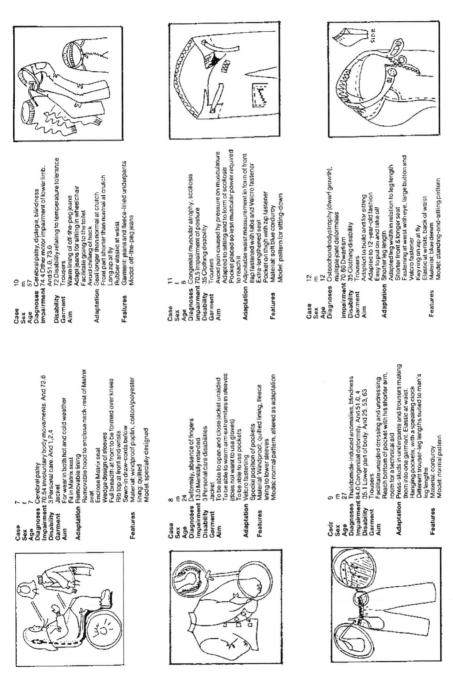

Case 7
Sex m
Age 7
Diagnoses Cerebral palsy
Impairment 70.54 Involuntary body movements. And 72.6
Disability 3 Personal care. And 1,2,4
Garment Jacket
Aim For wear in both hot and cold weather. Fit in Matrix seat
Adaptation Removable lining. Removable hood to enclose neck-rest of Matrix seat. Enclose Matrix seal. Wedge design of sleeves. Full breadth at front to be formed over knees. Rib top at front and wrists. Sewn-in draw-cords below
Features Material: windproof poplin, cotton/polyester lining, quilted. Model: specially designed

Case 8
Sex m
Age 24
Diagnoses Deformity, absence of fingers
Impairment 13.0 Mentally retarded
Disability 3 Personal care disabilities
Garment Jacket
Aim To be able to open and close jacket unaided. To be able to warm arm extremities in sleeves (does not want to use gloves). To be able to use pockets
Adaptation Velcro fastening
Features Special position of pockets. Material: Windproof, quilted lining, fleece lining to lower sleeves. Model: normal pattern, altered as adaptation

Case 9
Sex m
Age 27
Diagnoses Thalidomide-induced anomalies, blindness
Impairment 84.0 Congenital deformity. And 51.0, 4
Disability 35.1 Lower part of body. And 25, 53, 63
Garment Trousers
Aim Facilitate unaided dressing and undressing. Reach bottom of pocket with his shorter arm. Room for a technical aid
Adaptation Press-studs in underpants and trousers making them into one garment. Elastic at waist. Hanging pockets, with a speaking clock. Different trouser-leg lengths suited to man's leg lengths
Features Material: corduroy. Model: normal pattern

Case 10
Sex m
Age 57
Diagnoses Cerebral palsy, diplegia, blindness
Impairment 74.4 Other motor impairment of lower limb. And 51.0, 73.0
Disability 72 Disability relating to temperature tolerance
Garment Trousers
Aim Warming of off-the-peg jeans. Adapt jeans for sitting in wheelchair. Facilitate going to the toilet. Avoid chafing of back
Adaptation Seat longer than normal at crutch. Front part shorter than normal at fly. Long zip at fly. Rubber elastic at waist
Features Garment: jeans and fleece-lined underpants. Model: off-the-peg jeans

Case 11
Sex m
Age 8
Diagnoses Congenital muscular atrophy, scoliosis
Impairment 70.5 Impairment of posture
Disability 35 Clothing disability
Garment Trousers
Aim Avoid pain caused by pressure on musculature. Adapted to sitting and to form of scoliosis. Pocket placed so less muscular power required to reach it
Adaptation Adjustable waist measurement in form of front flap fastened with tabs and Velcro fastener. Extra-lengthened seat. Pocket on thigh with zip fastener
Features Material: soft blue corduroy. Model: pattern for sitting-down

Case 12
Sex m
Age 12
Diagnoses Osteochondrodystrophy (dwarf growth), multiple joint deformities
Impairment 70 80 Dwarfism
Disability 35 Clothing disability
Garment Trousers
Aim Adapted to build and for sitting. Adapted to 12-year-old fashion. Easy to pull on and take off. Shorter leg length
Adaptation Adapted to leg width in relation to leg length. Shorter front & longer seat. Fastening at waist with eye, large button and Velcro fastener. Key ring on zip at fly
Features Elastic at wrists, back of waist. Material: blue denim. Model: standing-and-sitting pattern

Figure 2.7 continued.

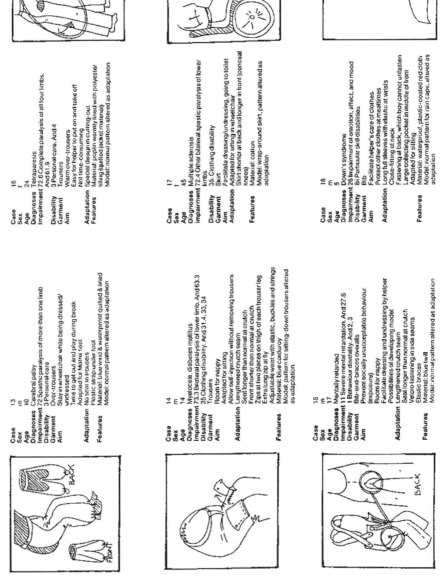

Case 13
Sex m
Age 10
Diagnoses Cerebral palsy
Impairment 72 Spastic paralysis of more than one limb
Disability 3 Personal care
Garment Over-trousers
Aim Stay in wheelchair while being dressed/undressed. Time to get out and play during break. Adapted for Matrix seat
Adaptation No seat to trousers
Features Plastic strap under foot. Material: blue wind & waterproof quilted & lined. Model: normal pattern altered as adaptation

Case 14
Sex m
Age 14
Diagnoses Myelocele, diabetes mellitus
Impairment 73.3 Bilateral paralysis of lower limb. And 63.3
Disability 35 Clothing disability. And 31.4, 33, 34
Garment Trousers
Aim Adapted for sitting. Allow self-injection without removing trousers
Adaptation Lengthened crutch seam. Front shorter than normal at crutch. Zips at two places on thigh of each trouser leg. Extra long zip at fly. Adjustable waist with elastic, buckles and strings
Features Material: blue corduroy. Model: pattern for sitting-down trousers altered as adaptation

Case 15
Sex m
Age 17
Diagnoses Mentally retarded
Impairment 11 Severe mental retardation. And 27.6
Disability 1 Behaviour disability. And 2, 3
Garment Bib-and-braces overalls
Aim Prevent socially unacceptable behaviour (exposing). Room for nappy. Facilitate dressing and undressing by helper. Possibilities of developing model
Adaptation Lengthened crutch seam. Seat longer than normal at crutch. Velcro fastening in side seams. Elastic braces
Features Material: blue twill. Model: normal pattern altered as adaptation

Case 16
Sex f
Age 24
Diagnoses Tetraparesis
Impairment 72.6 Complete paralysis of all four limbs. And 61.9
Disability 3 Personal care. And 4
Garment Trousers
Aim Warm over-trousers. Easy for helper to put on and take off. Not time-consuming
Adaptation Special design in cutting-out
Features Material: poplin warmly lined with polyester filling (quilted jacket material). Model: normal pattern altered as adaptation

Case 17
Sex f
Age 45
Diagnoses Multiple sclerosis
Impairment 72.4 Other bilateral spastic paralysis of lower limbs
Disability 35. Clothing disability
Garment Skirt
Aim Facilitate dressing/undressing, going to toilet. Adapted for sitting in wheelchair
Adaptation Skirt shorter at back and longer in front (conceal knees)
Features Material: cotton. Model: wrap-around skirt, pattern altered as adaptation

Case 18
Sex m
Age 5
Diagnoses Down's syndrome
Impairment 28 Impairment of emotion, affect, and mood
Disability 8ii Particular skill disabilities
Garment Bib
Aim Facilitate helper's care of clothes. Protect other clothes at mealtimes
Adaptation Long full sleeves with elastic at wrists. Close-fitting at neck. Fastening at back, which boy cannot unfasten. Large collecting pocket in middle of front. Adapted for sitting
Features Material: waterproof, plastic-coated red cloth. Model: normal pattern for rain cape, altered as adaptation

Figure 2.7 continued.

- Provide clothing that facilitates dressing, undressing and toileting during ADL. The client's and the caregiver's needs should be considered. Using garments with larger sleeves and trouser legs will make them easier to put on. Using elastic in the waist band of trousers makes toileting easier than when buttons or press-studs are used as fasteners.
- Use material that protects the client from becoming too cold, too hot or too wet, especially during outdoor activities. Frequently, individuals with disabilities are unaware of or unable to regulate their body temperature.
- Use materials that are smooth and non-abrasive so that the occurrence of pressure sores can be reduced.
- Use garments that are attractive and fashionable to increase the client's sense of well-being during social interactions.

Use of assistive devices and assistive technology in the home

People expect their home to be comfortable, safe and convenient. They also expect their home environment to support their health and well-being and to reduce the cost of living (Branson, 1991a). During the past century the use of electrical appliances to facilitate housework has become the standard for many households. For example, many homes have (a) microwave ovens for cooking and warming up food (Kondo et al., 1997); (b) electrostatic filters or Hepa air filters to reduce the dust, thereby reducing the possibility of asthmatic attacks; (c) automatic timers for electrical appliances, lights and watering devices; and (d) alarms to alert residents to fire, smoke or carbon monoxide. However, when people do not have access to these appliances, or the design of a specific appliance does not fit the individual's impairment, the occupational therapist, in consultation with the client, may recommend assistive technology devices or services.

The application of assistive devices or technology (AT) is mediated by the cognitive abilities of the individual, the task to be performed and the environment (Fuhrer et al., 2003). In this interaction, the impact of the disability or disease on the individual influences the ability to use assistive technology and to perform activities of daily living within home.

The relationship between the person, an activity, the environment and the assistive device or technology is described by three models (Ahmadi, 1997; Mace, 1998; Trachtman et al., 1999). In the Human Activity Assistance Technology Model (Cook and Hussey, 2002), the context of the person using the technology is important in determining whether the technology will be used. The Human Environment Technology Interface (HETI) (Smith, 1991) emphasizes the sensory input from the environment and the cognitive processes involved in decision-making with the functional use of the technology. The Human Interface Assessment (HIA) (Anson, 1994) model matches the abilities of the individual with the demands of the assistive technologies.

Under the Assistive Technology Act of 1998 (para. 2), assistive technology service is defined as:

> any service that directly assists an individual with a disability in the selection, acquisition, or use of an assistive technology device. Such term includes:
>
> A) the evaluation of the assistive technology needs of an individual with a disability, including functional evaluation of the impact of the provision of appropriate assistive technology and appropriate services to the individual in the customary environment of the individual;
>
> B) services consisting of the purchasing, leasing, or otherwise providing for the acquisition of assistive technology devices by individuals with disabilities;
>
> C) services consisting of selecting, designing, fitting, customizing, adapting, applying, maintaining, repairing, or replacing assistive technology devices;
>
> D) coordination and use of necessary therapies, interventions or services with assistive technology devices, such as [those] associated with education and rehabilitation plans, and programs;
>
> E) training or technical assistance for an individual with disabilities or, where appropriate, the family members, guardians, advocates or authorized representatives of such an individual;
>
> F) training or technical assistance for professionals (including individuals providing education and rehabilitation services), employers, or other individuals who provide services to, employ or are otherwise substantially involved in the major life functions of individuals with disabilities.

Although occupational therapists, physicians, nurses, physiotherapists and other caregivers by law have rights and obligations to prescribe assistive technology, country or state law determines what assistive technology or assistive technology services should be available for people with disabilities and at what cost (Kornblau et al., 2000). For example, in the United States, all new televisions must have accessibility to closed captions or availability to TTY (text telephone for the hearing impaired) (Americans with Disabilities Act of 1990, 1991).

Writing a prescription for assistive technology requires the occupational therapist to recommend the most appropriate assistive technology equipment based on the client's specific disability, functional status, habits, roles and the environment in which the device is being used (American Occupational Therapy Association, 1991; Deterding et al., 1991; Mann et al., 1995; Stein and Roose, 2000). Consideration of the quality, safety and installation of the equipment, as well as instructions and follow-up on how to use the assistive device or technology, is also important. This process may be performed by home visits or scheduled phone contacts.

Occupational therapists commonly prescribe orthoses to clients who have a static loss of body function or body structure (Belkin and Yasuda, 2001). Decisions about which orthoses or splints should be used are dependent on the functional capacity and disability of the client. The ergonomically appropriate decision will be based on (a) physical criteria (i.e. weight, material, size and shape); (b) functional criteria (i.e. stability, textures); and (c) aesthetics. Many assistive devices and assistive technologies are readily available on the market and hence occupational therapists are urged to consider commonly used objects when making clinical decisions about assistive devices (Nordenskiöld, 1997). Other assistive devices include walkers, reachers and dressing aids (Chen et al., 1998; Gitlin and Burgh, 1995; Mann and Lane, 1998; Mann et al., 1993a; Mann et al., 1993b; Mann et al., 1995).

Although the lines between categories are somewhat fuzzy, AT devices are often referred to as 'low-tech' or 'high-tech'. Low-tech devices include built-up handles, while high-tech devices include such devices as the Hoyer lifting system (Edlund et al., 1998a; Edlund et al., 1998b), electrical or pneumatic gripping systems (Davis et al., 1999; Saxena et al., 1995), powered feeding devices for individuals with cerebral palsy (Herrman et al., 1999), augmentative or alternative communication (Angelo and Smith 1993) and computers. Many high-tech devices involve computerized programming. An occupational therapist in collaboration with a computer consultant, can devise individual control systems to help people with a cognitive or physical disability to monitor (a) open or unlocked doors and windows; (b) stoves or electric appliances which have not been turned off; (c) running water; (d) daily schedules; and (e) recognition tasks, such as operating doors and windows (Cowan and Turner-Smith, 1999; Lindberg et al., 1999; Watzke, 1997).

One example of a computerized control system is the Imperium 200H, illustrated in Figure 2.8 (InterAct Plus, 2000–2002). This system enables an individual to control his or her environment by using a switch. Another example of an AT programme is the Mobility and Activity Assistance System for the Disabled (MOVAID) (Dario et al., 1999), available in Italy. Using two fixed workstations, the MOVAID is a personal robot that provides assistance to individuals with disabilities and elderly people in everyday activities of daily living. 'Typical tasks for the system, defined on the basis of identified users' needs are: to warm up some food in a microwave oven and serve it at user's bed, to clean the kitchen surface, to remove dirty sheets from a bed' (MTech Lab Research, 2000, para 3).

Assistive technology organizations

Many industrialized countries have organizations that develop, test and supply information about assistive technology to the general population.

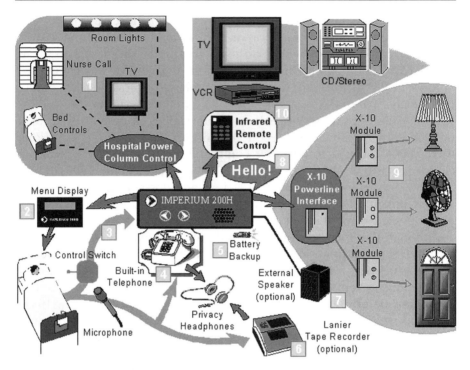

Figure 2.8 The Imperium(r) 200H environmental control unit.

1. Hospital facility controls: Control the Nurse Call, reading and room lights, TV, and electronic bed adjustments (via the Imperium 200AA Bed/Hospital Room Adapter).

2. Control menus: The top-level menu has sub-menus for: telephone, X-10, infrared, room controls, tape recorder, accessories, limited augmentative communication and clock. Menu items scan on the display and are spoken.

3. Dual-switch control: The system is usually operated by dual-switches, although two single switches can be used via a 'Y' connector adapter. Attendants can use the two switches on the unit's front panel.

4. Telephone: The built-in, hands-free speaker telephone holds a personal directory for speed-dialing, can be used with headphones for privacy, and electronically filters out background noises. The user controls the volume and, if using headphones, can mute the system speaker.

5. Battery backup: An internal battery/charger works continuously. If AC power is lost, the system switches to battery power and the green LEDs on the main unit and display unit will flash. When configured for a health care facility, the nurse call automatically activates after five minutes of battery operation.

6. Optional tape recorder: This provides note-taking capability for personal, educational and work purposes.

7. External speaker: An optional external speaker can be put nearby, if the Imperium 200H (with its built-in speaker) is situated some distance away.

8. Speech scanning: Using a recorded voice, the unit speaks each menu item as it is scanned on the LCD display.

9. X10 controls: Imperium 200H controls regular, unmodified lights and appliances using X10 technology through existing AC wiring.

10. Infrared controls: Up to five infrared devices may be controlled via the ONE FOR ALL 6 remote control unit.

11. Auxiliary equipment: Operate up to two switch-closure devices (e.g. automatic door openers, curtain controls, page turners) through a control function on the main menu.

Reprinted by permission from 'Diagram of Imperium 200H Functions' by InterAct Plus, 2000, available at http://www.interactplus.com/functional_diagram.htm

The following paragraphs describe some of these organizations:

- 'The Swedish Handicap Institute aims at improving the quality of life for people with disabilities. Its major tasks are to ensure access to high quality and well-functioning assistive technology and to work for an increased access to society. The Institute's work includes stimulation of research and development, analyses of needs and testing of assistive technology. It also gives out information and performs training to professionals regarding assistive technology for different categories of disabilities. The Institute is also involved in international research and co-operative projects in the field of assistive technology and accessibility' (The Swedish Handicap Institute, nd, para 1).
- Developed in 1971, the Trace Research and Development Center, a part of the College of Engineering, University of Wisconsin-Madison, has as its mission 'To prevent the barriers and capitalize on the opportunities presented by current and emerging technologies, in order to create a world that is as accessible and usable as possible for as many people as possible' (Trace Research and Development Center, nd, para 2)
- In Australia, the Australian Rehabilitation and Assistive Technology Association (ARATA) 'is a national association whose purpose is to serve as a forum for issues in rehabilitation and assistive technology' (Australian Rehabilitation and Assistive Technology Association, 2004, para 1).
- In the United Kingdom, the Foundation for Assistive Technology is an independent networking organization funded by the British Department of Health (FAST, 2002). Their mission is to work 'with users of assistive technology to maximise their independence. We bring together people who use assistive technology, researchers, developers, manufacturers and service providers to build effective partnerships. Our aim is to ensure that development of assistive technology and improvements to service delivery are led by the needs and wishes of users' (Guide Information Services, 2003, para 1).
- The Rehabilitation Engineering and Assistive Technology Society of North America (RESNA) is 'an interdisciplinary association of people with a common interest in technology and disability. Our purpose is to improve the potential of people with disabilities to achieve their goals through the use of technology. We serve that purpose by promoting research, development, education, advocacy and provision of technology; and by supporting the people engaged in these activities' (Rehabilitation Engineering and Assistive Technology Society of North America, nd, paras 1–3).

Case study example

An example of how ergonomics can be applied to the prescription of assistive technology (Anson, 1994) is described by Larsson et al. (1995).

Case study Bertil describes the application of computer technology as a way of compensating for difficulties in cognitive functions relating to impaired short-term memory, concentration difficulties and loss of initiative. The aim of the computer instruction for Bertil was to adapt the software and computer environment to his needs to enable him to engage in computer games and to operate a word-processing program.

Initial assessment
The results of the interview revealed that Bertil has a positive attitude towards computers. The evaluation instruments used for Bertil showed that he needed a programme compensating for his loss of initiative, poor concentration and impaired short-term memory to be independent with his computer. Bertil has good vision and relatively unaffected motor control.

Equipment
The software has to be adapted in the simplest possible way for Bertil's specific needs. The equipment obtained for Bertil was an IBM-type computer with a colour dot-matrix printer and the software program Hangman. This program is a computer game in the form of a word-guessing game. The task is to work out a predetermined word without being 'hanged'. The game is simple in design in clear graphics and both audio and visual feedback.

Supervision
Bertil received instruction once a week for 18 weeks. Each learning session was divided into short practical exercises lasting about three hours. Before the supervision the computer was set up for four weeks in the staff office to give the staff an opportunity to familiarize themselves with the computer so that they would be able to help Bertil. The computer was then, at the beginning of the supervision period, placed in Bertil's living room in a prominent place so that he would be reminded that it was there and thus, hopefully, would be inspired to work at it.

The computer 'screen-saver' displayed a recurring, scrolling encouragement in large text (Times New Roman 48 pt) 'PRESS ANY KEY, BERTIL'. This screen saver was turned on automatically after two minutes when the computer was not being used, which was a reminder for Bertil to take the initiative in using the computer. Bertil could find the on/off switch without help when it was adapted with a coloured, self-adhesive sticker placed over the switch showing up clearly against the grey tone of the computer. Bertil had problems relating the pointer movements on the screen to his own hand movements with the mouse. Therefore, a simpler menu program than Windows was produced with a limited number of possible one keystroke options. Here function keys F1–F12 were used with an associated choice of activity. Thus the activity 'writing' was selected by pressing F2. The menu program was arranged so that it was automatically the first, and only one, to be opened when the computer was started. The program included the option of entering new functions in the menu and the option of rapidly returning to the Windows program controller. The menu program included an 'initiative supporting' command in large letters 'CHOOSE WHAT YOU WANT TO DO, BERTIL'.

When Bertil tried to write he spent much time identifying keyboard letters. While scanning the screen he often lost the point of what he was doing, which meant that he got stuck in his writing. The keyboard letters were then enlarged so that he could scan and find them more quickly. An enlarged heading was also designed for the word-processing program. The purpose was to remind Bertil to continue the activity if and when his concentration or endurance faltered. The heading was phrased as a command 'WRITE SOMETHING HERE, BERTIL'.

The Hangman game was also installed in Bertil's computer. Here he was given the command 'CHOOSE A LETTER'. Bertil needed help to get into the program but, once there, he had no problems in handling it.

Goal attainment scaling

During the supervision, goal attainment was measured continuously. Bertil worked towards five different sub-goals working on two or three at a time . . . The evaluation showes that all the sub-goals were attained because a T value of over 50 was achieved (T = 57.77).

Summary of GAS sub-goals for case study B

Goal	Adaptations	Activity	Instructions
1	Start computer		
2	Handle computer after technical adaptation		
3			Compensate for impaired initiative
4		To write on his own a number of words in sequence	
5		To play a game independently	

Conclusion

During the supervision period, Bertil rarely sat at the computer of his own accord. According to the staff, relatives and the supervising occupational therapist, Bertil did show interest in the computer when he had someone's attention and encouragement. He also reacted positively to what he had completed, e.g. when he wrote a letter or succeeded in finding a word in the game.

The teaching-learning process

The outcome of the dynamic interaction process between the person, the environment and the task being performed in accordance with ergonomic principles is influenced by the occupational therapist's ability to teach and the person's ability to learn new strategies. As a part of this teaching-learning process the occupational therapist structures the components of the interaction, the environment and the tasks so that they are adapted to the individual's capabilities for performing daily occupations.

There are four steps to the teaching-learning process: acquisition, proficiency, maintenance and generalization. Initially during the teaching-learning process, the occupational therapist provides instruction in how to perform the task or in the use of an assistive technology device. At this stage the client acquires the knowledge or skill. For example, a client may be shown how to get in and out of a wheelchair. A caregiver may be given instruction on assisting the client into a bed from the wheelchair. Learning the skill is dependent on the client's active participation and understanding of the skill. Once the client has acquired the skill, then he or she must perform the task proficiently or automatically. Over time, with continued use, the skill is maintained. Finally, generalization involves using the skill in a new place, at a new time, with different people and with different materials.

Skill generalization is affected by a number of factors. The client's ability to generalize the skill is affected by his or her active participation and by the positive intrinsic or extrinsic feedback obtained. Generalization must also occur in a naturalistic setting. Thus, a client who automatically uses ergonomic principles to get in and out of a chair will generalize that skill to any situation in which he or she finds him- or herself. The intrinsic reward of being independent will further the use of the skill.

Strategies in the teaching-learning process

'Strategies are organized plans or sets of rules that guide action' (Sabari, 2001, p. 86). These strategies are combinations of (a) kinetic (movement) linkages (Sabari, 2001); (b) cognitive plans for recognizing, understanding, remembering and performing tasks in a logical order (Söderback, 1988a, 1988b); (c) interpersonal learned habits used in the social interaction with other people (Sabari, 2001); and (d) problem-focused coping behaviour for handling stress-reactions (Nätterlund, 2001; Nätterlund and Ahlström 1999). 'People develop strategies through a process of encountering problems, implementing solutions, and monitoring the effects of these solutions' (Sabari, 2001, p. 86). The occupational therapist promotes the development and learning of these strategies during the task performance process (Söderback, 1988a).

There are at least two types of strategies:

1 *Therapeutic strategies* involve supporting clients to be in control of their own lives. These strategies may include building a relationship with their clients, finding the right way to motivate clients, supporting the setting of goals and providing positive occupational experience by

adjusting training to the needs of the client (rather than focusing on teaching clients how to use technical and compensatory strategies) (Guidetti and Tham, 2002).

2 *A compensating strategy* teaches the client to compensate for impairments by using existing functions or by positioning the object so that an advantage is taken of gravity. This puts less demand on muscles and joints. For example, an individual with a unilateral upper extremity amputation can compensate by using his lower extremities to assist in opening a jar by placing and stabilizing the jar between his legs and using one hand to open the jar.

The strategies used to perform daily activities throughout the lifespan involve a long-standing teaching-learning process. Client's former habits may not work when an impairment suddenly occurs and they may be resistant to changes. The occupational therapist teaches new strategies to clients and must encourage them to use the strategy as part of their repertoire of behaviour. Appropriate individual strategies should be generalized and become a habit in one's everyday life. Individuals who slowly develop increased impairments such as muscular dystrophy, post-polio syndrome or amyotrophic lateral sclerosis sometimes develop their own strategies and figure out independently how to do something. Sometimes unorthodox movements and body parts are used, such as using teeth to open a package. In such cases the role of the occupational therapist is to encourage the client to become aware of these strategies and to encourage and generalize their use. These individually performed strategies are the person's unique way of coping with environmentally focused problems when performing occupations. For example, a person may be able to pick up a piece of paper from the floor, but because of muscle weakness cannot get up. That person may develop a strategy for sitting up again by using his or her other hand to pull themselves up (Nätterlund, 2001). Another person may have difficulties retrieving words, but develops a strategy of writing the first letter in his or her palm order to retrieve the word (Söderback, 1988c). Individual strategies commonly used by occupational therapists with clients having progressive muscle disease or dysfunction are identified below (Nätterlund, 2001; Nätterlund and Ahlström, 1999):

- using an unusual body part for an activity, such as using the toes as a gripping tool
- increasing ability to open objects (e.g. cans, jars, windows) by using both hands, using a lever or optimal positioning
- using gravity as a force. For example, if opening a window is difficult from waist-level due to lack of leverage, the individual might find it easier to get above the window.

Summary

In this chapter a dynamic integrative process based on ergonomic principles has been presented for working with clients in the home environment. Detailed descriptions of strategies and interventions are presented to help the reader develop the expertise and clinical reasoning skills to work effectively with the client with a disability to function in the home. Finally, home interventions using ergonomic principles are presented from a research perspective. These interventions include environmental strategies to prevent injuries in the home, to foster independence in the client and to assist the caregiver in helping the client optimally. In this process the occupational therapist uses compensation, adaptation and arrangement of the home environment, prescription of assistive technology and strategies concerning the teaching-learning process. In summary, a conceptual model for the occupational therapist has been presented to assist the client to become as independent as possible as using occupation in the home.

Review questions

1 How is the home environment defined?
2 What are the main components of home environment interventions?
3 How can ergonomic principles be applied to interventions in the home environment?
4 What are the major goals in applying the ergonomic model in the home?
5 How can we evaluate the outcome of the interventions applied to the home?
6 What effect does the disability in an individual have on functional independence in the home?
7 How can we help an individual with a disability to become independent in the home environment?
8 How can we teach the client biomechanical principles and functional strategies necessary to become as independent as possible in self-care and home-making tasks?

References

Acheson-Cooper, B. and Stewart, D. (1998). The effect of a transfer device in the homes of elderly women. Physical and Occupational Therapy in Geriatrics, 15, 61–76.

Ahmadi, R.T. (1997). Keys to independence: A universal design approach. Focus on Geriatric Care and Rehabilitation, 1, 1–38.

ADA Accessibility Guidelines for Buildings and Facilities (1991, 26 July). Federal Register, 56(144), 35633-35636. Retrieved 29 December 2004, http://www.cs.wright.edu/bie/rehabengr/ramps/adaramp.htm

Adaptive Environments Center (1996) The Consumer's Guide to Home Adaptation. Boston: AEC. Available from Adaptive Environments, 374 Congress St., Ste. 301, Boston, MA, 02240. 617-695-1225.

American Occupational Therapy Association (1991). Position paper: Occupational therapy and assistive technology. American Journal of Occupational Therapy, 45, 1076–1045.

Americans with Disabilities Act of 1990 (1991). 28 CFR Part 36: ADA standards for accessible design (Rev. 1 July, 1994). Retrieved 24 January 2004, http://www.usdoj.gov/crt/ada/adastd94.pdf

Aminzadeh, F., Plotinkoff, R. and Edwards, N. (1999). Development and evaluation of the Cane Cognitive Mediator Instrument. Nursing Research, 48, 269–275.

Angelo, J. and Smith, R.O. (1993). An analysis of computer-related articles in occupational therapy periodicals. American Journal of Occupational Therapy, 47, 25–29.

Anson, D. (1994). Finding your way in the maze of computer access technology. American Journal of Occupational Therapy, 48, 121–129.

Assistive Technology Act 2001. 29 U.S.C. §3002 (2001). Definitions: Assistive technology. Retrieved 28 December 2004, http://www.section508.gov/docs/AT1998.html#3

Australian Rehabilitation and Assistive Technology Association (2004). ARATA. Retrieved 29 December 2004, http://www.e-bility.com/arata/index.php

Barris, R. (1982). Environmental interactions: An extension of the model of occupation. American Journal of Occupational Therapy, 36, 637–644.

Barris, R., Cordero, J. and Christiansen, R. (1986). Occupational therapists' use of media. American Journal of Occupational Therapy, 40, 679–684.

Bashford, G.M., Steele, J.R., Munro, B.J., Westcott, G. and Jones, M.E. (1998). Ejector chairs: Do they work and are they safe? Australian Occupational Therapy Journal, 45, 99–106.

Belkin, J. and Yasuda, L. (2001). Orthotics. In L.W. Pedretti and M.B. Early (Eds). Occupational Therapy. Practice Skills for Physical Dysfunction (5th edn; pp. 529–567). St. Louis: Mosby.

Benktzon, M. (1993). Designing for our future selves: The Swedish experience. Applied Ergonomics, 24, 19–27.

Branson, G.D. (1991a). The Barrier Free Housing. Convenient Living for the Elderly and Physically Handicapped. White Hall, VA: Betterway Publications.

Branson, G.D. (1991b). The Complete Guide to Barrier Free Housing. White Hall, VA: Betterway Publications.

Breines, E.B. (2001). Occupational therapy interventions. The biomechanical approach. In L.W. Pedretti and M.B. Early (Eds). Occupational Therapy: Practice Skills for Physical Dysfunction (5th edn; pp. 503–529). St. Louis: Mosby.

Brodwin, MG., Cardoso, E. and Star, T. (2004). Computer assistive technology for people who have disabilities: Computer adaptations and modifications. Journal of Rehabilitation, 70, 28–33.

Bronfenbrenner, U. (1977). Toward an experimental ecology of human development. American Psychologist, 32, 513–531.

Brus, H.L.M., van de Laar, M.A.F., Oosterveld, F.G.J., van Bussel, A., Rasker, J.J. and Salmans, D. (1997). Development of a brief observation method for measuring joint protective behaviours: Reliability. Journal of Occupational Rehabilitation, 7, 167–172.

Burke, C.E. (1999). Summary of reliability study of matrices. Technology and Disability, 10, 181–185.

Burns, S.P. and Betz, K.L. (1999). Seating pressures with conventional and dynamic wheelchair cushions in tetraplegia. Archives in Physical and Medical Rehabilitation 80, 566–571.

Callinan, N.J. and Mathiowetz, V. (1996). Soft versus hard resting hand splints in rheumatoid arthritis: Pain relief, preference, and compliance. American Journal of Occupational Therapy, 50, 347–353.

Calkins, M. and Namazi, K. (1991). Caregivers' perception of the effectiveness of home modification for community living adults with dementia. Journal of Alzheimer's Care and Related Disorder Research, 6, 25–29.

Chen, L.P., Mann, W.C., Tomita, M. and Burford, T.E. (1998). An evaluation of reachers for use by older persons with disabilities. Assistive Technology, 10, 113–125.

Christenson, M.A. (1999). Embracing universal design. Occupational Therapy Practice, 8, 12–15.

Christophersen, J. (Ed.) (2002). Universal design: 17 ways of thinking and teaching. Oslo: Husbanken.

Chung, C., Mann, W.C., Mulloch, A. and Tomita, M. (1997). Comparisons of cane handle designs for use by elders with arthritic hands. Technology and Disability, 7, 183–198.

Clemson, L. and Martin, R. (1996). Usage and effectiveness of rails, bathing and toileting. Occupational Therapy in Health Care, 10, 41–59.

Clemson, L., Cusick, A. and Fozzard, C. (1999). Managing risk and exerting control: Determining follow through with falls prevention. Disability and Rehabilitation, 21, 531–541.

Collins, F. and Shipperley, T.F. (1999). Assessing the seated patient for the risk of pressure damage. Journal of Wound Care, 8, 123–126.

Cook, A.M. and Hussey, S.M. (2002). Assistive Technologies: Principles and Practice (2nd edn). St Louis: Mosby.

Cooper, B.A., Cohen, U. and Hasselkus, B.R. (1991). Barrier-free design: A review and critique of the occupational therapy perspective. American Journal of Occupational Therapy, 45, 344–350.

Cooper, R.A., Robertson, R.N., Boninger, M.L., Shimada, S.D., VanSickle, D.P., Lawrence, B. and Singleton, T. (1997). Wheelchair ergonomics. In S. Kumar (Ed.), Perspectives in Rehabilitation Ergonomics (pp. 246–272). Bristol, PA: Taylor and Francis.

Cowan, D.M. and Turner-Smith, A.R. (1999). The user's perspective on the provision of electronic assistive technology: Equipped for life? British Journal of Occupational Therapy, 62, 2–6.

Cutter, N.C. and Blake, D.J. (1997). Wheelchairs and seating systems: Clinical applications. Physical Medicine and Rehabilitation: State of the Art Reviews, 11, 223–226.

Dario, P., Guglienlmelli, E., Laschi, C. and Teti, G. (1999). MOVAID: A personal robot in everyday life of disabled and elderly people. Technology and Disability, 10, 77–93.

Davis, R., Mulcahey, M.J. and Betz, R.R. (1999). Making freehand their hand: The role of occupational therapy in implementing FES in tetraplegia. Technology and Disability, 11, 29–34.

Deterding, C., Youngstrom, M.J. and Dunn, W. (1991). Position paper: Occupational therapy and assistive technology. American Journal of Occupational Therapy, 45, 1076.

Dunn, P.A. (1996). Government policy innovations and trends in barrier-free housing, accessible transportation and personal supports. Canadian Journal of Rehabilitation, 10, 113–123.

Dunn, P.A. (1997). A comparative analysis of barrier-free housing: Policies for elderly people in the United States and Canada. Journal of Housing for the Elderly, 12, 37–53.

Eberhardt, K. (1998). Home modifications for persons with spinal cord injury. Occupational Therapy Practice 3, 24–27.

Edlich, R.F. (1995). Burn rehabilitation forum . . . Effective pressure ulcer prevention in burn centers. Journal of Burn Care and Rehabilitation, 16, 65–66.

Edlund, C.K., Harms-Ringdahl, K. and Ekholm, J. (1998a). Properties of person hoist spreader bars and their influence on sitting/lifting position. Scandinavian Journal of Rehabilitation Medicine, 30, 151–158.

Edlund, C.K., Harms-Ringdahl, K. and Seiger, A. (1998b). Lift/transfer and technical aids for persons with severe acquired brain injury: An inventory of problems. Scandinavian Journal of Caring Sciences, 12, 154–159.

Fänge, A. and Iwarsson, S. (2003). Accessibility and usability in housing: Construct validity and implication for research and practice. Disability Rehabilitation, 25, 1316–1325.

Forrest, G. and Gombas, G. (1995). Wheelchair accessible housing: Its role in cost containment in spinal cord injury. Archives of Physical Medicine and Rehabilitation, 76, 450–452.

Foti, D. (2001). Activities of daily living. In L.W. Pedretti and M.B. Early (Eds), Occupational Therapy: Practice Skills for Physical Dysfunction (5th edn; pp. 124–171). London: Mosby.

Fougeyrollas, P. (1995). Documenting environmental factors for preventing the handicap creation process. Disability and Rehabilitation, 17, 14153.

Foundation for Assistive Technology (FAST) (2002). Foundation for Assistive Technology. Retrieved 7 February 2004, http://www.fastuk.org/

Fricke, J. and Worrell, D. (1991). Hotel lounge chairs: Suitability for the elderly tourist. Australian Occupational Therapy Journal, 38, 93–99.

Frisk, M., Blomqvist, A., Stridh, G., Sjoden, P. and Kiviloog, J. (2002) Occupational therapy adaptation of the home environment in Sweden for people with asthma. Occupational Therapy International, 9, 294–311.

Fuhrer, M.J., Jutai, J.W., Scherer, M.J. and Deruyter, F. (2003). A framework for conceptual modeling of assistive technology device outcome. Disability and Rehabilitation, 25, 1243–1251.

Garber, S.L. and Dyerly, L.R. (1991). Wheelchair cushions for persons with spinal cord injury: An update. American Journal of Occupational Therapy, 45, 550–554.

Gignac, M. and Cott, C. (1998). A conceptual model of independence and dependence for adults with chronic physical illness and disability. Social Science and Medicine, 47, 739–753.

Gitlin, L.N. (1998a). The role of social science research in understanding technology use among older adults. In G. Ory and G.H. DeFriese (Eds), Self-care in Later Life. Research, Program, and Policy Issues (pp. 142–168). New York: Springer.

Gitlin, L.N. (1998b). Testing home modification interventions: Issues of theory, measurement, design, and implementation. Annual Review of Gerontology and Geriatrics, 18, 190–246.

Gitlin, L.N. and Burgh, D. (1995). Issuing assistive devices to older patients in rehabilitation: An exploratory study. American Journal of Occupational Therapy, 49, 994–1000.

Gitlin, L.N., Swenson Miller, K. and Boyce, A. (1999). Bathroom modifications for frail elderly renters: Outcomes of a community based program. Technology and Disability, 10, 131–149.

Guide Information Services (2003). Foundation for Assistive Technology (FAST). Retrieved 29 December 2004, http://www.guide-information.org.uk/guide/search_index_detail.lasso?RecID=G12781

Guidetti, S. and Söderback, I. (2001). Description of self care training in occupational therapy: Case studies of five Kenyan children with cerebral palsy. Occupational Therapy International, 8, 34–48.

Guidetti, S. and Tham, K. (2002). Therapeutic strategies used by occupational therapists in self-care training: A qualitative study. Occupational Therapy International 9, 257–276.

Gunningberg, L., Lindholm, C., Carlsson, M. and Sjödén, P.O. (2000). Effect of visco elastic foam mattressess on the development of pressure ulcers in patients with hip fractures. Journal of Wound Care, 9, 455–460.

Hagsten, B.E. and Söderback, I. (1994). Occupational therapy after hip fracture: A pilot study of the clients, the care and the costs. Clinical Rehabilitation, 8, 142–148.

Harlowe, D. (2001). Occupational therapy for prevention of injury and physical dysfunction. In L.W. Pedretti and M.B. Early (Eds), Occupational Therapy: Practice Skills for Physical dysfunction (5th edn; pp. 69–82). St. Louis: Mosby.

Hastings, J.D. (2000). Seating assessment and planning. Physical Medicine and Rehabilitation Clinics of North America, 11, 183–207.

Hefzy, M.S., Nemunaitis, G. and Hess, M. (1996). Design and development of a pressure relief seating apparatus for individuals with quadriplegia. Assistive Technology, 8, 14–22.

Hermenau, D.C. (1995). Seating. In K. Jacobs and C. Bettencourt, M. (Eds), Ergonomics for Therapists (pp. 137–155). Boston: Butterworth-Heinemann.

Herrman, R.P., Phalangas, A.C., Mahony, C. and Alexander, M.A. (1999). Powered feeding devices: An evaluation of three models. Archives of Physical Medicine and Rehabilitation, 80, 1212–1242.

InterAct Plus (2000–2002). Imperium 200H environmental control unit (ECU), an assistive technology for spinal cord injuries. Retrieved 28 December 2004, http://www.interactplus.com/functional_diagram.htm

Jackson, J., Carlson, M., Mandel, D., Zemke, R. and Clark, F. (1998). Occupation in lifestyle redesign: The well elderly study occupational therapy program. American Journal of Occupational Therapy, 52, 326–336.

Jacobs, K. and Bettencourt, C.M. (1995). Ergonomics for therapists (1st edn). Boston: Butterworth-Heineman.

Kang, T.E.T. and Mak, A.F.T. (1997). Development of a simple approach to modify the supporting properties of seating foam for pressure relief. Journal of Rehabilitation Research and Development, 9, 47–54.

Kanyer, B. (1992). Meeting the seating and mobility needs of the client with traumatic brain injury. Journal of Head Trauma Rehabilitation, 7, 81–93.

Kerr, K.M., White, J.A., Mollan, R.A.B. and Baird, H.E. (1991). Rising from a chair: A review of the literature. Physiotherapy, 77, 15–19.

Kondo, T., Mann, W.C., Tomita, M. and Ottenbacher, K.J. (1997). The use of microwave ovens by elderly persons with disabilities. American Journal of Occupational Therapy, 51, 739–747.

Kornblau, B.L., Shamberg, S. and Klein, R. (2000). Occupational therapy and the Americans with Disabilities Act (ADA). American Journal of Occupational Therapy, 54, 622–625.

Kratz, G. and Söderback, I. (1990). Individualised adaptation of clothes for impaired persons. Scandinavian Journal of Rehabilitation Medicine, 22, 163–170.

Kratz, G., Söderback, I., Guidetti, S., Hultling, C., Rykatkin, T. and Söderström, M. (1997). Wheelchair users' experience of non adapted and adapted clothes during sailing, quad rugby or wheel walking. International Disability Studies, 19, 26–34.

Lange, M. (1996). The challenge of fall prevention in home care. A review of the literature. Home Healthcare Nurse, 14, 198–206.

Larsson, Å., Nyström, C., Vikström, S., Walfridsson, T. and Söderback, I. (1995). Computer assisted cognitive rehabilitation for adults with traumatic brain damage: Four case studies. Occupational Therapy International, 2, 166–189.

Law, M., Cooper, B.A., Steward, D., Letts, L., Rigby, P. and Strong, S. (1994). Person environment relations. Work. A Journal of Prevention, Assessment and Rehabilitation, 4, 228–238.

Law, M., Cooper, B.A., Strong, S., Stewart, B., Rigby, P. and Letts, L. (1997). Theoretical contexts for the practice of occupational therapy. In C. Christiansen and C. Baum (Eds), Occupational Therapy. Enabling Function and Well-being (2nd edn; pp. 72–102).Thorofare, NJ: SLACK.

Leonard, R.B. (1997). Seating and mobility issues for polio survivors. Rehabilitation Management: The Interdisciplinary Journal of Rehabilitation, 10, 44–46.

Levine, R.E. and Glitin, L.N. (1990). Home adaptations for persons with chronic disabilities: An educational model. American Journal of Occupational Therapy, 44, 923–929.

Levine, R.E. and Gitlin, L.N. (1993). A model to promote activity competence in elders. American Journal of Occupational Therapy, 47, 147–153.

Liebig, P.S. (1999). Using home modifications to promote self maintenance and mutual care: The case of old age homes in India. Physical and Occupational Therapy in Geriatrics, 16, 79–99.

Lindberg, C., Bartfai, A., Granqvist, A., Söderström, M., Occhi, E., Spagnolin, A. and Panighetti, F. (1999). FACILE: Support tools for housing and management, integrated with telematic systems and services, devoted to disabled and elderly people. FACILE Project De 3207 Deliverable D6.4 FACILE system demonstration report. Stockholm: Danderyd Hospital, Sweden; Moelli Hospital, Italy.

Mace, R.L. (1998). Universal design in housing. Assistive Technology, 10, 21–28.

Mahoney, J. (1998). Immobility and falls. Clinics in Geriatric Medicine, 14, 699–726.

Mann, W.C. and Lane, J.P. (1998). Introduction. Home modifications. Technology and Disability, 8, 1–97.

Mann, W.C., Hurren, D. and Tomita, M. (1993a). Comparison of assistive device use and needs of home based older persons with different impairments. American Journal of Occupational Therapy, 47, 980–987.

Mann, W.C., Karuza, J., Hurren, M. and Tomita, M. (1993b). Needs of home based older persons for assistive devices. Technology and Disability, 2, 1–11.

Mann, W.C., Hurren, D. and Tomita, M. (1995). Assistive devices used by home based elderly persons with arthritis. American Journal of Occupational Therapy, 49, 810–820.

Marks, D. (1997). Models of disability. Disability and Rehabilitation, 19, 85–91.

Michlovitz, S., Hun. L., Ersala, G.N., Hengehold, D.A. and Weingand, K.W. (2004). Continuous low-level heat warp therapy is effective for treating wrist pain. Archives of Physical Medicine and Rehabilitation, 85, 1409–1416.

Minkel, J.L. (2000). Seating and mobility considerations for people with spinal cord injury. Physical Therapy, 80, 701–709.

MTech Lab Research (2000). MOVAID – Mobility and activity assistance system for the disabled. Retrieved 7 February 2004, http://www-arts.sssup.it/research/projects/MOVAID/default.htm

Müllersdorf, M. and Söderback, I. (2002). Occupational therapists' assessments of adults with long term pain: The Swedish experience. Occupational Therapy International, 9, 1–23.

Murata, J., Shimizu, J.I., Inoue, K. and Matsukawa, K. (2001). The effect of hand-rim position on torque development for wheelchair population. Scandinavian Journal of Occupational Therapy, 8, 79–84.

National Library of Medicine (2005). MeSH subject headers. Retrieved 10 April 2005, http://www.nlm.org/cgi/mesh/2005/MB_cgi

Nätterlund, B. (2001). Living with muscular dystrophy. Illness experience, activities of daily living, coping, quality of life and rehabilitation. Acta Universitatis Upsaliensis: Comprehensive Summaries of Uppsala Dissertations from the Faculty of Medicine, 1025, Uppsala University, Sweden.

Nätterlund, B. and Ahlström, G. (1999) Problem-focused coping and satisfaction in individuals with muscular dystrophy and post-polio. Scandinavian Journal of Caring Science 13, 26–32.

Nielsen, C.W. and Ambrose, I. (1999). Lifetime adaptable housing in Europe. Technology and Disability, 10, 11–19.

Nordenskiöld, U. (1997). Daily activities in women with rheumatoid arthritis: Aspects of patient education, assistive devices, and methods for disability and impairment assessment. Scandianavian Journal of Rehabilitation Medicine, 37 (Suppl. 1), 1–72.

Northen, J.G., Rust, D.M., Nelson, C.E. and Watts, J.H. (1995). Involvement of adult rehabilitation patients in setting occupational therapy goals. American Journal of Occupational Therapy, 49, 214–220.

Olsen, R.V., Hutchings, B.L. and Ehrenkrantz, E. (1999). The physical design of the home as a caregiving support: An environment for persons with dementia. Care Management Journals: Journal of Case Management: The Journal of Long Term Home Health Care, 1, 125–131.

Owens, T.R., Hoffman, G.L. and Kumar, S. (1996). An ergonomic perspective on accommodation in accessibility for people with disability. Disability and Rehabilitation, 18, 402–407.

Patterson, K. and Michael, S. (1991). Correcting the sitting posture of a person with a hindquarter amputation. Australian Occupational Therapy Journal, 38, 237–240.

Pedretti, L.W. and Early, M.B. (2001). Treatment planning. In L.W. Pedretti and M.B. Early (Eds), Occupational Therapy: Practice Skills for Physical Dysfunction (5th edn; pp. 50–51). St. Louis: Mosby.

Pellow, T.R. (1999). A comparison of interface pressure readings to wheelchair cushions and positioning: A pilot study. Canadian Journal of Occupational Therapy, 66, 140–149.

Permobil (2000). Innovated powered wheelchairs: About us. Retrieved 25 January 2004, http://www.permobilusa.com/about.htm

Prangrant, T., Mann, W.C. and Tomita, M. (2000). Impact of unilateral neglect on assistive device use. Technology and Disability, 12, 53–69.

Price, J.D., Hermans, D.G. and Grimley Evans, J. (2001). Subjective barriers to prevent wandering of cognitively impaired people. The Cochrane Library, Issue 4. Oxford: Update Software.

Rader, J., Jones, D. and Miller, L. (2000). The importance of individualized wheelchair seating for frail older adults. Journal of Gerontological Nursing, 15, 34–47.

Redford, J.B. (1993). Seating and wheeled mobility in the disabled elderly population. Archives of Physical Rehabilitation, 74, 877– 875.

Rehabilitation Engineering and Assistive Technology Society of North America (nd). RESNA Mission Statement. Retrieved 29 December 2004, http://www.resna.org/AboutRESNA/Mission/Mission.html

Rogers, J.C. (1983). Eleanor Clarke Slage Lectureship 1983; Clinical reasoning: The ethics, science, and art. American Journal of Occupational Therapy, 37, 601–616.

Sabari, J.S. (2001). Teaching activities in occupational therapy. In L.W. Pedretti and M.B. Early (Eds). Occupational Therapy. Practice Skills for Physical Dysfunction (5th edn; pp. 83–91). St. Louis: Mosby.

Sandberg, K., Ahlgren, G., Einarsson, L., Hellgren, M., Holmgren, F., Fors, B., Fredriksson, A., Jansson, E., Landin Lorentzon, L., Levander, S., Lindgren, L., Olsson, T., Ottosson, J., Mattson, R., Mattson, S., Person, H., Pettersson, R., Pålsson, K., Söderström, M., Westerberg, Y. and Winnberg Lindqvist, P. (2000). Möjligheternas trädgård, en trädgård för alla [The possibility garden, a garden for all people] (2nd edn). Stockholm: Hjälpmedelsinstitutet och Sveriges utbildningsradio AB [The Swedish Handicap Institute and The Swedish Educational Radio].

Saxena, S., Nikolic, S. and Popovic, D. (1995). An EMG controlled grasping system for tetraplegics. Journal of Rehabilitation Research and Development, 32, 17–24.

Smith, R.O. (1991). Technological approaches to performance enhancement. In C. Christiansen and C. Baum (Eds), Occupational Therapy. Overcoming Human Performance Deficits. Thorofare NJ: SLACK.

Söderback, I. (1988a). A housework based assessment of intellectual functions in patients with acquired brain damage. Development and evaluation of an occupational therapy method. Scandinavian Journal of Rehabilitation Medicine, 20, 57–69.

Söderback, I. (1988b). Intellectual function training and intellectual housework training in patients with acquired brain damage. A study of occupational therapy methods. Doctoral dissertation, Karolinska Institute, Stockholm, Sweden.

Söderback, I. (1988c). The effectiveness of training intellectual functions in adults with acquired brain damage. An evaluation of occupational therapy methods. Scandinavian Journal of Rehabilitation Medicine, 20, 47–56.

Söderback, I. (1999). Validation of the theory: Satisfaction with time delimited daily occupations. Work. A Journal of Prevention, Assessment and Rehabilitation, 12, 165–174.

Söderback, I. and Lassfolk, A. (1993). The usefulness of four methods of assessing the benefits of electrically adjustable beds in relation to their costs. International Journal of Technology Assessment in Health Care, 9, 573–587.

Söderback, I., Caneman, G. and Ekholm, J. (1993). Causes of dependence in personal care three years after stroke. A study in the home environment. NeuroRehabilitation, 3, 60–72.

Söderback, I., Krakau, I., Gruvsved, Å., Härtull, M., Kratz, G., Lind, A., Lassfolk, A., Pekkanen, K. and Riedel, D. (1994). The quality of occupational therapy evaluated in six outpatients. Occupational Therapy International, 1, 122–138.

Söderback, I., Söderström, M. and Schälander, E. (2004). Horticulture therapy: The 'healing garden' and gardening in rehabilitation measures at Danderyd Hospital Rehabilitation Clinic, Sweden. Pediatric Rehabilitation, 7, 245–260.

Stein, F. and Roose, B. (2000). Pocket Guide to Treatment in Occupational Therapy. San Diego: Singular.

Steultjens, E.M., Dekker, J., Bouter, L.M., Jeltema, S., Bakker, E.B. and van den Ende, C.H. (2004). Occupational therapy for community dwelling elderly people: A systematic review. Age and Aging, 33, 453–460.

Stinnett, K.A. (1997). Geriatric seating and positioning within a wheeled mobility frame of reference in the long term care setting. Topics in Geriatric Rehabilitation, 13, 75–84.

Swedish Handicap Institute (nd) The Swedish Handicap Institute. Retrieved 29 December 2004, http://www.hi.se/english/institute.shtm

Sweeney, G.M. and Clarke, A.K. (1992). Easy chairs for people with arthritis and low back pain: Results from an evaluation. British Journal of Occupational Therapy, 55, 69–72.

Tibbitts, M.G. (1996). Patients who fall: How to predict and prevent injuries. Geriatrics, 51, 24–31.

Trace Research and Development Center (nd) About the TRACE Center. Retrieved 29 December 2004, http://trace.wisc.edu/about/

Trachtman, L.H., Mace, R.L., Young, L.C. and Pace, R.J. (1999). The universal design home: Are we ready for it? Physical and Occupational Therapy in Geriatrics, 16, 1–16.

Tuleja, C. and DeMoss, A. (1999). Babycare assistive technology. Technology and Disability, 11, 71–78.

Watzke, J.R. (1997). Older adults' responses to an automated integrated environmental control device. The case of the Remote Gateway. Technology and Disability, 7, 103–114.

Williams, C. (2000). Product focus. The Flo tech Adjuster chair from Medical Support Systems. British Journal of Nursing, 9, 12–25.

Wong, C.K. and Wade, C.K. (1995). Reducing iliotibial band contractures in patient with muscular dystrophy using custom dry flotation cushions. Archives of Physical Rehabilitation, 76, 695–700.

Woodcock, K. (1997). Ergonomics and automatic speech recognition applications for deaf and hard-of-hearing users. Technology and Disability, 7, 147–164.

World Health Organization (1980). ICIDH II International Classification of Impairments, Disabilities and Handicaps II. A manual for classification relating to the consequences of disease. WHO 29.35 of the Twenty-ninth World Health Assembly, May 1976. Geneva: WHO.

World Health Organization (2000). Literature review on environmental factors: The role of environmental factors in functioning and disability. Retrieved 4 January 2004, http://www3.who.int/icf/icftemplate.cfm?mytitle=Literature%20review%20on%20environmental%20factors&myurl=litreview.html

World Health Organization (2001a). International Classification of Functioning, Disability and Health [ICF]. Geneva, Switzerland: WHO.

World Health Organization (2001b). ICF classification: Hypertext version. Retrieved 10 January 2001, http://www3.who.int/icf/onlinebrowser/icf.cfm

Yuen, H.K. and D'Amico, M. (1998). Improved feeding ability in adults with acquired brain damage: Two case studies. Australian Occupational Therapy Journal, 45, 43–45.

CHAPTER 3

The case study of Ben: Prescription and use of a wheelchair

There are five major goals of wheelchair prescription: (1) maximization of the efficient independent mobility, (2) prevention/minimization of deformity or injury, (3) maximization of independent functioning, (4) projection of a healthy, vital, attractive 'body image', and (5) minimization of short-term and long-term equipment costs.

N.C. Cutter and D.J. Blake, 1997, p. 107

Learning objectives

By the end of this chapter the learner will:

1 Understand the steps of the Socratic Case Study Method (SCSM).
2 Be able to apply the SCSM in clinical reasoning to a specific case study or clinical situation.
3 Be able to use a literature review to solve a clinical case study based on the SCSM.
4 Understand the justification and ethical considerations related to prescribing a wheelchair and its components.
5 Understand the factors related to prescribing and adapting a wheelchair.
6 Understand the significance of using wheelchairs in a population.
7 Write a scientific report on prescribing a wheelchair.

Definition of the Socratic Case Study Method

According to Gilbert Highet (1950), there are three methods of teaching: lecturing, classroom discussion and the Socratic Method. During a lecture, students are usually passive, having little or no opportunity to apply their learning to a real-case situation. During a classroom discussion, which students have prepared for prior to the class session, 'the lesson is then explained to them more fully and clearly by the teacher, who examines the pupils to make sure that they have assimilated it fully' (Highet, 1950, p. 88).

With the Socratic Method, students can be presented with a situation or a problem and asked to formulate hypotheses that might lead to possible solutions. The process of working through the situation or problem is called active learning (Johannessen, 2000). The student is not given the solution, but is asked to develop possible solutions by applying the theory to the situation. Thus, the theory is internalized and learning takes place.

One way to engage in active learning is through the Socratic Case Study Method (SCSM) (Lynn, 1999; Sudzina, 2000). SCSM is characterized by question-and-answer analysis of a problem. Students are given a simulated, actual or clinical problem and asked to determine a solution by investigating the scientific literature. The teacher presents questions and the student thinks through possible solutions. The questions are designed so that the student is made aware of the possible options in a problem and can determine the best solution based on this analysis. Use of this method teaches students to apply clinical reasoning to specific situations and evidence-based learning (Gassner and Wotton, 1998; Jones and Sheridan, 1999; Sudzina, 2000).

In this chapter, a case study is presented that is related to wheelchair prescription for a person with paraplegia. The purpose of this analysis is to help the student to apply (a) clinical reasoning for solving a client-centred problem in accordance with ergonomic principles; (b) critically evaluate the research literature; and (c) identify ergonomic principles to use in evidence-based practice. This example of a case study using SCSM is in three parts (1) an overview of the content; (2) the background history of the clinical case; and (3) the synthesis of the content related to the clinical case describing one of many possible solutions (Lynn, 1999).

Part one: Overview of the content

The theme of this case is the adaptation of a wheelchair. In the initial presentation of the case, the student is introduced to the use of the wheelchair. The students' tasks include (a) finding information about the history, distribution, population of wheelchair users and reasons for prescribing the use of a wheelchair; (b) identifying the main components and principles to be considered when prescribing wheelchairs, including purposes, types and adjustable parts of the wheelchairs; (c) locating, selecting and analysing the research literature related to wheelchairs; and (d) synthesizing the information into a report.

As a starting point, students should use the following list of references to gather background information. Selected references are listed here; others can be found at the end of this chapter.

- Cook, A.M. and Hussey, S.M. (2002). Technologies that enable mobility. In A.M. Cook and. S.M. Hussey (Eds), Assistive Technology: Principles and Practices (2nd edn, pp. 329–373). St. Louis: Mosby.

- Cooper, R.A., Robertson, R.N., Boninger, M.L., Shimada, S.D., VanSickle, D.P., Lawrence, B. and Singleton, T. (1997). Wheelchair ergonomics. In S. Kumar (Ed.), Perspectives in Rehabilitation Ergonomics (pp. 246–272). Bristol, PA: Taylor & Francis.
- Cutter, N.C. and Blake, D.J. (1997). Wheelchairs and seating systems: Clinical applications. Physical Medicine and Rehabilitation: State of the Art Reviews, 11, 107–132.
- Ferrarin, M., Andreoni, G. and Pedotti, A. (2000). Comparative biomechanical evaluation of different wheelchair seat cushions. Journal of Rehabilitation Research and Development, 37, 315–324.
- Hastings, J.D. (2000). Seating assessment and planning. Physical Medicine and Rehabilitation Clinics of North America, 11, 183–207.
- Kilkens, O.J., Post, M.W., Dallmeijer, A.J. Seelen, H.A. and van der Woude (2003). Wheelchair tests: a systematic review. Clinical Rehabilitation, 17, 418–430.
- Samuelsson, K.A.M, Tropp, H., Nylander, E. and Gerdle, B. (2004). The effect of rear-wheel position on seating ergonomics and mobility efficiency in wheelchair users with spinal cord injuries: A pilot study. Journal of Rehabilitation Research and Development, 41, 65–74.

Sample case report

How did wheelchairs evolve based on recorded history?

The first known recorded information about wheelchairs comes from a Chinese engraving on a sarcophagus dated at about AD525, which depicts a chair with wheels (Garber and Krouskop, 1997). Aristocrats in Europe used custom-made wheelchairs in the sixteenth century (Kamenetz, 1969). According to Cooper et. al. (1997), the development of the modern wheelchair was introduced in the early eighteenth century. This wheelchair had two large front wooden wheels and a caster in the rear. During the American Civil War-wooden wheelchairs were constructed for war related injuries (Garber and Krouskop, 1997). Later after the Civil War and into the twentieth century the wheelchair was refined with metal tubing, adjustable arm rests, footrests and large spoked wheels.

Significant progress in American wheelchairs arose out of a mining accident that left Herbert A. Everest a paraplegic in 1918. Unable to get around in the cumbersome wooden wheelchair that weighed 75–90 pounds, he spurred the design of a light metal wheelchair by his friend Harry C. Jennings, Sr. By 1932 demand for this type of wheelchair led Everest and Jennings, mechanical engineers, to found a company to manufacture wheelchairs (Davis, 1973).

Simultaneously, and without knowledge of the achievement of Everest and Jennings, Sam Duke, a Chicago supplier of rental equipment, responded to requests for rental of wheelchairs by constructing a few from bicycles and wagon wheels. He produced a folding wheelchair in 1931 and a lightweight folding chair in 1937. So great was customer demand that Duke founded the American Wheelchair Co. Currently, there are many manufacturers of manual and power-driven wheelchairs that have evolved over the years.

Power-driven wheelchairs, folding wheelchairs, sports wheelchairs custom-designed ergonomic wheelchairs, and wheelchairs with micro-processors have revolutionized the manufacture and adaptability of wheelchairs to meet the individual needs of the client (Woods and Watson, 2003). The impetus for changing the designs of wheelchairs has been the First and Second World Wars, accidents, worldwide infectious epidemics such as polio, and the advocacy of individuals with disabilities in sports and the Olympic Games (Garber and Krouskop, 1997).

What is the distribution of wheelchair users?

Approximately ten per cent of the world population has a disability, with many of these individuals having a mobility impairment requiring a wheelchair. The relationship between one's need for a wheelchair and owning one is unknown, but there is an imbalance at least in the developing countries (Kim and Mulholland, 1999). In 1992 there were 1,411,000 wheelchair users in the United States of America, which is about four per cent of individuals with disabilities (Burke, 1999; Cutter and Blake, 1997). About half of the individuals needing wheelchairs use them all the time, while the other half uses them intermittently.

What is the population of individuals with disabilities who are wheelchair users?

Children or teenagers with physical disabilities, middle-aged individuals who have sustained any type of traumatic disorders or diseases, and five per cent of elderly adults aged over 70 years, use wheelchairs. Impairments of these individuals include restricted range of motion, muscle weakness, muscle paralyses and pareses, physical deformities and respiratory restrictions. Individuals diagnosed with cerebral palsy, traumatic brain injury, spina bifida, spinal cord injuries resulting in quadriplegia, rheumatoid arthritis and lower limb amputation commonly use wheelchairs (Cooper et al., 1997). Hence, the indications for prescribing a wheelchair are a loss of lower limb body functions, postural instability and general debilitation (Cutter and Blake, 1997), or cardiovascular and neuromuscular movement-related impairments (World Health Organization, 2001).

What knowledge is required to prescribe a wheelchair adequately?

Prescribing a wheelchair adequately requires knowledge in the following areas (Kim and Mulholland, 1999):

- Pathology of physical conditions or diseases.
- Anthropometrics and body positioning when transporting oneself in a seated position.
- Skills for completing an activity analysis that will enable the wheelchair user to function optimally in the specific environments where the wheelchair will be used.
- Familiarity with cultural, social and physical environments where the wheelchair will be used.
- Knowledge of technical aspects of design, construction, available materials and qualities of available wheelchairs, seat cushions and attachments.
- Collaboration, mediation and advocacy for wheelchair users and other involved individuals.
- Teaching and research skills.

What are the purposes for prescribing a wheelchair?

There are three major purposes for prescribing a wheelchair (Cutter and Blake, 1997; Garber and Krouskop, 1997; Kim and Mulholland, 1999; Minkel, 2000): (1) to increase client mobility; (2) to meet the physiological and psychological needs of the client; and (3) to apply ergonomic principles and cost considerations.

Increase mobility

The aim is to:

- maximize efficient independent mobility and activity. The optimal wheelchair allows the user to have independent mobility by using as little strength and energy as possible.
- promote the individual's sense of value and place in the world by enabling independence in mobility.

Physiological and psychological needs

The wheelchair should:

- be comfortable when the individual is seated
- support the body in the neutral sitting position and allow for circulatory function in the buttocks
- prevent postural abnormalities, joint and tension contractures, pressure ulcers, respiratory restrictions and injury
- protect a healthy, vital, attractive 'body image' by using cosmetically acceptable wheelchairs

Ergonomic principles and costs

When choosing a wheelchair, consider the following:

- ergonomic fit and comfort in use

- size such that the individual can get around easily in buildings
- manoeuvrability in streets
- power-driven chair battery life and methods of recharging the battery
- short- and long-term equipment costs
- weight involved when transporting the wheelchair
- storage when not in use
- maintenance and repair
- transferability from chair to bed and chair to bath.

What types of wheelchairs are available?

Cooper et al. (1997) have categorized wheelchairs into the following types:

- manually powered or electrically (battery) powered
- ultra-light manual wheelchairs used for recreation and self-transport
- manual or electrically powered wheelchairs designed to support body balance and compensate for deformities
- manual amputee wheelchairs
- power-driven wheelchairs for standing position.

What are the components of a wheelchair?

The three main parts of a wheelchair are the frame (including the wheels), the seat base and the seat back. The main components of the manual wheelchair are the backrest, seat rail, axle plate, caster housing, caster stern bolt, caster fork and the cushions of the seating system (Hastings, 2000) (see Figure 3.1.).

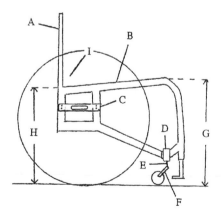

Figure 3.1 Components of the manual wheelchair; A = backrest; B = seat rail; C = axle plate; D = caster housing; E = caster stern bolt; F = caster fork; G = front seat to floor height; H = rear seat to floor height; I = inside back to seat angle. Adapted with permission from 'Seating assessment and planning', J.D. Hastings, 2000, Physical Medicine and Rehabilitation Clinics of North America, 11, 197.

The power-driven wheelchair contains the same components as a manual wheelchair and in addition has an electric motor and a joystick.

The advantages and disadvantages of different kinds of armrests, front riggings, backrests, rear wheels, front casters, frame style, rear axle, brakes and accessories have been extensively researched and should be taken into account when prescribing a wheelchair for an individual client (Cooper et al., 1997; Cutter and Blake, 1997; Garber and Krouskop, 1997; Hastings, 2000; Kim and Mulholland, 1999).

What are the adjustable parts of a wheelchair?

The material for this section was obtained from the following references: Cooper et al. (1997), Cutter and Blake (1997), Garber and Krouskop (1997), Hastings (2000) and Kim and Mulholland (1999).

- The frame axle: The rear axle of the frame is the most important adjustable part and allows the therapist to manipulate the user's centre of gravity both horizontally and vertically by changing the wheeled camber and wheelbase width seat height.
- The seat: The height of the front and rear parts of the seat to floor and the seat angle are adjustable.
- Seat back rests: These should be adjustable in height and angle.
- The seating system: One of the most important parts of a wheelchair is the selection of seating systems and cushions. The material and configuration of the cushion are of vital importance for preventing pressure sores in the buttocks. It is possible to choose products that are air-, fluid- or gel-filled or made of foam.
- Foot-plates: The vertical direction and lengths of the foot-plates should be adjusted to the individual's hip, knee and ankle joint positions.
- The design: The recommended weight of a wheelchair should be less than 20 pounds in order for the individual to be able to use it independently.
- The elbow rests: these should be adjusted in relation to activities performed.

How to prescribe a wheelchair

The processes for determining which wheelchair should be prescribed for a client are cited in the following references: Burke (1999), Cooper et al. (1997), Garber and Krouskop (1997), Kanyer (1992), Kim and Mulholland (1999) and Minkel (2000). 'Many factors influence selection of the correct wheelchair' (Everest and Jennings, Inc, 1979, p. 1); however, no standard criteria exist for determining the appropriate seating positioning and wheeled mobility systems (Burke, 1999). Here are some recommendations:

1 When prescribing a wheelchair the client and therapist jointly:
   a decide who will operate and assist the client in using and maintaining the wheelchair – the owner, the caregiver or both?
   b perform a needs assessment. Information about the client, such as age, time since the onset of illness occurred, prognosis and severity of the disease are especially important. Moreover, the user's occupation and prior lifestyle should also be considered.

   c determine the user's physical status and, if relevant, cognitive status.

   d determine the wheelchair user's anthropometric dimensions (seating and shoulder height, leg, foot and arm length, shoulder, chest, waist, pelvic, knee and overall width and seating depth). These measurements, combined with biomechanical principles, are used to control posture stability, while neurodevelopment is addressed to control tone, reflexes, weight lifting and movement, and sensorimotor dysfunction. The wheelchair user's seated postural stability and control may be measured according to the technique of Kamper et al. (2000) and used to obtain optimal adaptation of the adjustable parts of the wheelchair.

   e determine the user(s) attitudes for using the wheelchair.

2 Identify the environmental situation for using the wheelchair by:

   a determining the contexts in the home, work, school and leisure situations where the wheelchair will be used.

   b determining where in the environment the wheelchair will be used (i.e. indoors or outdoors or both). If it is to be used primarily out of doors, identify the ground surface.

   c determining the environmental accessibility needed for the wheelchair (e.g. dimensions of the bedroom, kitchen, doorways, bathroom).

3 Choose the wheelchair based on the individual's needs and by examining the following:

   a durability of the wheelchair

   b optimal seating position based on the postural support needed

   c maximum pressure relief

   d relationship between the cost of the wheelchair and the expected use.

Part two: The background history of the clinical case study

In part two of the SCSM, specific details of the case are presented. First, the student is asked to read material specifically related to the clinical case study. While some material may be provided by the instructor, the student develops a reference list by performing a database search using the following keywords: wheeled mobility or wheelchair combined with cushions, ergonomics, pressure distribution, positioning evaluation, posture technology, seated body position, seat. The content from the literature search will be discussed with seminar participants. Some references are listed at the end of this section; however, this list should be updated with more recent primary sources. Following the initial discussion, the pertinent information about the case is presented. The student uses his or her knowledge to (a) apply ergonomic principles to occupational therapy practice, and (b) describe the content appropriate for designing an intervention protocol, including theory, assessment, treatment and outcome. This information is summarized in a report.

The use of a wheelchair: The case of Ben

Ben is 44 years old. His present height is 180 cm (about 6 feet) and his weight is 66 kg (about 146 pounds). Ben was born in India and then emigrated to the United States where he grew up in New York City under poor circumstances. He finished the ninth grade, but has had no further education. He is a member of a large family with close relationships. He lives alone in a modern apartment on the seventh floor, and uses the lift. For many years he worked as a taxi driver in midtown Manhattan.

Slowly, over a one-year period, Ben has developed pareses in both legs. When a physician finally examined him, he was diagnosed with a cancerous tumour that had infiltrated the spinal cord. The tumour was successfully removed during an operation six months ago, and the prognosis indicated minimal risk for relapse.

Six months post-surgery, Ben was in an accident and sustained a complete spinal cord injury at the thoracic level (T4–T5), resulting in lack of sensitivity in his buttocks or thighs. He has hypertonicity (spasticity), which is typical for this level of spinal cord injury (Ditunno et al., 1994).

A manual wheelchair had been prescribed during his visits to a rehabilitation clinic, but no consideration had been given to the choice of a cushion. Ben could transport himself independently in the wheelchair. Prior to his present injury, Ben was socially active; however, since the injury he has limited his social participation. He no longer goes on family visits or to the East Indian club which he had formerly visited once a week. This is because, as he said, he feels stigmatized because of the impairment. Consequently Ben sits indoors in his wheelchair in the same position for long periods of time.

Currently, Ben is a day-care client at the same rehabilitation clinic where he was treated previously. At the clinic the clients are taught to routinely inspect their skin near their buttocks in order to prevent pressure sores. During an individual session, the nurse found a red necrotic area over his right ischial part below the hip. Ben was referred to the 'Seat and Positioning Lab' so that a therapist could check whether Ben's wheelchair was optimally adapted to his seating body position and to prescribe a wheelchair cushion that would give him maximum seating relief. Other preventative interventions for eliminating pressure sores in the buttocks area were requested, such as frequently moving off the seat. Follow-up and re-evaluation for Ben's condition was requested after three months.

The task of the student is to develop an intervention strategy with Ben that helps him holistically by applying ergonomic principles. In determining solutions to this case study, using SCSM, the student is encouraged to begin a literature search by making a list of relevant questions related to the case study. For example, the student might ask what biopsychosocial aspects of this case should be considered. Second, the student will apply ergonomic principles to develop possible solutions. For example, the student might consider which aspects of the wheelchair should be changed to enable Ben to be most functional in the home and at work. The final report should be a process-oriented plan related to the short- and long-term goals, including an intervention protocol comprised of assessment tools, treatment methods and procedures to measure outcome. References should provide the rationale for assessments and interventions.

The student's report: Example of a clinical report

The following guiding questions have been identified as important in developing possible solutions in this case study. These questions were generated from the references found in the literature search:

- What are the key words in this case study?
- What areas of the body are vulnerable to pressure sores in wheelchair users and how can they be prevented?
- What are the important issues and goals when choosing an appropriate cushion to provide comfort and prevent pressure sores?
- What is the research-based evidence for selecting wheelchair cushions?
- Which assessments are used to determine an appropriate wheelchair cushion?
- What are the advantages and disadvantages of various types of wheelchair cushions in preventing pressure sores?
- How can pressure sores be prevented through behavioural strategies?
- What theoretical models are the most appropriate for intervention related to this case?
- Which pre-intervention assessments are planned?
- What are the short- and long-term goals for Ben?
- How can Ben improve his social interactions?
- How can Ben increase his participation in leisure activities?
- How can Ben be helped to comply with an intervention programme?
- What instruction is needed to foster independence?

What are the major definitions and concepts used in the case?

Among possible concepts, the understanding of pressure sores is of prime concern in this case. A pressure sore might cause Ben to have major discomfort and disrupt his ability to lead an independent and productive life (Pellow, 1999). The main factors involved in the formation of pressure ulcers are:

- insufficient vascularization in the tissues subjected to high pressure (mainly under bone prominences) due to occlusion of blood and lymphatic vessels, resulting in tissue death
- stagnation of perspiration on the skin as a result of inadequate air ventilation

- presence of local areas of high temperature
- shearing stressors on the skin (Ferrarin et al., 2000).

Which body parts commonly get pressure or ulcer sores?

For wheelchair users, the prominent parts of the buttocks such as under and posterior to the ischial tuberosities and the sacrum are at risk for pressure sores. Therefore, these areas need to be inspected frequently by Ben.

What are the most important issues and goals when choosing an appropriate cushion?

Development of pressure sores are influenced by physical mechanical factors, comfort and pressure management of the seating system, perpendicular stresses of pressure and the parallel stresses of shearing. The interacting variables are the person's body weight and the seating surface area. If these stressors are not balanced for the seating cushion, blood circulation can be reduced, lymphatic vessels can be blocked and tissue necrosis may occur causing a pressure sore (Cutter and Blake, 1997). Other physical factors that increase the risk for development of pressure sores are the amount of moisture (e.g. perspiration, humidity) and skin temperature (Garber and Krouskop, 1997). Preventing pressure sores is achieved by the combination of reducing perpendicular pressure (i.e. weight) and increasing the distributed pressure of the cushion surface. The lowest perpendicular pressure refers to the distribution of weight on the wheelchair seat. Preventing pressure sores to the buttocks is based on biomechanical principles of seating including the controlling of body posture through forces applied to the body, support for comfort and restraining undesirable movements (Garber and Krouskop, 1997).

Body postural control or trunk balance is a function of muscle strength and sensory feedback. The effect of body posture on prevention of pressure sores on the buttocks depends on the tilt of the body in space and the wheelchair backrest recline, which affects the pressure distribution. Staying in neutral body position for long periods of time causes unnecessary weight-bearing on the ischial tuberosities (Pellow, 1999). In custom-designing a wheelchair, the therapist would take standard anatomic dimensions, as noted in Figure 3.2 (Kamper et al., 2000) using an anatomical goniometer according to the checklist recommended by Hastings (2000).

Table 3.1 describes in detail the anatomical dimensions used in custom-designing a wheelchair. The client should be in a dynamic position while carrying out activities of daily living when the measuring takes place. The custom-designing of a wheelchair is critical in preventing pressure sores. A computer-aided wheelchair prescription system is available for the therapist to use (Axelson, 1996).

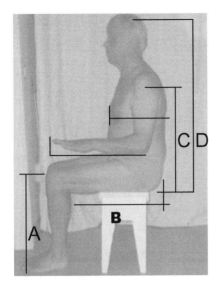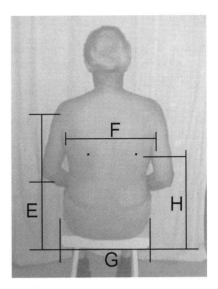

Figure 3.2 Standard anatomic dimensions necessary for the determination of the seating system and the wheelchair. Left picture: (A) shank length; (B) seat depth, (C) back height (middle length for back support); (D) head, neck and back height (full length for back support): Right picture: (E) elbow rest height; (F) back wide; (G) back seat width; (H) body side length (short length for back support). (Adopted from Cutter and Blake, 1997). (Photo and design: Second author)

Table 3.1 Evaluation of posture for sitting in a wheelchair

Remember to record what is SEEN, not what one thinks should be seen

1 Observe short sitting in the wheelchair in the frontal plane

Anterior view
- Shoulder height
- Sternum orientation
- Anterior superior iliac spine (ASIS) height
- Knee height
- Hip position (rotation, adduction [ADD], abduction [ABD])
- Ankle position
- Rib to iliac crest clearance posterior view

Posterior view
- Shoulder height
- Scapular orientation
- Posterior superior iliac spine height
- Spine for curvature
- Ribs for humps
- Posterior skin for signs of backrest pressure/shear

Sagittal view
- Observe for curvature: lumbar, thoracic, cervical curves
- Orientation of head to cervical (C) spine
- Note the backrest height relative to a bony landmark (scapula)

Table 3.1 Evaluation of posture for sitting in a wheelchair (continued)

2 Repeat all of the anterior and posterior observations in short sitting on a mat
   edge. (The firmer the mat the better – if client must be supported, make it a very
   light support.)
      Do not do sagittal plane evaluation because the person will C-sit into spinal
   flexion for stability – do not allow them to prop with arms.
      With the patient out of the wheelchair, note the parameters of the wheelchair
   set-up.
   • Note the seat plane angle to the floor (slope-rise over run)
   • Note the angle of the seat to the backrest
   • Note the state of the upholstery (slung out? Worn or torn on the front aspect?)
   • Note the angle of the footrest drop relative to the seat plane
   • Note the width of the wheelchair relative to the supine width of the patient

3 Repeat all of the anterior observations in supine

4 Do a passive range of motion evaluation (PROM) (especially those tightened by
   sitting or impacting sitting) and leg lengths

5 Assess the flexibility in trunk
   • Lower trunk rotation
   • Lateral bending
   • Flexion and extension of the lumbar spine

6 Determine the flexibility of any deformity

7 Synthesize the findings and do empirical trials.

Adapted from 'Seating assessment and planning', J.D. Hastings, 2000, Physical Medicine and Rehabilitation
Clinics of North America, 11, 193.

Hastings (2000) describes the desired alignment necessary when
designing a wheelchair for the body positioning compensating for loss of
vestibular reflexes, muscle power and sensation below the level of the
spinal cord injury. He recommends that the adjustments of the body position in the wheelchair include the following:

• Floor-to-foot clearance should be 1–2 inches
• The seat's depth should allow 1–2 inches of clearance between the
  edge of the seat pan and the popliteal fold, near the back of the knee
• The seat's width should allow 1–2 inches of clearance on each side of
  the hips
• The height at the back of the seat depends on the client's trunk control. Therefore Ben's trunk control at the T4–T5 injury level should be
  carefully checked
• The wheelchair seat and back should be adjusted so that the body orientation in space (tilt) and posture minimize pressure distribution on
  the buttocks. In addition, important adaptations of the wheelchair

include tilting the seat back to 65 degrees for significant pressure relief. Individuals who cannot tolerate this amount of tilting can benefit from as little as 20 degrees tilting. Furthermore, a reclined backrest of 120 degrees reduces internal body pressure by about ten per cent (Pellow, 1999).

Another area to consider is the seating system. The wheelchair cushion seating is an interacting system between the design and material of the cushion and the person's functioning, positioning and movement habits. The prevention of pressure sores depends both on the person moving himself or herself in the wheelchair (i.e. changing body position to relieve pressure to the buttocks), and the covering and filling material of the cushion (Garber and Krouskop, 1997; Pellow, 1999). Choices of cushions include different fillings, such as air, foam, gel and fluid flotation. The advantages and disadvantages are shown in Table 3.2 (Garber and Krouskop, 1997).

Table 3.2 Advantages and limitations of various seating systems

Product class	Advantages	Disadvantages
Air-filled products	Lightweight Easy to clean Effective with many people Promotes even distribution of pressure Reduces shear	Subject to puncture Difficult to repair Inflation must be monitored routinely May compromise user stability May exacerbate postural deformities
Fluid-filled products	Easy to clean Effective with a broad group of users Promotes even distribution of pressure Skin temperature control	Often heavy May compromise user stability May exacerbate postural deformities Subject to puncture Difficult to repair
Gel-filled products	Effectively reduces shear Easy to clean Shock absorbency	Weight Must be stored flat Susceptible to puncture
Foam products	Lightweight Cost Can be easily modified Many variations	Life expectancy is short Not washable Support properties change with time
Combination products	Easily modified Easily customized	Components may be lost Fitting Weight

From 'Technical advances in wheelchairs and seating systems', S. Garber and T. Krouskop, 1997, Physical Medicine and Rehabilitation: State of the Art Reviews, 11, 98. Reprinted with permission from Elsevier Ltd.

Which assessments are used to determine an appropriate wheelchair cushion?

The physical assessments related to prevention of pressure sores include pressure peaks, the shape of the buttocks and skin temperature. The relative dampness of the seat due to perspiration should be taken into consideration in measuring these variables. The decision-making process for selecting cushions could be partly guided by the algorithm for seat cushion selection (Cutter and Blake, 1997) (see Figure 3.3). Collins (2004) also provides a practical guide for seating assessment and selection of the most appropriate wheelchair cushion.

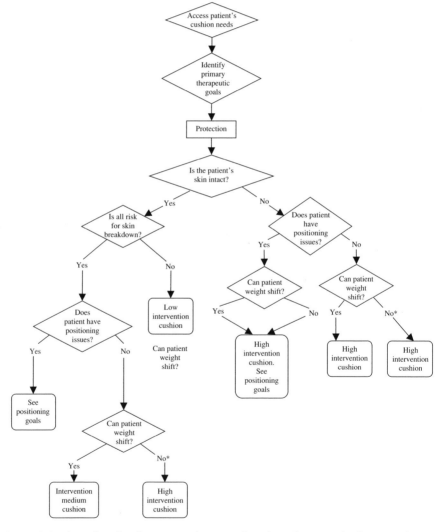

Figure 3.3 Algorithm for decision-making used in the selection of selecting wheelchair cushions. From 'Wheelchairs and seating systems: clinical applications', N.C. Cutter and D.J. Blake, 1997, Physical Medicine and Rehabilitation: State of the Art Reviews, 11, 125. Reprinted with permission from Elsevier Ltd.

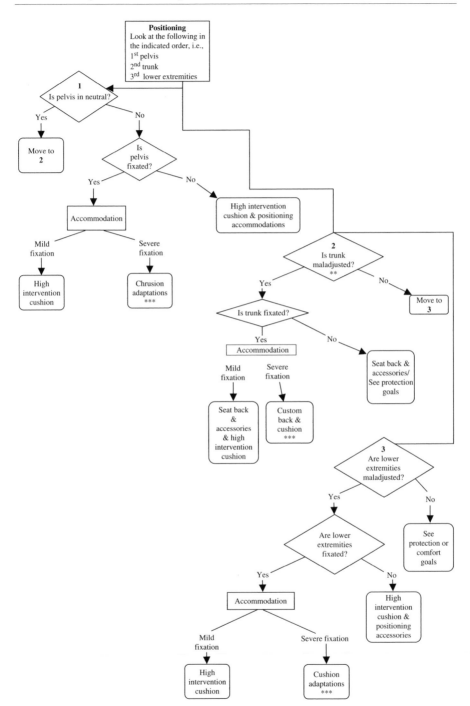

Figure 3.3 continued.

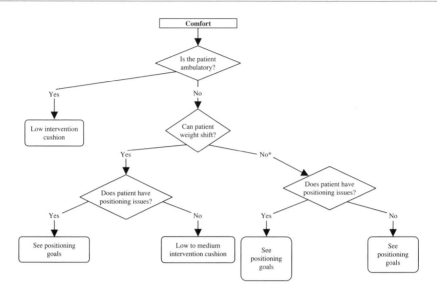

Cushion Intervention Level

Low	Medium	High
Alimed Sit Straight	Avanti Personal Soal	Jay cushion
Avanti Foam Contour	Joy Active	Jay J2
Avanti Foam Support	Joy Care	Roho Enhancer
Jay Combi	Roho Low Protects	Roho High Profile
Naxi Generation Ulrahan	Roho Naxus	Roho Cutanro
SHS Comfort Mase	Varitile Module System	Varitile Pro Foam
	Vartilo Solo	

* Patient will need assistance with weight shifts via caregiver or equipment
** Evaluation for trunk support or cushion backs may be necessary
*** Consult seating specialist regarding cushion adaptations necessary

Figure 3.3 continued.

Pressure peaks

The most clinically effective assessment instrument in measuring pressure peaks is a computerized sensor matrix. This measures the distribution in terms of maximum peaks of sitting pressure and their location between the buttocks and the cushion (Ferrarin et al., 2000) (see, for example, Figure 3.4). Some computerized systems for measuring the pressure exerted by a person's body on another surface include The Texas Interface Pressure Evaluator, The Tally Oxford Pressure Monitor, The QA Pressure Measurement System and The Force Sensing Array (Garber and Krouskop, 1997; Kang et al., 1997; Pellow, 1999). Ferrarin et al. (2000) describe a protocol for using the Tekscan Inc., manufactured in Boston. This system uses a 'matrix of piezoresistive pressure system of 42 rows and 48 columns of sensors,

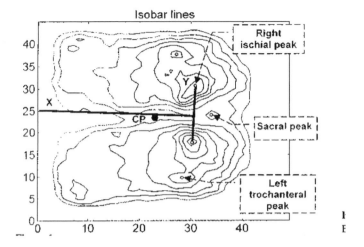

Figure 3.4 Measurement of the seating position showing a pressure map with isobars lines and the anatomical reference system (X = longitudinal axis, Y = transversal axis) defined on the basis of the position of ischial tuberosities. Centre of Pressure (CP) is displayed as well as sacral, trochanteral and ischial pressure peaks. Note that X and Y are not parallel to matrix rows and columns: it depends on the orientation of the sensing pad in relation to the pelvis. From 'Comparative biomechanical evaluation of different wheelchair seat cushions', M. Ferrarin, G. Andreoni and A. Pedotti, 2000, Journal of Rehabilitation Research and Development, 37, 318. Reprinted with permission.

giving a total of 2016 sensors' (p. 316). Ferrarin et al. found that 'it is not possible to identify a single cushion type that is effective in all subjects or in a specific category of subjects' (p. 323). By using computerized procedures, an appropriate cushion for a specific client could be developed.

Shape of the buttocks

A frequently used measure for wheelchair cushions is a Computer Aided Design/Computer Aided Manufacture (CAD/CAM) system. This type of system is used to digitize the measurement of the wheelchair user's back and/or buttocks to design the shape of the wheelchair cushion. One example is the Otto Back Shape System (Lemaire et al., 1996). Lemaire et al. (1996) compared the CAD/CAM system with traditional hand-sculpturing designing of a wheelchair cushion. There was no significant difference ($p < 0.05$) in the clients' (N = 25/9) satisfaction regardless of whether the cushion needed minor (10%), intermediate (11–25%), excessive (26–50%) or total modification.

Skin temperature and relative dampness of the seat because of perspiration

These can be measured using an infrared thermographic system (Ferrarin et al., 2000). The cushion cloth material should be chosen to avoid unnecessary force and friction between the client and the cushion and facilitate movement when transferring between the wheelchair and other furniture. Cutter and Blake (1997) suggested that gel-filled cushions maintain more constant skin temperature (two-degree increase during two hours of constant sitting) than other materials. Underpants and trousers should be made of soft material that absorbs perspiration in order to obtain less friction with the cushion surface. Edges or seams in clothing should be avoided or should be flexible to prevent pressure to the skin.

What is the effectiveness of different cushions in preventing pressure sores?

An effective cushion reduces interface between the pressure and the buttocks, promotes sitting balance and stability, and provides comfort. An interface pressure below 32 mm Hg is necessary to ensure adequate blood and lymphatic flow in the capillaries (Garber and Krouskop, 1997), and 20–33 mm Hg is recommended. Pellow (1999) tested the High Profile Roho (airfilled rubber cells on a flat rubber base), the Jay2 Gel cushion (a contoured, firm foam base, covered in the ischial area by a silicon gel pad) and the Ultimate Cushion. The High Profile Roho (47/54 mm Hg) provided the lowest pressure over the ischial tuberosities. Ferrarin et al. (2000) compared four cushions, including two polyuretanic gel-filled foam-based cushions from different manufacturers, a Roho Low Profile, and Jay2 cushions in ten individuals who had sustained spinal cord injuries at the thoracic level. The Roho Low Profile and the Jay2 cushion had significantly lower peak pressure (p < 0.05) over the ischial tuberosities compared with the other cushions.

What instruction is needed to foster independence?

The client has personal responsibility for preventing pressure sores. Lifestyle factors that help to prevent pressure sores include the level of continence of bladder and bowel and the client's diet. How independent the wheelchair user becomes affects his or her responsibility and self-efficacy (Garber and Krouskop, 1997). Regularly changing one's body position is extremely important to prevent pressure sores.

The client using a wheelchair needs education specifically adapted to his or her appropriate learning strategy and cognitive level of understanding.

Computer-assisted or interactive programmes (Garber and Krouskop, 1997) are recommended. These programmes contain information about skin care and inspection, pressure relief techniques, proper use of the wheelchair and positioning of the wheelchair cushion (Pellow, 1999).

Garber and Krouskop (1997) suggested the use of an alarm during initial habit training to help the wheelchair user shift weight on a regular basis. However, use of the alarm should not be a long-term solution, as the individual may become habituated to the alarm resulting in the device becoming ineffective.

What models of practice are the most appropriate in this case study?

The client-centred model or the person-environment-occupation model is used to involve the client actively in the intervention process (Canadian Association of Occupational Therapists, 1993; Sumsion, 1993).

What are the goals related to the solution of Ben's case?

Six major goals are identified:

1 The wheelchair should be appropriately adapted for Ben according to body positioning using biomechanical principles.
2 A wheelchair cushion should be prescribed with emphasis on relieving pressure and using neurophysiological principles to prevent pressure sores.
3 Ben should be responsible for moving his body and increasing the number of times he lifts his buttocks from the wheelchair cushion.
4 Ben should be encouraged to participate in occupational therapy group activities to increase social interactions.
5 Ben's quality of life and satisfaction will be increased by use of assistive technology.
6 Ben and the occupational therapist will identify vocational goals and leisure activities that are feasible for a wheelchair user.

Which pre-intervention assessments are planned?

Some of the required information is available in Ben's medical record, but other suggested assessments (see Table 3.3) will be completed during Ben's visit to the 'The Seat and Positioning Lab'. Information from these assessments is planned as part of the clinical decision-making process designed to choose an appropriate intervention for Ben.

Table 3.3 Suggested assessments to use for intervention planning when prescribing a wheelchair cushion

Assessment purpose	Assessment method/instrument
Body functions	
Muscle tone function of trunk and legs	Reflex hammer
Sensations related to muscles and movements	Standard neurological investigation of pin pricks and light touch.
Standard anatomical measure (Kamper et al., 2000) compared to measurements on the parts of the wheelchair	Goniometer measuring body parts according to a checklist (Hastings, 2000) that is compared to measurements of a wheelchair
The interface between the person and the wheelchair cushion surface	
The amount of pressure of Ben's buttocks on the wheelchair cushion	Tekscan Inc. computerized measuring system for the maximum pressure peak value, the peak values of the ischial tuberoses (which is Ben's critical anatomical areas), total mean pressure and standard deviation plus the total contact surface parameter registered for one second at 1, 5, 10 and 15 minutes.
Skin temperature	Thermographic system

What interventions are suggested?

The main interventions (Cutter and Blake, 1997; Pellow, 1999) include modifying the interface between Ben and his wheelchair and promoting social participation. The following interventions will be recommended:

1 Wheelchair: The wheelchair will be ergonomically adapted by adjusting the parts of the wheelchair to allow Ben's body to recline at the best tilting position.
2 Seating system. The prescription of an ergonomically sound seating system for Ben will bring about maximum pressure relief under the ischial tuberosities. The choice will be based on Ben's individual initial measurement of the pressure peaks and repeated measures during the follow-up period of Ben's status on his buttocks. The primary selection might be a Jay2 cushion, a contoured, firm foam base, covered in the ischial area by a silicon gel pad (Flolite®).
3 Teaching. Ben will be prescribed a two-week use of an alarm system promoting regular shifting and movement of his body. This intervention is

aimed at developing regular movement habits when sitting in the wheel-chair. An interactive computerized programme will help with his understanding of his responsibility for prevention of pressure sores.

4 Socialization. Ben will be encouraged to participate in group activities in the day-care treatment programme, which he presently attends and participate in activities where occupations are used as intervention media. Social participation with the group members will increase Ben's quality of life and occupational roles.

5 Vocational and leisure activities. Ben will receive vocational counselling and explore opportunities for leisure activities in the community.

What type of outcome design is appropriate for evaluating follow-up at three-months?

An interrupted time series design repeating Pellow's (1999) study is sug-gested. The dependent variable is improved skin status over the ischial tuberosities with no indicators for risk of new pressure sores. The inde-pendent variables are the interventions, including changing body position, choice of cushion and teaching new ways to move the body.

The following assessment instruments will be used:

- The Norton Scale (Norton et al., 1962), aimed at skin inspection for use every day.
- The Tekscan Inc. system aimed at measuring pressure relief to the but-tocks, will be used if the cut-off scores of the Norton scale is above the recommended limits.
- The computerized alarm system measuring shifting in body positioning during a two-week period will be used to give Ben continuous feed-back and help him to remember to shift his body.
- The Quebec User Evaluation of Satisfaction with Assistive Technology scale (Demers et al., 1999) is a self-assessment of client satisfaction for assistive technology.

Summary

In this chapter the Socratic Case Study Method (SCSM) is introduced. SCSM enables the learner (a) to apply principles and concepts to specific cases; (b) become actively involved in the application of ergonomic principles to specific situations and problems; (c) develop skills to iden-tify the relevant key issues in ergonomics by providing different solutions or scenarios; (d) examine literature for each of the key issues; and (e) apply critical thinking skills needed in clinical practice. The case study of Ben has been presented to demonstrate the application of the SCSM method to an individual with a spinal cord injury.

Review questions

1 How can SCSM help in clinical reasoning to solve problem in the perspective of the ergonomic model (e.g. discharge from hospital to home)?
2 What is the learner's role in SCSM?
3 How does the case of Ben help the learner to understand SCSM?
4 What are the justification and ethical considerations related to pre-scribing a wheelchair and its components?
5 What factors are related to prescribing and adapting a wheelchair?.
6 How would you write a scientific report for a clinical case study?

References

Axelson, P. (1996). The 14th annual survey of lightweight wheelchairs: It's the wheel thing. Sports-N-Spokes, 23, 73–86.

Burke, C.E. (1999). Summary of reliability study of matrices. Technology and Disability, 10, 181–185.

Canadian Association of Occupational Therapists (1993). Occupational Therapy Guidelines for Client-centred Mental Health Practice. Toronto, ON: CAOT.

Collins, F. (2004). Seating: Assessment and selection. Journal of Wound Care, 13, 9–12.

Cook, A.M. and Hussey, S.M. (2002). Technologies that enable mobility. In A.M. Cook and. S.M. Hussey (Eds), Assistive Technology: Principles and Practices (2nd edn, pp. 329–373). St. Louis: Mosby.

Cooper, R.A., Robertson, R.N., Boninger, M.L., Shimada, S.D., VanSickle, D.P., Lawrence, B. and Singleton, T. (1997). Wheelchair ergonomics. In S. Kumar (Ed.), Perspectives in Rehabilitation Ergonomics (pp. 246–272). Bristol, PA: Taylor & Francis.

Cutter, N.C. and Blake, D.J. (1997). Wheelchairs and seating systems: Clinical applications. Physical Medicine and Rehabilitation: State of the Art Reviews, 11, 107–132.

Davis, A.B. (1973). Triumph over Disability: The Development of Rehabilitation Medicine in the USA. Washington, DC: The National Museum of History and Technology, Smithsonian Institute.

Demers, L., Wessels, R.D., Weiss-Lambrou, R., Ska, B. and De-Witte, L.P. (1999). An international content validation of the Quebec User Evaluation of Satisfaction and Assistive Technology [QUEST]. Occupational Therapy International, 6, 159–175.

Ditunno, J.F., Yung, W., Donovan, W.H. and Creasey, G. (1994). The international standards booklet for neurological and functional classification of spinal cord injury. Paraplegia, 32, 70–80.

Everest and Jennings, Inc (1979). Modification and Accessory Analysis. [Brochure]. Available from Everest and Jennings, Inc, 3233 E. Mission Oaks Boulevard Camarillo, CA 93010.

Ferrarin, M., Andreoni, G. and Pedotti, A. (2000). Comparative biomechanical evaluation of different wheelchair seat cushions. Journal of Rehabilitation Research and Development, 37, 315–324.

Garber, S. and Krouskop, T. (1997). Technical advances in wheelchairs and seating systems. Physical Medicine and Rehabilitation: State of the Art Reviews, 11, 93–106.

Gassner, L.A. and Wotton, K. (1998). Nursing students' integration of theory and practice: The development and implementation of a practice and theoretical framework for teaching – A case study. Higher Education Research and Development, 17, 239–249.

Hastings, J.D. (2000). Seating assessment and planning. Physical Medicine and Rehabilitation Clinics of North America, 11, 183–207.

Highet, G. (1950). The Art of Teaching. New York: Vintage.

Johannessen, L.R. (2000). Encouraging active learning with case studies. Paper presented at the Annual Spring Meeting of the National Council of Teachers of English, New York, March.

Jones, D.C. and Sheridan, M.E. (1999). A case study approach: Developing critical thinking skills in novice pediatric nurses. Journal of Continuing Education in Nursing, 30, 75–78.

Kamenetz, H.L. (1969). The Wheelchair Book. Springfield, IL: Charles C. Thomas.

Kamper, D.G., Adams, T.C., Reger, S.I., Parnianpour, M., Barin, K. and Linden, M.A. (2000). A technique for quantifying the response of seated individuals to dynamic perturbations. Journal of Rehabilitation Research and Development, 37, 81–88.

Kang, T.E., Eng, B., Phil, M. and Mak, A.F.T. (1997). Evaluation of a simple approach to modify the supporting property of seating foam cushion for pressure relief. Assistive Technology, 9, 47–54.

Kanyer, B. (1992). Meeting the seating and mobility needs of the client with traumatic brain injury. Journal of Head Trauma Rehabilitation, 7, 81–93.

Kilkens, O.J., Post, M.W., Dallmeijer, A.J. Seelen, H.A. and van der Woude, L.H. (2003). Wheelchair tests: A systematic review. Clinical Rehabilitation, 17, 418–430.

Kim, J. and Mulholland, S.J. (1999). Seating/wheelchair technology in the developing world: Need for a closer look. Technology and Disability, 11, 21–27.

Lemaire, E.D., Upton, D., Paialunga, J., Martel, G. and Boucher, J. (1996). Clinical analysis of a CAD/CAM system for custom seating: A comparison with hand-sculpting methods. Journal of Rehabilitation Research and Development, 33, 311–320.

Lynn, L.E. (1999). Teaching and Learning with Cases: A Guidebook. New York: Seven Bridges.

Minkel, J.L. (2000). Seating and mobility considerations for people with spinal cord injury. Physical Therapy, 80, 701–709.

Norton, D., McLaren, R. and Exton-Smith, A.N. (1962). An Investigation of Geriatric Nursing Problems in Hospitals. Edinburgh: Churchill Livingstone.

Pellow, T.R. (1999). A comparison of interface pressure readings to wheelchair cushions and positioning: A pilot study. Canadian Journal of Occupational Therapy, 66, 140–149.

Samuelsson, K.A.M, Tropp, H., Nylander, E. and Gerdle, B. (2004). The effect of rear-wheel position on seating ergonomics and mobility efficiency in wheelchair users with spinal cord injuries: A pilot study. Journal of Rehabilitation Research and Development, 41, 65–74.

Sudzina, M.R. (2000). Case study considerations for teaching educational psychology. Paper presented at the Annual Meeting of the American Educational Research Association, New Orleans, April 24–28.

Sumsion, T. (1993). Client-centred practice: The true impact. Canadian Journal of Occupational Therapy, 60, 6–8.

Woods, B. and Watson, N. (2003). A short history of powered wheelchairs. Assistive Technology, 15, 164–180.

World Health Organization (2001). International Classification of Functioning, Disability, and Health [ICF]. Geneva, Switzerland: WHO.

CHAPTER 4

The case study of Emmy: Preventing accidental falls among older adults

All falls occur somewhere. Environmental risk factors at the location of a fall have been repeatedly recognized as contributing to falls in older people. The extent that environmental conditions play a role in falls ... offers an appealing approach to falls prevention. In general, the ease, cost and feasibility of modifying environmental conditions relevant to falls are likely to compare favorably with those of interventions that target other types of fall risk factors such as health factors and risky behaviours.

Betty Rose Connell, 1996, p. 859

The assessment of risk factors for falls and the implementation of interventions that address primary, secondary, and tertiary activities prevent falls from occurring.

Margie Lange,1996, p.198

Learning objectives

By the end of this chapter the learner will:

1 Understand the risk factors for falls in the elderly.
2 Become familiar with strategies and interventions used to prevent accidental falls in elderly persons.
3 Understand how to apply ergonomic principles to formulate goals in the home environment.
4 Apply ergonomic principles regarding the use of assistive devices, environmental accessibility and adaptations.
5 Identify suitable residential placements for the elderly.

Definition of falls

An accidental fall is a slip to the floor, whether or not injury is sustained (Benson and Lusardi, 1995). Falls can occur in many cases because of a relatively minor misstep that makes the person's centre of gravity move outside the effective base of support. These missteps often occur when standing on one foot. This task is difficult for elderly persons. Standing on one foot is necessary for skills such as walking on slippery surfaces, reaching for objects on a high shelf, turning quickly and climbing stairs (Richardson and Hurvitz, 1995). In addition, these tasks may be difficult for elderly persons who are at risk of falls because of problems with balance (Suzuki et al., 2004), poor vision (Sihvonen et al., 2004), side effects of psychoactive medication (Kallin et al., 2004a; Monane and Avorn, 1996), low bone mass (Toofanny et al., 2004), a vestibular hypofunction (Hall et al., 2004) or muscle weakness in the lower extremities due to arthritis (Sturnieks et al., 2004).

Background and description of the case

A governmental health and welfare organization in Sweden has been developed to decrease accidental falls among the elderly by applying ergonomic principles to (a) reduce risk factors; (b) maximize clients' functioning (i.e. mobility); (c) maintain or improve clients' daily activities (i.e. personal care and social participation); and (d) improve quality of care. The Socratic Case Study Method (SCSM) in the case of Emmy will illustrate the application of ergonomic principles in preventing accidental falls in the elderly.

Description of the case

Emmy is 79 years old. She lives alone in a one-room apartment (see Figure 4.1) on the first mezzanine floor. From the front door seven steps were required to get to her apartment, and no handrails or lift were available. Every morning Emmy went to the convenience store in the same block as her home. Every week Emmy had participated in a mixed T'ai-Chi group (Kessenich, 1998) for an hour.

A year ago, Emmy suffered a slight stroke from a transient ischaemic attack (TIA). During her acute three-day stay at the hospital, she had fallen from her bed to the ground as she attempted to transfer from her bed to an easy chair three metres away. On this hospital ward double side-rails were used routinely at night-time on all beds (Capezuti et al., 1998). Emmy had access to an alarm warning system, but had not used it. After this incident, Emmy used a cane in her right hand when walking. She also had minor problems with incontinence. For safety she uses incontinence-protection.

Within a six-month period, Emmy had fallen a second time when she attempted to leave her bed to go to the toilet at 5 am. She said she did not put on her glasses because she needed to go to the toilet immediately and then had difficulties finding her way. Furthermore, this time she did not reach for her cane. Her friend had moved it the previous afternoon while visiting Emmy. Emmy was very embarrassed

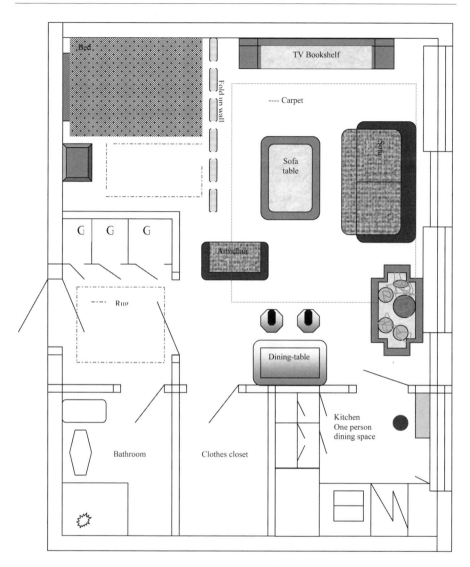

Figure 4.1 Drawing of Emmy's apartment.

and scared about falling, subsequently she avoided moving around in her flat.

Lynn is 53 years old and Emmy's closest friend. She has been worried about Emmy and strongly suggested that Emmy should move to a nursing home; however, Emmy does not want to do this.

Clinical reasoning

You, as an occupational therapist, have visited Emmy's home. There you met Emmy and Lynn. Together you, Emmy and Lynn have brainstormed some possible solutions which are the most feasible for the present situation and most convenient to Emmy's quality of life. How would you set goals using a client-centred model? Which goals, interventions and outcome evaluations would be considered while applying ergonomic principles?

Relevant literature review

Economics

Prevention of accidental falls among the elderly is very cost-effective. Costs of prevention are based on the expenditures for ergonomics and environmental arrangements that decrease the number of accidental falls. The cost of prevention is compared with the cost of having an accidental fall. When there is a fall, the direct and indirect costs include the additional probability of an accidental fall with a treatable injury, the medical cost of intervention and rehabilitation, and the client's fearfulness of having a fall, which reduces the client's functional activities and social participation. Since the healthcare system seldom reimburses for preventative medicine the clients are left on their own to prevent falls in the home (Englander et al., 1996).

Epidemiology statistics and outcome

Injuries caused by accidental falls are the sixth leading cause of death in older persons. Approximately 70 per cent of all deaths due to falls (some 10,000 per year in the United States of America) occur in the 13 per cent of the population aged 65 and older. Both injurious and non-injurious falls are associated with subsequent functional decline (Edelberg, 2001).

The rate of incidental falls increases with age (Cumming, 1998), with the ratio of falls in males to females about 40–60 per cent (Englander et al., 1996). Twenty-five per cent of individuals over 65 years old who still live in their homes fall at least once each year. For those individuals over 75 years old, the rate increases to more than 30 per cent. This rate increases to about 40 per cent of individuals living in a nursing home. Ninety per cent of individuals over 80 years old suffer from an accidental fall at least once a year. Those who are over 90 years old fall more than once a year (Edelberg, 2001; Englander et al., 1996).

One accidental fall may be predictive for the second fall (Steinweg, 1997). Within six months a second fall may occur in about two-thirds of individuals over 80 years old. Accidental falls among those individuals older than 80 can be fatal or lead to conditions that cause death (Mahoney, 1998; Tideiksaar and Kay, 1986). Approximately two per cent of those clients over 80 who are admitted to a hospital die as a result of an accidental fall (Tideiksaar and Kay, 1986).

Aetiology of accidental falls

Accidental falls occur more often in individuals with a medical diagnosis such as stoke (Mahoney, 1998; Tideiksaar, 1996), Parkinson's disease (Grimbergen et al., 2004a), osteoarthritis, arthritis of lower limb and joints, osteoporosis (Cumming, 1998; Tideiksaar, 1996), hypothyroidism (Kramer and Achiron, 1993), peripheral neuropathy (Richardson and Hurvitz, 1996) psychosis, dementia and acute illness (Mahoney, 1998) than in a healthy elderly population. Accidental falls in elderly people can be explained by a model that contains medical, psychological, social and environmental factors that interact with physiological age-related factors (Cwikel and Fried, 1992; Kallin et al., 2004b).

A literature review (Rawsky, 1998) that included more than 100 publications revealed that the main risk factors for accidental falls are both intrinsic and extrinsic. Intrinsic risk factors, caused by factors within the individual, occur more often among people with dementia-related symptoms with decreased cognitive skill and confusion (Benson and Lusardi, 1995; Mahoney, 1998), or with physical impairments such as decreased muscle strength, immobility, imbalance or vertigo (Mahoney, 1998; Rigler, 1996; Tideiksaar, 1996); incontinence (Capezuti et al., 1998); visual impairment (e.g. inability to detect edges of steps) (Cumming, 1998; Tideiksaar, 1996); fatigue (Rigler, 1996); and behaviours, such as 'stops walking when talking' (Henderson et al., 1998).

Extrinsic factors that contribute to the incidence of accidental falls include hazards such as obstacles in the environment; uneven, rough or slippery walking surfaces; presence of stairs or thresholds; absent or poor lighting (Mahoney, 1998; Studenski et al., 1994; Tideiksaar, 1996); or unfamiliar environments (Mahoney, 1998). Inappropriate shoes (Mahoney, 1998), neglecting to use bed rails with individuals prone to fall out of bed (Everitt and Bridel-Nixon, 1997), and furniture with wheels preventing the use of the furniture for stability when standing or sitting (Connell, 1996) may also result in accidental falls.

Although drugs or medications are usually classified as extrinsic, they also interact with intrinsic factors such as cognitive and physical functions, causing dizziness, muscle weakness, poor judgement, limited range of motion and imbalance (Kallin et al., 2004a; Kallin et al., 2004b). Environmental hazards can contribute to risk factors for healthier elderly people, while behavioural and situational factors are of greater danger among frail elderly people (Cutson, 1994; Steinweg, 1997; Wilson, 1998).

Consequences of accidental falls

Approximately 85 per cent of individuals involved in a single accidental fall do not suffer from any physical injury or any physical consequences; however, the fear of falling again may lead to emotional problems such as depression and fear, or cognitive and physical decline (Tideiksaar, 1996, 2003). This in turn may interfere with the person's habitual activity pattern leading to deceased activity and possible death (Cumming et al., 1999; Edelberg, 2001; Tideiksaar, 1996, 2003). The remaining 15 per cent need medical consultation. Among these persons, biological complications (e.g. head and soft tissue trauma, musculoskeletal sprains) are seen in about 5–10 per cent, while bone fractures (e.g. hip, wrist, neck or upper arm) occur in about 3–5 per cent (Cumming, 1998). Hip fractures are the most serious outcome of falls (Cumming, 1998; Edelberg, 2001; Tideiksaar, 1996; White, 1988).

Whether an accidental fall causes a fracture or not depends on the person's muscle strength, bone density and biomechanical factors. Factors include (a) the nature of the fall direction (sidewards, backwards or forwards); (b) the energy in the fall (dependent on the height of the fall); (c) the quality of the landing surface (the harder the floor, the greater risk for fracture); and (d) the body mass index (e.g. ratio of fat to muscle) (Cummings and Nevitt, 1994; Henderson et al., 1998). Injuries in accidental falls can be prevented by examining the relationships between these factors.

An accidental fall causes neuromusculoskeletal and movement-related impairments. Only one-half of people sustaining a hip fracture are able to walk and move around independently without having surgery such as a hip replacement. Many of the elderly require a cane or a walker and/or personal assistance (Tideiksaar, 1996). The heightened risk of falling can cause worry and stress to relatives, spouses and close friends. In addition, many people who have sustained an accidental fall are fearful of falling again (Tideiksaar, 1996, 2003) and may experience pain that restricts their activity (Hagsten and Söderback, 1994).

Individuals who sustain a hip fracture frequently avoid performing daily activities and tasks that involve walking or moving about (Cumming, 1998; Englander et al., 1996; Hagsten and Söderback, 1994; Henderson et al., 1998; Tideikssar, 1996). This, in turn, decreases bone, joint and muscle functions (Englander et al., 1996; Henderson et al., 1998; Tideiksaar, 1996). Hagsten and Söderback (1994) found that participation in occupational therapy for 4–10 days post-operation resulted in greater independence in dressing, mobility and hygiene/bathing during the following 120 days. The most difficult activities reported by the 14 participants in the study were washing hair, making beds and grocery shopping. The relationship between an accidental fall causing a hip fracture and the individual's participation in social activities needs further research.

Applying ergonomic principles to the home environment in a case of accidental falls

Assessment

The primary purposes for assessments are (a) to identify individuals who are at a high risk of having accidental falls (Cwikel et al., 1998; Lange, 1996) and (b) to identify factors to minimize these risks. The occupational therapist's responsibility in a 'Fall and Balance Clinic' is to assess the client's ability to perform IADL and PADL and to assess his or her home environment (Hill et al., 1994). A system-oriented approach is recommended when evaluating ways to prevent accidental falls. Intrinsic, extrinsic and social-epidemiological factors relevant for the actual client should be identified. Functioning and contextual environmental factors should also be examined. This information will help the therapist to develop an appropriate intervention plan for the client who is at risk of falling (Rawsky, 1998; Wilson, 1998). The assessment procedure should incorporate (a) a physical examination; (b) information about the pre-existing activity level; and (c) an evaluation of the person's home environment. The latter can be accomplished through a home visit aimed at identifying the environmental risks related to falling (Cwikel and Fried, 1992; Hill et al., 1994; Rigler, 1996, Studenski et al., 1994).

Interventions

Three different forms of interventions are used in the application of ergonomic principles: (a) teaching ergonomically safe practices to clients; (b) making changes within the environment to prevent accidental falls; and (c) supplying assistive devices to provide a safe environment so that the client can be more active on a daily basis.

Teaching ergonomically safe practices

Accidental falls can be prevented by teaching ergonomically safe practices in several different formats. Direct instruction of skills to the elderly and those involved in the care of the elderly is one format. Clients who are at risk of accidental falls must be taught to use ergonomically safe practices in ambulation. Various aspects of ambulating are demonstrated to the client and include transporting from sitting to standing, standing still after rising until one's balance is stable and strategies for getting up from the floor (Henderson et al., 1998; Rubenstein et al., 1996). Other interventions include providing visual feedback-based balance training (Sihvonen et al., 2004) and balance exercises, giving the client an understanding of the major uses of falls, and documenting situations in which falls have occurred (Edelberg, 2001). Individuals who are responsible for designing an ergonomic environment, such as nursing home staffs, should be educated in both ergonomically safe practices in ambulation and in the development of ward routines that will prevent accidental falls (Lange, 1996; Rubenstein et al., 1996).

Interventions other than just direct instruction have been developed; however, these have not been found to be as effective as when the client and caregivers are provided practice in ergonomically safe techniques. Cwikel and Fried (1992) developed a programme for use with individuals and groups that included videos and audio tapes. The Frailty and Injuries Cooperative Studies of Intervention Techniques (FICISIT research project) demonstrated that providing brochures such as 'Decreasing Your Risk of Falls' (Steinweg, 1997, p. 1823) was helpful for both older people and their significant others. The result of using these handouts reduced the falls up to 30 per cent for the intervention group (Steinweg, 1997).

Participation in physical training is another intervention that may reduce accidental falls (Grimbergen et al., 2004b). Higher levels of habitual daily activities in the elderly are associated with lower prevalence of risk factors ($r = 0.41$ for men, $r = 0.76$ for women; Henderson et al., 1998). Therapists should encourage elderly clients to implement daily habitual routine programmes and to participate in gymnastic groups (Mahoney, 1998).

Participation in social group activities can increase self-confidence (Wilson, 1998) and lower stress. Deforche and De Bourdeaudhuij (2000) found that elderly adults involved in structured exercise classes were more active and reported higher self-confidence than those who did not participate in an organized social group. The authors concluded that 'stimulating older adults to join a structured activity programme in the company of family or friends in order to enhance supporting social influences and perceived competence could be an important intervention strategy' (p. 362).

Modifying the home environment

Because environmental conditions contribute to the occurrence of accidental falls (Connell, 1996), the removal of home hazards is strongly recommended if accidents are to be prevented (Cwikel and Fried, 1992). In short, a supportive and accessible home environment should be designed. Rooms should be minimally furnished to allow for free passage around the furniture. The remaining furniture should be ergonomically designed and stable because elderly people often use it as supports. Furnishings, such as rugs and thresholds that may cause an individual to stumble, should be removed (Connell, 1996; Lange, 1996). The bed should not be on wheels, should be at the level of the individual's hip to facilitate standing and should be accessible from both sides (Capezuti et al., 1998; Everitt and Bridel-Nixon, 1997).

Ergonomic and adaptive changes inside homes and buildings include modifying and adapting lighting, floors and hallways, rugs, bathrooms, stairways, furniture (e.g. chairs, beds) or storage (Capezuti et al., 1998; Mahoney, 1998; Rigler, 1996). There should be optimal lighting at all times in stairways, halls and bathrooms. Floor surfaces should be non-slippery. Handrails should be present in the bathrooms and storage should be easily accessible (Capezuti et al., 1998; Everitt and Bridel-Nixon, 1997; Mahoney, 1998; Rigler, 1996).

The prescription of underwear that has been padded with soft materials is helpful for people at high risks for accidental falls. When an individual falls, the padding will moderate the fall (Dubey et al., 1999).

Intervention studies have shown disappointingly small effects and the effects are difficult to interpret on falls-related outcomes (Connell, 1996; Lange, 1996). Connell (1996) identified studies that examined the environmental risk factors associated with falls among the elderly living in the community. 'The first group of studies suggests an approach to falls prevention centered on hazard removal; the second group suggests an approach centered on the provision of more supportive environments that reduce excessive environmental demands' (Connell, 1996, p. 859). Rubenstein et al. (1996) reported a situation in which the nursing home environment was arranged based on the principles of total quality management (TQM system). Everitt and Bridel-Nixon (1997) conducted a study aimed at creating a safer outdoor environment. Factors considered included (a) commonly used mobility aids; (b) location of incidents (e.g. falls and missteps); and (c) descriptions of pavement, street or pathway surface conditions (e.g. uneven, wet, broken, slippery, littered). While this information is useful for healthcare professionals and city planners responsible for removing hazards and reconstructing the environment, publicizing this in the daily newspapers is not always effective (Cwikel, 1992).

Prescribing assistive technology

Clients who have sustained a hip fracture are regularly offered assistive technology in Sweden (Hagsten and Söderback, 1994). For example, bed blocks, cushions, reachers, stocking aids, raised toilet seats, bath seats, shower benches, canes, walking frames and/or mounting bathroom assist rails are commonly prescribed. These devices are designed to increase the client's independence in self-care but are also used in preventing further accidental falls. The use of a personal alarm warning system can alert staff or family members that the client needs immediate help (Studenski et al., 1994; Weiner et al., 1998). It is also important to *compensate for visual deficits* because the clients' feeling of being safe when waking in the morning and moving around in the home can depend on the client's vision (Studenski et al., 1994).

When assistive technology is combined with follow-up activities, such as home visits by the occupational therapist, clients may be influenced to maintain a high level of activity (Cumming et al., 1999; Hagsten and

Söderback, 1994), and may be more compliant in using the devices (Henderson et al., 1998; Hill et al., 1988).

Significant landmark studies

Capezuti, E., Talerico, K.A., Strumpf, N. and Evans, L.K. (1998). Individualized assessment and intervention in bilateral siderail use. Geriatric Nursing, 19, 322–330.

Abstract: The use of bilateral side rails, similar to physical restraints, can be safely reduced by comprehensive assessment process. This article presents an individualized assessment for evaluating side rail use to guide the caring staff in managing resident characteristics for falling out of bed and intervening for high-risk residents. The individualized assessment is consistent with federal resident assessment instrument requirements and includes risk factors specific to falls from bed.

Everitt, V. and Bridel-Nixon, J. (1997). The use of bed rails: Principles of patient assessment. Nursing Standard, 12(6), 44–47.

Abstract: Bed rails are often used to prevent patients from injuring themselves through falling, but they may not always have the desired effect. In this literature review, the authors demonstrate that patients must be assessed in relation to clearly defined risk factors to prevent indiscriminate use of bed rails.

Hill, K.D., Dwyer, J.M., Schwarz, J.A. and Helme, R. (1994). A falls and balance clinic for the elderly. Physiotherapy Canada, 46, 20–27.

Abstract: A falls and balance clinic for the elderly has been developed with the aim of identifying those at risk of subsequent falls, and recommending intervention strategies to reduce this risk. The physical and functional status of 149 clients referred to the clinic are reported. Neurological and musculoskeletal pathologies were identified as the cause of falls in the majority of clients. Measures of gait velocity and stride length, and ability to stand on one leg were markedly reduced compared with normative data for healthy elderly. A number of other measures of balance, strength and function are also reported. The results of a questionnaire about home environment indicated that only 28 per cent of those referred had been assessed in their own home in the previous year. Home environment was considered a potential risk in a further 28 per cent of clients and a home visit was instituted in these cases. Other intervention strategies included referral for further investigations (36 per cent), Day Hospital (33 per cent), provision of a home programme of balance or strengthening exercises (27 per cent), and medication change (15 per cent). Issues related to the establishment, operation and long-term evaluation of the effectiveness of a specialist falls and balance clinic for the elderly are discussed.

Mahoney, J.E. (1998). Immobility and falls. Clinics in Geriatric Medicine, 14, 699–726.

Abstract: Immobility is a common problem for hospitalized older adults. Excessive bed rest results in multiple adverse physiological consequences and may contribute to functional decline and increased risk for falls in the hospital setting. About 2 per cent of hospitalized older adults fall during hospitalization. Risk factors for in-hospital falls includes cognitive impairment, mobility impairment, specific diagnoses, multiple comorbidities and psychotropic medications. Appropriate actions to prevent immobility and falls include increasing exercise and activity levels, improving the hospital environment and decreasing the use of psychotropic medications. Bed alarms and increased supervision for high-risk patients also may help prevent falls.

Tideiksaar, R. (2003). Best practice approach to fall prevention in community-living elders. Topics in Geriatric Rehabilitation, 19, 199–205.

Abstract: Falls among adults aged 65 and older are a major health problem. Approximately 35 per cent to 40 per cent of community-living elders fall annually. Falling is associated with considerable mortality and morbidity. Falls generally result from an interaction of multiple intrinsic and extrinsic factors. The ability to reduce falls depends on understanding (1) fall preventative strategies, particularly evidence-based strategies, and most important, on (2) turning evidence-based strategies into 'best practices' under real-world conditions.

Wilson, E.B. (1998). Preventing patient falls. AACN Clinical Issues, 9, 100–108.

Abstract: Falls are among the most common, yet potentially preventable, adverse events experienced by patients in hospitals. Such serious outcomes as physical and emotional injury, increased dependence, admission to a long-term care facility and poor quality of life can result from falling. Traditionally, elderly patients have been at highest risk for falling, with many falls resulting in serious injury. These injuries cost billions of dollars and expose hospitals and their staff to liability. As the elderly population continues to increase, it is imperative that falls and associated injuries be prevented whenever possible identification of non-traditional patients at high risk for falls is emerging in the professional literature. Educating professionals about risk factors, prevention strategies and application of fall index and fall injury statistics can improve the safety of fall-prone patients. Refining, modifying and individualizing fall risk factors and prevention interventions for traditional and non-traditional high-risk groups are a necessary focus for future research.

Effectiveness of interventions

Studies have shown that participation in exercise programmes improves mobility and balance, but whether these programmes prevent accidental falls is still an open question (Buchner et al., 1997). Elinge et al. (2003) examined whether the effects of a group learning programme would influence participants' perceived activity performance and ability to participate in social life after a hip fracture intervention. Participants, randomized into an intervention group (n = 21) or control group (n = 14), had completed ordinary care and rehabilitation after their hip fractures. The participants' perception of their activity performance and ability to participate in social life was measured at the end of the intervention period and 12 months thereafter. Results showed no significant difference between either group in their ability to perform ADL activities measured by the Barthel ADL Index. The only significant difference between groups was in the increased participation in social activities for the intervention group. These results relate to the efficacy of ergonomic intervention that sometimes appear inconsistent because of the differences in research methodology (King and Tinetti, 1996; Studenski et al., 1994), resulting in difficulties in generalizing the results (Connell, 1996; Söderback, 1995).

Summary

The occupational therapist plays a significant role in preventing, assessing and developing interventions of accidental falls especially in elderly people. This chapter has presented the case of Emmy and has given some background information about an individual who has had accidental falls. In the case of Emmy, the interventions used in preventing falls through the application of ergonomic principles include (a) teaching ergonomically safe practices to clients to prevent accidental falls; (b) making adaptations in the home environment; and (c) prescribing assistive devices. These intervention programmes are appropriate whether Emmy decides to continue living in her home or moving to a nursing home. It is hoped that the reader will now develop an intervention for Emmy that applies the ergonomic principles.

References

Benson, C. and Lusardi, P. (1995). Neurologic antecedents to patient falls. Journal of Neuroscience Nursing, 27, 331–337.

Buchner, D.M., Cress, M.E., de Lateur, B.J., Esselman, P.C., Margherita, A.J., Price, R. and Wagner, E.H. (1997). The effect of strength and endurance training on gait, balance, fall risk, and health services use in community-living older adults. Journal of Gerontology: Biological Sciences: Medical Sciences, 52, M218–224.

Capezuti, E., Talerico, K.A., Strumpf, N. and Evans, L.K. (1998). Individualized assessment and intervention in bilateral siderail use. Geriatric Nursing, 19, 322–330.

Connell, B.R. (1996). Role of the environment in falls prevention. Clinics in Geriatric Medicine, 12, 859–880.

Cumming, R.G. (1998). Epidemiology of medication-related falls and fractures in the elderly. Drugs and Aging, 12, 43–53.

Cumming, R.G., Thomas, M., Szonyi, G., Salkeld, G., O'Neill, E., Westbury, C. and Frampton, G. (1999). Home visits by an occupational therapist for assessment and modification of environmental hazards: A randomized trial of falls prevention [see comments]. Journal of the American Geriatric Society, 47, 1397–1402.

Cummings, S.R. and Nevitt, M.C. (1994). Non-skeletal determinants of fractures: The potential importance of the mechanics of falls. Study of Osteoporotic Fractures Research Group. Osteoporosis International, 4, 67–70.

Cutson, T.M. (1994). Falls in the elderly. American Family Physician, 49, 149–156.

Cwikel, J. (1992). Falls among elderly people living at home: Medical and social factors in a national sample [see comments]. Israel Journal of Medical Science, 28, 446–453.

Cwikel, J.G. and Fried, A.V. (1992). The social epidemiology of falls among community-dwelling elderly: Guidelines for prevention. Disability Rehabilitation, 14, 113–121.

Cwikel, J.G., Fried, A.V., Biderman, A. and Galinsky, D. (1998). Validation of a fall-risk screening test, the Elderly Fall Screening Test (EFST), for community-dwelling elderly. Disability Rehabilitation, 20, 161–167.

Deforche, B. and De Bourdeaudhuij, I. (2000). Differences in psychosocial determinants of physical activity in older adults participation in organised versus non-organised activities. Journal of Sports Medicine and Physical Fitness, 40, 362–372.

Dubey, B.A., Koval, K.J. and Zuckerman, J.D. (1999). Hip fracture prevention: A review. American Journal of Orthopedics, 28, 190–194.

Edelberg, H.K. (2001). Falls and function: How to prevent falls and injuries in patients with impaired mobility. Geriatrics, 56, 41–45.

Elinge, E., Löfgren, B. Gagerman, E. and Nyberg, L. (2003). A group learning programme for old people with hip fracture: A randomized study. Scandinavian Journal of Occupational Therapy, 10, 27–33.

Englander, F., Hodson, T.J. and Terregrossa, R.A. (1996). Economic dimensions of slip and fall injuries. Journal of Forensic Science, 41, 733–746.

Everitt, V. and Bridel-Nixon, J. (1997). The use of bed rails: Principles of patient assessment. Nursing Standard, 12(6), 44–47.

Grimbergen, Y.A,. Munneke, M. and Bloem, B.R. (2004a) Falls in Parkinson's disease. Current Opinion in Neurology, 17, 405–415.

Grimbergen, Y.A., Munneke, M., Bloem, B.R., Sherrington, C., Lord, S.R. and Finch, C.F. (2004b). Physical activity interventions to prevent falls among older people: Update of the evidence. Journal of Science and Medicine in Sport, 7 (1 Suppl), 43–51.

Hagsten, B.E. and Söderback, I. (1994). Occupational therapy after hip fracture: A pilot study of the clients, the care and the costs. Clinical Rehabilitation, 8, 52–58.

Hall, C.D., Schubert, M.C. and Herdman, S.J. (2004). Prediction of fall risk reduction as measured by dynamic gait index in individuals with unilateral vestibular hypofunction. Otology and Neurotology: Official Publication of the American Otological Society, American Neurotology Society [and] European Academy of Otology and Neurotology, 25, 746–751.

Henderson, N. K., White, C. P., and Eisman, J. A. (1998). The roles of exercise and fall risk reduction in the prevention of osteoporosis. Endocrinology and Metabolic Clinics of North America, 27, 369–387.

Hill, B.A., Johnson, R. and Garrett, B.L. (1988). Reducing the incidence of falls in high risk patients. Journal of Nursing Administration, 18, 24–28.

Hill, K.D., Dwyer, J.M., Schwarz, J.A. and Helme, R. (1994). A falls and balance clinic for the elderly. Physiotherapy Canada, 46, 20–27.

Kallin, K., Gustafson, Y., Sandman, P.O. and Karlsson, S. (2004a). Drugs and falls in older people in geriatric care settings. Aging, Clinical and Experimental Research, 16, 270–276.

Kallin, K., Jensen, J., Olsson, L. L., Nyberg, L. and Gustafson, Y. (2004b). Why the elderly fall in residential care facilities, and suggested remedies. Journal of Family Practice, 53, 41–52.

Kessenich, C.R. (1998). T'ai Chi as a method of fall prevention in the elderly. Orthopedic Nursing, 17, 27–29.

King, M.B. and Tinetti, M.E. (1996). A multifactorial approach to reducing injurious falls. Clinical Geriatric Medicine, 12, 745–759.

Kramer, U. and Achiron, A. (1993). Drop attacks induced by hypothyroidism. Acta Neurologica Scandinavica, 88, 410–411.

Lange, M. (1996). The challenge of fall prevention in home care: A review of the literature. Home Health Nurse, 14, 198–206.

Mahoney, J.E. (1998). Immobility and falls. Clinics in Geriatric Medicine, 14, 699–726.

Monane, M. and Avorn, J. (1996). Medications and falls. Causation, correlation, and prevention. Clinical Geriatric Medicine, 12, 847–858.

Rawsky, E. (1998). Review of the literature on falls among the elderly. Image: The Journal Nursing Scholarship, 30, 47–52.

Richardson, J.K. and Hurvitz, E.A. (1995). Peripheral neuropathy: A true risk factor for falls. Journal of Gerontology: Biological Sciences: Medical Sciences, 50, 211–215.

Rigler, S. (1996). Instability in the older adult. Comprehensive Therapy, 22, 297–303.

Rubenstein, L.Z., Josephson, K.R. and Osterweil, D. (1996). Falls and fall prevention in the nursing home. Clinics in Geriatric Medicine, 12, 881–902.

Sihvonen, S., Sipila, S., Taskinen, S. and Era, P. (2004). Fall incidence in frail older women after individualized visual feedback-based balance training. Gerontology, 50, 411–416.

Söderback, I. (1995). Effectiveness in rehabilitation. Critical Reviews in Rehabilitation Medicine, 7, 275–286.

Steinweg, K.K. (1997). The changing approach to falls in the elderly. American Family Physician, 56, 1815–1823.

Studenski, S., Duncan, P.W., Chandler, J., Samsa, G., Prescott, B., Hogue, C. and Bearon, L.B. (1994). Predicting falls: The role of mobility and nonphysical factors. Journal of American Geriatrics Society, 42, 297–302.

Sturnieks, D.L., Tiedemann, A., Chapman, K., Munro, B., Murray, S.M. and Lord, S.R. (2004). Physiological risk factors for falls in older people with lower limb arthritis. Journal of Rheumatology, 31, 2272–2279.

Suzuki, T., Kim, H., Yoshida, H. and Ishizaki, T. (2004). Randomized controlled trial of exercise intervention for the prevention of falls in community-dwelling elderly Japanese women. Journal of Bone and Mineral Metabolism, 22, 602–611.

Tideiksaar, R. (1996). Preventing falls: How to identify risk factors, reduce complications. Geriatrics, 51, 43–46, 49–50, 53–55.

Tideiksaar, R. (2003). Best practice approach to fall prevention in community-living elders. Topics in Geriatric Rehabilitation, 19, 199–205.

Tideiksaar, R. and Kay, A.D. (1986). What causes falls? A logical diagnostic procedure. Geriatrics, 41, 32–50.

Toofanny, N, Maddens, M.E., Voytas, J. and Kowalski, D.J. (2004). Low bone mass and postfall fracture risk among elderly nursing home men. Journal of the American Medical Directors Association, 5, 367–370.

Weiner, D.K., Hanlon, J.T. and Studenski, S.A. (1998). Effects of central nervous system polypharmacy on falls liability in community-dwelling elderly. Gerontology, 44, 217–221.

White, H.C. (1988). Post-stroke hip fractures. Archives of Orthopedic Trauma Surgery, 107, 345–347.

Wilson, E.B. (1998). Preventing patient falls. AACN Clinical Issues, 9, 100–108.

CHAPTER 5

Applying ergonomic principles to the worker and work environment

How can empirical findings about human work actually help designers create systems that fit how people work and think? Ergonomics research uses method, argument and rhetoric (or verbal strategies of persuasion) to justify the relevance of their findings to systems-to-be-designed.

S.W.A. Dekker and J.M. Nyce, 2004, p. 1624

Industrial urbanism is largely a work culture. It puts the engineer and the manager ahead of the artist and social scholar. It is a culture that judges man by his will to work, the efficiency of his work, and what he gets out of his work above mere subsistence.

N. Anderson, 1964, p. vii

Learning objectives

By the end of this chapter the learner will:

1 Understand the meaning and theory of work and its relationship to ergonomics.
2 Discuss the major occupational work injuries.
3 Describe the major interventions in the work setting.
4 Describe the major components in the Occupational Rehabilitation Process.
5 Describe the occupational therapist's role in work hardening.
6 Define work conditioning.
7 Describe stress management and pain management.
8 Define job simulation and on-site job analysis.
9 Explore the issues in client discharge and follow-up.
10 Define job analysis.
11 Discuss the US Department of Labor's analysis of worker functions (data, people, things).
12 Define and describe functional capacity assessment.
13 Describe the types of work samples used in occupational rehabilitation programmes.

14 Define and give examples of Commercial Work Evaluation Sample Systems.
15 Identify tasks, vulnerabilities and preventive strategies for specific occupations.
16 Discuss anthropometry and its relationship to ergonomics.

Purposes of this chapter

The purposes of this chapter are to enable occupational therapists to develop a systematic plan to prevent work injuries and to design comprehensive work adjustment programmes for individuals with disabilities. What knowledge or skills does the occupational therapist need to have to work in this area? The occupational therapist should:

* have a good concept of the meaning of work
* understand the causes of the major musculoskeletal injuries that occur on the job
* become familiar with current occupational rehabilitation programmes for preventing on-the-job work injuries
* implement an individualized occupational rehabilitation programme to restore employability for an individual with a work-related injury
* be able to carry out an on-site ergonomic job analysis
* contribute as a team member to a work conditioning or work hardening programme.

In accomplishing these tasks, the occupational therapist should be familiar with the purposes and functions of the major governmental and private agencies that play key roles in worker safety and worker rehabilitation In the USA, these include the Occupational Safety and Health Administration (OSHA; http://www.osha.gov/), National Institutes of Occupational Safety and Health (NIOSH; http://www.cdc.gov/niosh/homepage.html), Americans with Disabilities Act (ADA, 1990; http://www.usdoj.gov/crt/ada/adahom1.htm and http://www.usdoj.gov/crt/ada/adastd94.pdf), Commission on Accreditation of Rehabilitation Facilities (CARF; http://www.carf.org/default.aspx). It is also important for the occupational therapist to be familiar with current literature on ergonomics research.

Definitions of work and occupational choice

Neff (1985) defines work as 'an instrumental activity carried out by human beings, the object of which is to preserve and maintain life, which is directed at a planned alteration of certain features of man's environment' (p. 78). Work can be a paid or unpaid activity or occupation in which one is engaged to sustain life and to provide meaning to one's existence. In general work is a purposeful occupation or activity that leads to a product or service (Söderback et al., 1993). People continue to work during an extensive part of their lifetime because (a) they need to earn money to survive (extrinsic motivation); (b) work establishes a career that fulfils a need for self-actualization (Maslow, 1970), such as a mathematician who continues to work with numbers because of an ability to conceptualize mathematical concepts; (c) the work itself gives one satisfaction (intrinsic motivation) such as an artist who works to express oneself without immediate reward; (d) work provides opportunities to be part of a social group that fulfils a need for social interactions; and (e) work may define the meaning and purpose of one's life such as volunteering to help others who are needy (Synnerholm et al., 1995).

> Work has been written about by theologians and philosophers, by poets and novelists, by historians, economists, and sociologists, by biologists and naturalists, by politicians, by essayists and journalists. It has been described as both a blessing and a curse, and a ravager of our natural environment.
>
> Neff, 1985, p.1

Questions regarding work behaviour have generated many theories regarding occupational choice, including why an individual selects a specific job or occupation. A number of theories have been developed to explain occupational choice. For example, Super (1957) proposed that an individual selects an occupation through developmental stages that begin in early childhood. Self-concept is an important component of Super's theory. He believed that an individual selects an occupation that is congruent with a belief in the ability to take on a specific occupational role. The person's attitudes, interests and aspirations influence the choice of an occupation (Neff, 1985). Other theorists have applied psychoanalytic theory to explain occupational choice. For example, Erikson (1963), in his eight stages of development, proposed that at a critical point the adolescent develops an identity and attitude towards work that affects occupational choice. Hendrick (1943), another psychoanalyst, believed that humans work to fulfil an instinctual need to master the environment.

There are still many unanswered questions regarding occupational choice and personality. Do individuals with certain personality characteristics select jobs that are congruent with their personality? For example, do those who are very systematic lean towards such jobs as accountants, mathematicians or engineers? Does cognitive style such as being field independent (objective view of the world) or field dependent (subjective view of the world (Stein, 1968)) motivate an individual towards a specific occupational area? In general, why do individuals who are field dependent select occupations such as social workers, therapists and teachers while individuals who are field independent select occupations such as engineers, physicists and chemists?

On the other hand, many individuals in developing countries who are born into poverty have little choice in how they will spend their time and work. In these instances, where unemployment is widespread and work, if available, is equated with subsistence there are few opportunities to be educated into an occupational role. Occupational choice, then, is a sociological issue where economics will affect how an individual will live and work.

There are also issues of gender. In some countries females are unable to work in certain jobs and are discriminated against. Ideally, the goal for humanity is to encourage every individual regardless of gender, race or ethnic origin to actualize one's abilities and to have freedom of choice in selecting an occupation. The variables in occupational choice should be based on aptitudes, motivation, interests, personality and work values.

Human needs met by work in the twenty-first century

In our contemporary society, does work fulfil a biological, social or psychological need? In other words, do we work because of a biological urge, because it makes our lives meaningful and purposeful, or because we want to? Is work a precondition of physical, mental and social health? If an individual became independently wealthy, would that person continue to work? Does the definition of meaningful and purposeful work change for individuals who retire from full-time work at 65 when life expectancy is more than 80? Why do some individuals spend their retirement years in leisure pursuits while others who are past retirement age continue to work at a profession or occupation even though they do not need additional money? What is the difference between work and leisure (De Grazia, 1964)? Is work therapeutic? At on the other extreme, how do you motivate an individual who feels hopeless and is not motivated to work?

The work environment

Does a good job and work environment motivate an individual to perform at the highest level? Pehr G. Gyllenhammar (2002), former senior manager for VOLVO, proposed that keeping workers healthy on the job results in maintaining the workers' job motivation and job satisfaction and increases product quality while decreasing costs. In addition the worker's performance on the job will be affected by a healthy balance in the time one spends in work, family, and leisure activities (Söderback, 1999). Ideally, the workplace should be a supportive and learning environment, where the worker's safety and health are priorities. Ideally, a healthy physical and psychological work environment is created when the work methods, workstations, tools and equipment are ergonomically designed, and the worker has control over the work tasks and can cope with their demands in a way that reduces the effects of stress (Karasek and Theorell, 1990). The worker should have knowledge about the connection between his or her work effort and the results of that effort. He or she should receive support from supervisors and colleagues and feel like a respected member of the work team (Johnson et al., 1989). In addition there should be an opportunity to participate in health promotion training programmes.

In the twenty-first century in developed countries, work is linked to an individual's educational attainment. For example, most skilled jobs in Western countries require at a minimum a high school education while almost all professional positions require a college degree. Job satisfaction is a result of an individual's match of aptitudes, skills, education, related experiences and interests. Occupational stress, boredom, feelings of job alienation, job dissatisfaction and 'burn-out' are risk factors for injuries on the job. How can the occupational therapist using ergonomic principles prevent and intervene in occupational injuries and occupational stress? In the following sections the major factors in occupational rehabilitation that enable a worker to achieve maximum job satisfaction and prevent occupationally related injuries are explored.

Most common occupational injuries

The US Bureau of Labor Statistics (BLS) (2004a) reported that a total of 4.4 million injuries and illnesses that occurred in private industry workplaces during 2003 represented a rate of 5 cases per 100 full-time workers. In general, occupational injuries have a significant impact on the worker and family and on economic costs to society.

In March 2003, the reporters on the (US) Public Broadcasting Service documentary programme *Frontline* stated that there is a growing problem of occupational injuries in the workplace (Docherty and Rummel, 2003). The following quote from the programme summarizes the findings:

- Roughly 6371 job-related injury deaths, 13.3 million nonfatal injuries, 60,300 disease deaths, and 1,184,000 illnesses occurred in the US workplace in 2002.
- The total direct and indirect costs associated with these injuries and illnesses were estimated to be $155.5 billion, or nearly 3 per cent of gross domestic product (GDP).
- Direct costs included medical expenses for hospitals, physicians, and drugs, as well as health insurance administration costs, and were estimated to be $51.8 billion.
- The indirect costs included loss of wages, costs of fringe benefits, and loss of home production (e.g. child care provided by parent and home repairs), as well as employer retraining and workplace disruption costs, and were estimated to be $103.7 billion.
- Injuries generated roughly 85 per cent whereas diseases generated 15 percent of all costs.

- These costs are large when compared to those for other diseases. The costs are roughly five times the costs of AIDS, three times the costs of Alzheimer's disease, more than the costs of arthritis, nearly as great as the costs of cancer, and roughly 82 per cent of the costs of all circulatory (heart and stroke) diseases.
- Workers' compensation covered roughly 27 per cent of all costs. Taxpayers paid approximately 18 per cent of these costs through contributions to Medicare, Medicaid, and Social Security.
- Costs were borne by injured workers and their families, by all other workers through lower wages, by firms through lower profits, and by consumers through higher prices.
- [The survey results were the first] to use national data to produce estimates on costs for occupational injuries and illnesses. Prior studies have underestimated costs by ignoring non-disabling injuries, deaths, and workplace violence, by taking inadequate account of diseases, and, most importantly, by relying on only one or two sources of data.
- The Annual Survey of the Bureau of Labor Statistics (BLS) provides the most reliable and comprehensive data on nonfatal injuries. However, it misses roughly 53 per cent of job-related injuries. This omission, in part, is due to the exclusion of government employees and the self-employed and also, in part, due to illegal underreporting by private firms.
- Contrary to the Annual Survey data, we find small firms have exceptionally high injury rates.
- Occupations contributing the most to costs included truck drivers, laborers, janitors, nursing orderlies, assemblers, and carpenters. On a per capita basis, lumberjacks, laborers, millwrights, prison guards, and meat cutters contributed the most to costs.
- Occupations at highest risk for carpal tunnel syndrome include dental hygienists, meat cutters, sewing machine operators, and assemblers. Among well-paid professions, dentists face the highest risks.
- Any of the major sources of data, such as the Bureau of Labor Statistics, National Institute for Occupational Safety and Health, workers' compensation systems, or National Health Interview Survey, by themselves underestimate the numbers of injuries and illnesses.
- Greater efforts need to be directed toward gathering data on job-related injuries and illnesses. The United States needs a comprehensive data bank for fatal and nonfatal injuries and all illnesses. Future researchers should not have to investigate the over 20 sources of primary data and 300 sources of secondary data that [the authors] investigated.

Docherty and Rummel, 2003, para 2

Since the mid-1980s, the annual leading causes of occupational injuries were related to accidents involving motor vehicles, use of machines on the job, violence in the workplace, falls, accidents from electrical devices and being hurt by falling objects (Center for Disease Control [CDC], Division of Media Relations, 1997). In the workplace the leading causes of occupational injuries were due to (a) overexertion when pushing, pulling, holding, carrying or turning objects; and (b) repetitive motion in activities involving typing, key entry, using tools, and placing, grasping or moving objects other than tools. Most of these injuries affected the back and upper extremities.

Repetitive motion injuries occurring on the job are one of the major causes of musculoskeletal disorders (MSDs) affecting the nerves, tendons, muscles and supporting structures of the body (Bernard, 1997). The BLS estimates that over two million Americans suffer from repetitive motion injuries on the job every year. As reported by BLS (2004c), in 2004 repetitive motion injuries resulting from grasping tools, scanning groceries, typing and related job tasks resulted in the longest absences from work: 23 days (BLS, 2004b). In 2002, 40.3 per cent of repetitive motion injuries occurred in the manufacturing industries; 26.2 per cent in service corporations including finance, insurance and real estate; 18.8 per cent in wholesale and retail trade establishments; 8.6 per cent in transportation and public utilities such as telephone companies; 4.9 per cent in construction industries; and about 1.2 per cent in agriculture, forestry, fishing and mining. The parts of the body most affected by repetitive motion injuries include 49.5 per cent in the wrist; 18.7 per cent in the head, neck, trunk, back and shoulder; 2.1 per cent in the knee, foot, toe and other extremities; and 6.6 per cent in multiple areas of the body (BLS, 2004c).

MSDs were first identified as being caused by occupational injuries during the eighteenth century. Scientific studies initiated in the 1970s have linked occupational injuries and work-related accidents to faulty body mechanics and neglect of preventative measures. Since then, thousands of research studies have examined the causes of MSDs in the workplace (Bernard, 1997). The general descriptive terms for these disorders include repetitive motion injuries (RMI), cumulative trauma disorders (CTD), repetitive strain injuries (RSI) and occupational overuse disorder (OOD). These terms are interchangeable and denote an occupational injury that results from repeated movements or overuse of the same joints and muscles causing persistent discomfort, as well as pain in muscles, tendons and joints in the fingers, hands, wrist, arms, neck and shoulders.

The major disorders under the rubric repetitive motion injuries include low back disorders and upper extremity disorders. Upper extremity disorders are further divided into three areas: (a) muscle and tendon damage, (b) neurological injuries and (c) neurovascular disorders (Habes, 1996; Pascarelli and Quilter, 1992).

Low back disorders due to occupation related injuries

Low back pain (LBP) due to occupation-related injuries or repetitive motion is a significant problem in the United States of America and throughout the world (Guerriero et al., 1999). The following quote from the National Institutes of Health (1997) summarizes the impact of low back pain on health problems in general, and on work specifically:

> Low back pain continues to be a significant public health problem. Seventy to 85% of all people have back pain at some time in life, with the annual

prevalence of back pain ranging from 15–45%. Back pain is the most frequent cause of activity limitation in people below 45 years and is a common reason for visiting a health care provider. Symptoms are most common in middle-aged adults, with back pain equally common in men and women; however, back pain secondary to disc disorders is more common in men. Reported rates of low back pain are generally higher for Whites than Blacks or other racial groups.

The recurrence rate of low back pain is very high. Indeed, recurrences appear to be part of the natural history. One-year recurrence rates have been reported ranging from 20–44%. Lifetime recurrences of 85% have been reported. Fortunately, most patients with back pain recover quickly and without residual functional loss. Typically, 60–70% recover by 6 weeks and 80–90% by 12 weeks. After 12 weeks, further recovery is slow.

Each year, about 2% of the work forces have back injuries covered by workman's compensation. The total annual direct cost of treating this subgroup of low back pain patients rose from $4.6 billion in 1977 to $11.4 billion in 1994. Typically, 25% or fewer of low back cases are responsible for 75% or more of the cost.

There continues to be great variability in health care service utilization for low back pain. From 1979 to 1987, U.S. rates of back surgery increased 49–55%, while the rate of non-surgical hospitalization decreased 33%. Marked geographic variation in the rate of back surgery (twice as high in the South as compared to the Northeast) has been reported. The increase in surgical rates was especially marked for fusions, which increased 100% from 1979 to 1990. In addition, there is marked international variation in rates of back surgery. A recent study comparing the rates of back surgery in thirteen countries and provinces revealed that the rate of back surgery in the U.S. was 40% higher than in any other country or province. These differences in surgical rates were not felt to be due to underlying differences in the prevalence of low back pain. Complicating this variability in service utilization is the reality that only a small number of the commonly used non-operative and operative treatments have been scientifically validated for their effectiveness/outcomes.

National Institutes of Health, 1997, Research Objectives, para. 1–4

Low back pain is also the leading cause of emergency hospital admissions, visits to physicians' surgeries and outpatient clinics. It is second to upper respiratory infections as a cause of absences from work (Hedge, 2002). The economic costs of LBP are substantial with approximately 24 billion dollars per year spent in direct medical expenses and about 27 billion dollars a year in lost productivity. In general, low back symptoms are the most common cause of disability for persons less than 45 years of age. In addition, the average workers' compensation claim for a low back disorder is approximately $8300. It is estimated that '30% of American workers are employed in jobs that routinely require them to perform activities that may increase risk of developing low back disorders' (National Institute of Occupational Safety and Health (NIOSH), 1998, Additional Information, para. 1).

Certain occupations or jobs are associated with a high risk of developing low back disorders: (a) nurses, especially in situations when nursing personnel lift persons who are elderly or disabled (Yip, 2001); (b) male construction labourers engaged in heavy lifting activities (Pope et al., 2002); (c) agricultural workers who spend much of their day lifting and carrying awkward loads of fruits and vegetables (Park et al., 2001); (d) carpenters who handle large lengths of wood, and truck and tractor operators who sit for long hours in uncomfortable seats (Lings and Leboeuf-Yde, 1998); and (e) clerical workers who sit at their jobs (Hartvigsen et al., 2002).

Causes of low back pain

There are numerous studies in the literature examining the causes of LBP. In general the causes of low back pain can be analysed into (a) predisposing factors that place an individual at risk to low back pain, and (b) precipitating causes or factors that trigger symptoms of LBP in individuals at risk.

Research studies have examined the relationship between LBP and the following predisposing factors: (a) obesity (Leboeuf-Yde, 2000); (b) sedentary life style (Burdorf et al., 1993); (c) smoking (Levangie, 1999); (d) poor conditioning or lack of exercise (Quittan, 2002); (e) occupational stress (Pope, 1989); and (f) structural problems in the back e.g. cumulative lumbar disc compression (Kerr et al., 2001). Other predisposing factors can include congenital abnormalities of the spine (Deyo, 1998), such as scoliosis (lateral curvature of the spine) lordosis (convex curvature of lumbar spine), and kyphosis (angular hump in spine), as well as osteoarthritis (Hodge and Bessette, 1999).

Precipitating factors in the workplace are primarily due to the following:

- *Improper lifting techniques*, where the worker puts heavy pressure on the spine rather than using the large muscles of the quadriceps and abdominals. 'Occupational exposures such as lifting, particularly in awkward postures; heavy lifting; or repetitive lifting are related to LBP' (Pope et al., 2002, p. 49). Workers commonly experience injury to the low back when (a) lifting heavy objects repeatedly from the floor without bending their knees; (b) lifting and carrying bulky objects away from the body; (c) repeatedly lifting objects without rest intervals; and (d) pulling heavy objects rather than pushing them. There are numerous research studies in the literature implicating improper lifting and carrying of heavy objects as causative factors in the development of LBP (Kingma et al., 2001). Collins et al. (2004) found that applying mechanical lifts and repositioning aids and training employees on proper lifting techniques were effective in reducing musculoskeletal injuries in nursing personnel.
- *Poor posture position of the body* while (a) sitting for long periods of time, especially when using a chair that puts pressure on the lumbar vertebrae (Pope et al., 2002); (b) standing in a fixed position for sustained periods of time without rest intervals; or (c) during vibrational

loading (i.e. extensive shaking movement in a machine or vehicle), which can potentially cause damage to the spine (Lings and Leboeuf-Yde, 1998). Vibrational loading often occurs in truck drivers who spend long hours driving while being exposed to engine vibration and rough surfaces. Anannontsak and Puapan (1996) studied employees (n = 100) in a clothes factory and found that working activities such as lifting, pulling, pushing, bending and sitting were highly associated with back pain.

* *Psychological factors*, such as monotony, job dissatisfaction or 'burn-out' can aggravate LBP. Hoogendoorn et al. (2002) investigated the relationship between high physical workload, low job satisfaction and low back pain in 732 workers from 21 companies in the Netherlands. They concluded that job tasks involving extensive flexion and rotation of the trunk while lifting objects, when combined with low job satisfaction, were significantly related to absences from work because of LBP. In addition, low levels of social support from supervisors and co-workers contributed to sick leave. These results were confirmed in a prospective study of 327 workers with LBP (Miranda et al., 2002). The participants in the study were compared to a symptom-free control group of 2077 workers in Finland during a one-year follow-up. They concluded that mental stress and psychosocial factors were significantly related to the onset of sciatic pain for workers at risk.

Treatment of LBP caused by occupational hazards

The non-pharmaceutical treatments of LBP can be grouped under five major headings: (a) exercise programmes for primary and secondary prevention; (b) back schools and psycho-educational programmes to educate the client; (c) ergonomic solutions on the job such as job modification; (d) relaxation therapies; and (e) physical agent modalities, such as biofeedback or transcutaneous electrical nerve stimulation (TENS). In general a multi-modal approach to intervention is more effective than either surgery or pharmaceuticals used alone. 'Scientific evidence shows that an active approach to low back pain patients is effective' (van Tulder, 2001, p. 499).

The prevention, treatment and rehabilitation of persons with back injuries or vulnerability to back problems involve a multidisciplinary and multi-modal approach. Key (1996) identifies this approach as a team effort comprising the occupational therapist, physical therapist, vocational rehabilitation consultant, psychologist, physician, exercise physiologist, employer and attorney, working in conjunction with the client, family and co-workers. The primary goal of this approach is to help the worker with a back injury to return to the same job with accommodations or to a new job that matches one's aptitudes and interests. This systematic team approach includes (a) job analysis; (b) work conditioning; (c) work hardening; (d) functional capacity assessment; (e) job modification or job accommodation; and (f) special placement. In a multidimensional analysis of work-related outcomes in occupational low back pain Pransky et al. (2002) concluded that 'timing of return to work, occupational ergonomic risks, and appropriate job modifications appeared to be particularly important in a safe return to the job after an occupational low back injury' (p. 864).

When preparing a treatment plan for the client it is important to individualize the specific interventions used. For example, the client's cooperation and compliance may be the most important considerations in selecting techniques and strategies that work for that client. There are many research studies to support the effectiveness of several of the interventions. In a review of the most effective return-to-work interventions of low back pain, Staal et al. (2002) analysed 14 randomized controlled trials. They found that 'the most prevalent combination of components was the combination of physical exercises, behavioural treatment and education' (p. 251). Psychological factors play an important role in (a) the client's subjective reporting of the severity of the pain; (b) the areas where the pain exists; and (c) compliance with a back programme to reduce the pain. In a Swedish study, Linton and Buer (1995) compared individuals working full-time in spite of back pain (coping group) with a group of individuals who were not working because of the pain (dysfunctional group). The researchers found that 'dysfunctional subjects had stronger beliefs that pain was directly related to the activities, that they had little control over their pain, that their health was poor, and they tended to focus more on their pain' (p. 252). The researchers concluded that psychosocial factors are important in the workers' reactions to their pain and that these factors strongly influence whether the workers will take sick leave because of their back pain.

Upper extremity disorders due to repetitive motion injuries

Muscle and tendon disorders

Muscle and tendon disorders are primarily caused by damage to the muscles and tendons of joints without damage to accompanying nerves. In general these disorders are caused at work by (a) intense, repeated and sustained exertions; (b) awkward, prolonged or extreme postures; (c) insufficient rest periods between job tasks; (d) experiencing excessive vibration from hand tools and machines; and (e) working for prolonged periods in cold temperature environments (Bernard, 1997; Hansen, 1998; Medical Multimedia Group, 1999–2005; Pascarelli and Quilter, 1992).

The types of muscle and tendon disorders commonly encountered are given below.

- *Tenosynovitis* is an inflammation of a tendon sheath, a protective covering around tendons that secretes synovial fluid to protect the tendon from injury. Tenosynovitis is not uncommon in workers who use repetitive motions with their hands. For example, in a study of injured workers (mean age = 38; n = 485) with work-related pain, the majority of the pain experienced was in the upper extremity and affected mostly the hand. Seventy per cent of the workers were computer users and 28 per cent were musicians (Pascarelli and Hsu, 2001).

- *Trauma to the hand* can cause de Quervain tenosynovitis, or inflammation of the abductor pollicis longus and extensor pollicis brevis tendons located at the junction of the wrist and thumb. Injured workers feel acute pain when they move their thumb or when they perform a movement that involves twisting their wrist and thumb. This disorder is common when individuals work on a computer and use their thumbs on the space bar with too much force (Pascarelli and Quilter, 1992).

- *Flexor tenosynovitis*, commonly called 'trigger finger', is an inflammation of the tendons surrounding the ring or middle finger and occasionally the thumb (flexor carpi radialis tendinitis). Excessive finger motion or gripping a tool can also cause flexor tendinitis. Occupational tasks that involve overuse and/or excessive force of the fingers (e.g. using a hand drill or a vibrating tool with a switch that is operated by the middle finger) can cause this disorder. These conditions cause the fingers to lock in a bent position and it becomes very painful to straighten the finger joint. The immediate cause is a cyst that forms on the tendon.

- *Bicipital tendonitis* involves the tendons around the biceps muscle. Pain can be felt when moving the arms above the shoulders, such as when a worker is lifting objects for a prolonged time in an overhead bin.

- *Rotator cuff tendonitis* occurs when the group of muscles and tendons near the shoulder are overused. One example is throwing a baseball with velocity over an extended period of time or in playing tennis. Workers who forcefully use the shoulder joint in daily activities such as working at tasks that are above their heads are at risk for rotator cuff injuries.

- *Extensor tendonitis* may occur if the worker does a task such as pushing objects with the hands held for prolonged periods in dorsiflexion (hands bent backwards at the wrist).

- *Lateral and medial epicondylitis*, also called tennis elbow (lateral) and golfer's elbow (medial), are injuries to the elbow that can occur when tasks involve repetitive grasping and twisting the arm (e.g. assembly-line work).

Neurological disorders

Nerve disorders are due to damage to nerves causing sensory and motor problems such as numbness, muscle pain and muscle weakness. A common test used to diagnose upper extremity neuropathies is the nerve conduction velocity test (NCV), used to measure the speed of neuro impulses travelling along the median nerve or in the abductor pollicis brevis (Buschbacher, 1999). Impulses are slowed when the nerve is compressed or constricted. The NCV is sometimes combined with an electromyogram (EMG), such as when testing the muscles of the forearm controlled by the the ulnar nerve.

Carpal tunnel syndrome

Carpal tunnel syndrome (CTS) is a disorder of the median nerve in the wrist that creates reduced function in the fingers and hand. It is defined as a 'neuropathy syndrome resulting from entrapment of the median nerve within a narrowed carpal tunnel' (Hansen, 1998, p. 676). The carpal tunnel is comprised of the eight bones in the wrist that form a canal that is lined with flexor tendons controlling finger movements. This canal or tunnel provides a pathway for the median nerve as well as tendons, arteries, veins and connective tissue. Damage to the lining of the carpal tunnel causes swelling which results in compression to the median nerve. The median nerve serves as a sensory transmitter to the thumb, index, second and inner aspect of the third finger. Damage to the median nerve will cause (a) pain and sensory loss, such as soreness, numbness and tingling; and (b) motor deficits such as muscle weakness, difficulty in squeezing, pinching or gripping objects, and clumsiness in such daily tasks as tying one's shoes or picking up small objects.

CTS is a major problem in industrialized countries affecting as many as one per cent of the population (NIOSH, 1997). A major cause of CTS is repetitive and forceful movements of the wrist during work and leisure activities. Research conducted by NIOSH (1997) has indicated that 'job tasks involving highly repetitive manual acts, or necessitating wrist bending or other stressful wrist postures, are connected with incidents of CTS or related problems. The use of vibrating tools also may contribute to CTS. Moreover, it is apparent that this hazard is not confined to a single industry or job but occurs in many occupations' (para 5). The government, employers, unions and insurance companies recognize that CTS is a major problem among workers and that it is increasing worldwide. One explanation for the epidemic proportions of CTS is the increase in automation in many manufacturing industries with fragmented job tasks in which workers engage in repetitive motions on the same tasks without variation in the movements.

CTS can be reduced through use of the following preventative measures:

- Rotating jobs so the worker will have the opportunity to vary movements
- Providing short rest breaks in the morning and afternoon
- Using warm-up exercises before beginning work to stretch wrist and finger joints
- Redesigning tools and tool handles to maintain the worker's wrist in a neutral position

- Providing worker education focused on becoming aware of the causes of CTS and ways to prevent injury to the wrist
- Reducing the use of vibrating tools for extended periods of time
- Modifying the workstation to reduce awkward movements, such as extreme bending of the wrist in ulnar or radial deviation
- Using adapted devices, such as a palm or wrist rest so that the worker can keep his or her wrist in neutral position when using a computer (OSHA, nd)
- Prescribing hand splinting to reduce tendon swelling and as a night splint to reduce pain
- In severe cases anti-inflammatory medication, such as ibuprofen or aspirin, and carpal tunnel release or surgery may be indicated.

When treating CTS, an ergonomic job analysis is a good screening procedure to help the therapist select the solutions that fit the individual worker. O'Connor et al. (2003), in an extensive review of non-surgical treatment of CTS based on the research literature from 1966 to 2002, concluded that (a) splinting, (b) yoga, (c) ultrasound, (d) oral steroids and (e) carpal bone mobilization are effective in reducing the symptoms of CTS and in achieving significant short-term benefits.

Radial tunnel syndrome

This is caused by compression of the radial nerve (Barnum et al., 1996). The radial nerve originates in the neck and runs along the back of the arm, down the forearm into the hand. The impulses of the radial nerve move in a tunnel surrounded by muscles and bone. The nerve enables one to twist the hand clockwise such as in opening a jar lid or using a screwdriver. If damaged, the nerve can be compressed along this route. Repetitive motion involving activities using the forearm and forceful pushing and pulling of the arm, or prolonged bending of the wrist while gripping and pinching objects can further stretch and irritate the nerve. Sometimes a direct blow to the lateral side of the elbow may injure or damage the radial nerve. Constant use of the arm for twisting activities, such as might be found on an assembly-line, can cause irritation on the radial nerve. The symptoms of radial nerve damage include tenderness and pain at the lateral side of the elbow, loss of sensation on the dorsal radial surface of the hand, pain on both sides of the forearm just below the elbow, difficulty making a fist, and weakened fingers and thumb.

Prevention of radial tunnel syndrome on the job is similar to preventing carpal tunnel syndrome. These include (a) job rotation, (b) rest breaks, (c) muscle strengthening exercises before working, and (d) using a resting splint at night that is fitted by a therapist. In addition, the worker is advised to limit heavy and/or prolonged use of upper extremities in pushing, pulling or grasping of objects. Anti-inflammatory medications and/or surgery to relieve pressure on the radial nerve may be recommended by a physician.

Cubital tunnel syndrome

This is also known as flexor carpi ulnaris muscle syndrome, and is second to CTS as the most common compressive neuropathy in the workplace (Tetro and Pichora, 1996). The syndrome is caused by compression to the ulnar nerve where it passes through the back of the elbow. The ulnar nerve, like the radial nerve, originates at the side of the neck and runs along the arm and through the cubital tunnel to the hand and fingers. The nerve supplies sensations to the little finger and partly to the ring finger, as well as controlling the movements of the small muscles of the hand. The symptoms of cubital tunnel syndrome include pain occurring at the 'funny bone' area of the elbow and numbness on the inside of the hand and in the ring and little fingers. These initial symptoms, if prolonged, can lead to generalized hand pain and weakness and clumsiness in the hand and thumb causing major difficulties for a worker.

In jobs where there is frequent elbow flexion there is risk for cubital tunnel syndrome. Examples of such jobs include pulling levers, or lifting objects away from the body primarily by using arm movements. Computer workers can develop flexion symptoms of the elbow when they position their elbows on hard surfaces for long periods of time. Other workers vulnerable to cubital tunnel syndrome include (a) long-distance lorry drivers who may put pressure on their elbows while driving, (b) factory workers who operate machines while their elbows are positioned on a hard surface, and (c) workers experiencing cumulative trauma to the elbow such as prolonged positioning of their elbow on a vibrating machine.

Prevention and treatment for work-related cubital tunnel syndrome are similar to treating any nerve injury to the upper extremity. Prevention of cubital tunnel syndrome includes (a) having the worker take regular rest breaks; (b) altering work positions so as to avoid prolonged pressure on the elbow; (c) using protective elbow pads to prevent trauma to the elbow; (d) rotating jobs with tasks that reduce the stresses on the elbow; (e) modifying job to protect the elbows; (f) using warm-up exercises to increase range of motion and muscle strength around the elbow joint; (g) applying heat to the elbow joint to increase circulation and decrease inflammation; and (h) applying ice after there is noticeable swelling in the elbow joint. All of these interventions should be individualized to meet the needs of the worker. Anti-inflammatory medications are often prescribed by physicians to relieve the pain. In severe cases, surgery may be indicated to relieve the pressure on the ulnar nerve through release of the cubital tunnel (Tetro and Pichora, 1996).

Guyon's canal syndrome

Also known as ulnar tunnel syndrome, Guyon's canal syndrome involves compression of the ulnar nerve near the wrist area around the carpal tunnel (De Smet 2002). The syndrome is similar to carpal tunnel syndrome in terms of symptoms and treatment, but involves the ulnar nerve instead of the median nerve. The ulnar nerve supplies sensation to the little finger, half of the ring finger and intrinsic muscles of the hand. Symptoms of Guyon's canal syndrome begin with a sensation of pins and needles in the ring and little finger, starting in the early morning upon waking. Symptoms can further progress to a burning pain in the wrist and hand, followed by decreased sensation and eventual difficulty in grasping objects securely. The weakness in grasp is evidenced by the individual's inability to spread his or her fingers, and may include a weak pinch in the thumb. Overuse or repetitive motion involving the wrist especially in tasks bending the wrist down (hyperflexing) can cause the syndrome. Preventative interventions include frequent rest breaks, or limiting the amount of time spent performing tasks that require flexing and turning the wrist due to constant pressure on the palm. A wrist splint may be prescribed to be worn at night to decrease the 'pins and needles' sensation. Keyboard operators may find that use of a wrist rest to facilitate placement of the wrist in a neutral position may decrease symptoms. Anti-inflammatory medications are often prescribed by a physician to reduce the symptoms. If the symptoms persist in spite of behavioural changes and medications, surgery may be needed to relieve pressure on the ulnar nerve. The ligament that forms the roof of Guyon's canal is cut to relieve pressure on the nerve.

Neurovascular disorders

Neurovascular disorders are due to injuries to both nerves and blood vessels. The most common of these disorders include thoracic outlet syndrome, Raynaud's disease and cervical rediculopathy.

Thoracic outlet syndrome

This is a disorder of the upper extremity that is caused by compression of the brachial nerve plexus as it passes through the thoracic outlet, located behind the clavicle (collar bone), from the base of the neck to the axilla (Wilbourn, 1999). The primary symptoms of thoracic outlet syndrome are severe pain in the neck and shoulder region. Other prominent symptoms include numbness along the forearm and fingers; headaches at the back of the head; tingling sensations in the neck, shoulder region, arm and hand; coldness in the hands; weakness in the fingers, arms and hands; and a generalized swelling in the arms and hands.

In the workplace, the symptoms of thoracic outlet syndrome can cause difficulty in upper extremity tasks (e.g. driving a truck, gripping and holding tools, performing fine motor tasks, assembling objects, or lifting and carrying objects). Compression or irritation of the nerves can occur in the workplace from cumulative trauma to the neck or upper back due to repetitive motions that require overhead arm movements. Examples of such movements are seen in activities such as painting ceilings, plastering walls and installing electrical fixtures in ceilings or high walls.

Sometimes assembly-line workers, cash register operators and those who do needlework work in a static upper body position. The worker with a drooping shoulder and forward head posture that accompanies this position can develop thoracic outlet syndrome. Carrying heavy loads on the shoulder for prolonged periods of time can also put one at risk of injury to the brachial plexus. Athletes who hyper-abduct their shoulder muscles while performing a sport (e.g. pitching in baseball, playing tennis) are also at risk of injury to the brachial plexus. Other related injuries can occur in jobs that require heavy lifting and pressure on the muscles around the shoulder girdle and the shoulder and neck, resulting in pain in the clavicle and the ribs.

Prevention and treatment of thoracic outlet syndrome generally involve physical therapy and include moderate muscle strengthening, using a range of motion activities and physical agent modalities. These activities are helpful in keeping the joints mobile and muscles active and protect the individual from atrophy. Exercises prescribed by the occupational therapist can also be embedded in leisure activities such as weaving, playing the piano, using ceramics or working on models. Slow gentle exercises such as T'ai-Chi and Feldenkrais are better than painful stretching or using heavy weights.

Ergonomic techniques to prevent thoracic outlet syndrome in the workplace include frequent rest breaks, job rotation and workplace modification to prevent putting excessive stress on the shoulder muscles and joints. It is important that the worker perform tasks in a neutral position and avoid a stooped position. If the symptoms persist and conservative treatment doesn't work, medication and surgery are usually prescribed by a physician to reduce the symptoms.

Raynaud's syndrome (disease or phenomenon)

This is characterized by digital vasospasm or vasoconstriction in the hands and the feet causing continuous cold extremities (Hansen, 1998; Kaufman and All, 1996). Raynaud's symptoms are often sudden brief attacks that can be caused by (a) repetitive motion activities (e.g. computer typing, prolonged playing of the piano or guitar, sewing, chopping and dicing food), or (b) by using vibrating tools, such as a chainsaw, jackhammer or drill, for sustained periods of time. The attacks can last from five minutes to an hour. Changes in skin colour frequently occur with extremities turning white indicating a severe decrease in the blood circulation to the hands. In individuals with Raynaud's syndrome, blue hands may indicate a limited blood flow, while hands that turn red may indicate a sudden infusion of oxygenated blood bringing a burning, throbbing or tingling sensation with swelling. The severity, duration and frequency of these symptoms can vary and change over time. The disease may be in remission for many years, but it can recur suddenly in response to infection, fatigue or stress.

Treatment and interventions for Raynaud's syndrome are based on three strategies. First, the use of proper gloves, socks and clothing to keep warm. Gloves heated with a battery may be useful. Socks and gloves warmed in a microwave oven result in the heat lasting for about three hours. Second, the individual must avoid or reduce psychological stress that may cause cold, clammy hands. Stress management is an important skill that all workers at risk should learn (see Chapter 6). Finally, the use of cognitive control techniques, such as biofeedback with meditation in increasing warmth of fingers, is particularly appropriate. Birger, et al. (1997) indicated that the use of biofeedback combined with relaxation techniques, guided imagery and computer-assisted monitoring of sympathetic arousal may be effective in controlling the symptoms of Raynaud's syndrome. The efficacy of biofeedback for individuals with Raynaud's syndrome has been documented by many scientific studies (Freedman, 1989; Schwartz and Kelly, 1995), with symptomatic improvement maintained for nine weeks, one year and even three years after the start of training. (For additional information on biofeedback, see Chapter 6.)

The rationale for using biofeedback is that people can 'teach' their body to relax. One form of biofeedback is simply 'thinking' your hands warm. The other form of biofeedback is more specific. Starting in a warm room, hands are placed in a warm bowl of water for five minutes. The individual moves to a cold room or outdoors and again places hands in warm water, this time for 10 minutes. The procedure is repeated several times a day for as many days as necessary to produce a conditioned reflex that is the opposite of the normal one: when exposed to cold, the blood vessels in the fingers will open up rather than close down, without the aid of warm water.

Other methods to control the symptoms of Raynaud's syndrome are (a) avoidance of extremely cold work environments (e.g. meat-packing plant or outside work in extreme cold weather), and (b) use of a daily exercise regimen that emphasizes gentle movements to the hands and feet in order to increase blood flow. In all exercises it is critical to examine the hands and feet routinely since poor circulation can increase the risk of developing skin infections. Soaking in a warm bath for 20 minutes before bed can also be helpful in stimulating blood flow and improving circulation. In addition, it is important that the worker eliminate smoking since nicotine can act as a vasoconstrictor causing reduction of circulation in the extremities (Winniford et al., 1987).

Cervical radiculopathy

This is a nerve entrapment disorder similar to thoracic outlet syndrome where a nerve is compressed causing pain and numbness or tingling in the area that the sensory nerve serves (Malanga, 1997). The causes of cervical radiculopathy include a herniated cervical disc, where a disc between the cervical vertebrae protrudes and puts pressure on the nerve causing neck pain. Spinal stenosis is also a cause of pressure on the nerve and nerve roots because of the narrowing of the tunnel. Degenerative disc disease where the cervical discs shrink can also cause symptoms of neck pain.

Treatment of cervical radiculopathy consists of physical therapy entailing a cervical traction device, physical agent modalities including heat or cold therapies, electrical stimulation and exercises that include stretching. Occupational interventions include rest breaks, job rotation and workstation modifications that are appropriate. Medication may be prescribed to relieve pain and swelling, while specific rehabilitation strategies may be prescribed based on the patient's medical history and diagnostic findings (McClure, 2000).

On-site occupational interventions

In general occupational interventions can be classified into four independent methods: human, human environmental, equipment/facility and organizational control methods (Kohn, 1997).

1 *Human control methods* include teaching proper lifting techniques, training the worker in using special ergonomic equipment, such as adjustable chairs, stretching muscles at the beginning of the work shift, and introducing wellness programmes for workers.
2 *Human environmental control methods* reduce the effects of environmental stressors in the workplace. These include moderating extreme temperatures and excessive noise, preventing improper lighting, reducing harmful vibration to extremities and whole body, and pacing the amount of work during the day to accommodate for worker fatigue at the end of the shift.
3 *Equipment/facility control methods* include the design of protective equipment, ergonomically designed workstations and work facilities. Examples include using such devices as ergonomic keyboards and mouse, wrist rest, adjustable keyboard trays, document holders and anti-glare screens. Other equipment includes ergonomic chairs, sit/stand swivel chairs, lumbar support moulds, adjustable footrests, height-adjustable work tables and adjustable monitor arms. Protection can also be provided by using noise-reducing headsets, adjustable ergonomic tool handles to keep wrists in a neutral position, cushioned handles for scissors, goggles for eye protection, ear plugs, specially designed work gloves, tubing on tools to reduce vibrating effects, braces and splints to support upper extremity joints, shoe cushions, knee pads, anti-fatigue mats, back belts, hydraulic lifts and adjustable hand trucks.
4 *Organizational control methods* in the workplace include strategies to limit the amount of time a worker is exposed to a stressor such as repetitive motion. These strategies consist of rest breaks during the

morning and afternoon. A study of forest workers in New Zealand showed a positive relationship between fatigue, sleepiness and the risk for injuries and near-miss injuries (Lilley et al., 2002). The authors concluded that there is a need to reduce fatigue in the workplace that can be accommodated by appropriately spaced rest breaks.

Using job rotation is another ergonomic intervention used by the organization. This method allows the worker to alternate tasks in order to reduce repetitive motion, boredom and job burn-out. A unique study was carried out in a restaurant in Stockholm to reduce the risks of strain injuries by increasing the cooperation between the staff at the restaurant and decreasing the stress on the job (Haider, 1996). The employer received a grant from the Working Life Fund to improve the work environment of the kitchen and the dishwashing room, and to provide new equipment to reduce heavy lifting. 'The implementation of the project has been based throughout on the physical changes, which according to the plans led to a natural transition to increased job rotation and reduced stress' (Implementation, para. 11).

Occupational rehabilitation process

The occupational rehabilitation process encompassing work hardening is a comprehensive, interdisciplinary programme that includes (a) evaluation using functional capacity assessments and vocational tests; (b) job analysis; (c) work conditioning; (d) stress and pain management; (e) job simulation; and (f) return to work counselling for a worker injured on a job. The Commission on Accreditation of Rehabilitation Facilities (CARF, 2005) has been actively engaged since 1989 in spelling out guidelines for work hardening.

Work hardening

The major purpose of work hardening is to prepare the client physically and psychologically for returning to work (Lechner, 1994). It provides a transition between acute care and return to work (American Occupational Therapy Association, 1986; Brewer and Storms, 1993; Zeller et al., 1993). The emphasis in work hardening programmes is to integrate the client's return to work as an aspect of treatment while focusing on the client's functional capacities (Burt, 2001; Lacroix, 1995). Work hardening programmes utilize a goal-directed and solution-based therapy rather than focusing on the clients' perception of pain (Cockburn et al., 1997; Lacroix, 1995; Matheson and Brophy, 1997; Saunders, 1997). The approach used in pain-management rehabilitation incorporates several conceptual models, such as biomedical, psychiatric, insurance, labour relations and biopsychosocial (Schultz et al., 2000; Talo et al., 1996).

Work hardening programmes are intended to progressively improve the client's function in the following areas:

- *biomechanical*: such as muscle strength and range of motion
- *neuromuscular*: physical and lifting tolerance
- *cardiovascular and metabolic rate*: physical conditioning
- *psychosocial functions*: stress-management techniques
- *work endurance*: ability to work in a full-time job
- *productivity*: ability to fulfil an employer's goals (Chan et al., 2000; Cooper et al., 1997; Greenberg and Bello, 1997; Norris, 1996; Ogden-Niemeyer and Jacobs, 1989; Weir and Nielson, 2001; Zeller et al., 1993).

Other purposes of work hardening programmes include reducing risks of repetitive motion, excessive force and awkward posture. In the work-place, the employer needs to be aware of the work/rest cycles and how these impact on risk for occupational injury and worker productivity. Likewise, the work hardening programme tries to modify the client's work style (Feuerstein et al., 1993) in order to increase job satisfaction.

Clinical applications of work hardening programmes usually begin 10–14 weeks after an acute work-related injury (Gerardi, 1999; Saunders, 1997) and last approximately four to six weeks (Greenberg and Bello, 1997; King, 1998; Robert et al., 1995). Assessments are conducted in the areas of (a) vocational assessment (Söderback et al., 2000); (b) impairment and disability; (c) work feasibility; (d) employability (Ogden-Niemeyer and Jacobs, 1989); and (e) job and task analysis (Wyman, 1999). Job and task analysis were originally based on the *Dictionary of Occupational Titles* (US Department of Labor, Employment and Training Administration, 1991a), and are now based on the O*NET™ OnLine (http://online.onetcenter.org/).

The success of work hardening programmes using return-to-work as an outcome measure is generally positive, although great variability is noted (King, 1993; King et al., 1998; Niemeyer et al., 1994). Work hardening programmes have a return-to-work success rate of about 50–88 per cent (Scully Palmer, 2000). Jang et al. (1997) found that 48 per cent of the clients returned to competitive work, attended school, returned to home-maker activities or participated in vocational training within 90 days after completion of a work hardening programme. Most researchers have found a higher success rate. Lacroix (1995) found that 85 per cent of the workers returned to work within a forecasted time. Guerriero et al. (1999) found that 90 per cent of clients were able to return to work upon discharge from the programme. Significant improvements were demon-strated in pain tolerance (Joy et al., 2001), isometric strength and endurance, self-perceived performance competence and satisfaction with work performance (Chan et al., 2000), and speed of lifting objects (Lieber et al., 2000). In general, the effectiveness of work hardening programmes depends on the interventions used and the client characteristics, work history and work ethics. Work hardening programmes are generally successful in helping clients return to work who have had work-related injuries for six or more months.

There is incomplete evidence on what aspects of work hardening programmes are most helpful to the client. Work conditioning and work hardening may not improve the success rate for those individuals with chronic disabilities (Johnson et al., 2001; Weir and Nielson, 2001). Clients who demonstrated an internal locus of control (i.e. felt they were able to impact on their own performances) had a better success rate in work hardening programmes than those with an external locus of control (i.e. felt that they had little control over their performances) when physical functioning was measured (Johnson et al., 2001; Weir and Nielson, 2001; Wiegmann and Berven, 1998). Other predictors of success in a work hardening programme include age, gender, length of disability, emotional factors and type and duration of rehabilitation programme (Wiegmann and Berven, 1998). Correlation with success in work hardening programmes have also been found with (a) 'single' marital status; (b) lower perceived disability scores when entering the work hardening programme; (c) higher Barthel ADL index scores (Mahoney et al., 1992); (d) reduction in reported pain during programme duration; (e) client's opportunity to return to work with the pre-injury employer; (f) amount of time out of work before attending the work hardening programme; and (g) the employee's annual salary (Beissner et al., 1996; Jang et al., 1997; Johnson et al., 2001; Matheson et al., 2002; Voaklander et al., 1995).

Work hardening is an individualized intervention programme, which encourages the client to take an active role in his or her management (Beissner et al., 1996; Frost et al., 2000; Healy and Comerouskik, 1999). The client is involved in highly structured simulated or actual work tasks. The activities are graded by increasing the time and intensity of the client's ability to complete a job task. This is analogous to the psychopharmacology model of dose-and-response (Chan et al., 2000; Cooper and Stewart, 1997; Norris, 1996; Weir and Nielson, 2001).

Examples of occupational rehabilitation programmes

• *The Worker Assessment and Rehabilitation Center* (WARC) (Community Memorial Hospital, n.d.) in Menomonee Falls, Wisconsin is an example of a comprehensive occupational rehabilitation programme. The programme defines work hardening as 'an interdisciplinary outcomes-focused and individualized program, which addresses the medical, psychological, behavioral, functional and vocational components of employability and return to work' (p. 1). The primary outcome of the programme is to bridge the gap between the worker's initial acute injury on the job and the worker's return to work. The three major components of the programme are (1) job task simulation; (2) fitness-conditioning; and (3) client education regarding risk factors,

application of ergonomic principles to prevent injury, and understanding of body mechanics and the dynamics of occupational injuries.
The centre also provides on-site job analysis and ergonomic consultation, functional capacity evaluations, work adjustment counselling and
return to work vocational counselling. The average client spends
about three to four weeks in the programme. The stated success rate,
which is defined as the ability of the clients to return to work, is 88 per
cent. The Menomonee programme is a model interdisciplinary
approach demonstrating the cost benefits of an occupational rehabilitation programme enabling injured workers to successfully return to
work.

- *MVP Physical Therapy Orthopedic and Sports Rehabilitation* (nd) in
  the state of Washington similarly defines work hardening as an interdisciplinary, individualized, job-specific programme designed to
  improve biomechanical, neuromuscular, cardiovascular and psychosocial functioning of the worker with the goal of return to work. The
  required components of a work hardening or occupational rehabilitation programme as mandated by the State of Washington includes work
  conditioning, job simulation, education on body mechanics, pacing of
  work rate, occupational safety, job analysis and assessment of the need
  for job modifications, documented individual goals for each client,
  dedicated space for work hardening, quality assurance plan and outcomes reporting of the relative success of the programme, and a work
  adjustment component that includes evaluation of the client's timeli-
  ness, attendance, ability to follow directions, interpersonal relationships
  and overall work behaviour.

- *The Peak Performance Center in Oklahoma City* (Integris Health,
  2002) incorporates a work hardening programme as part of the Jim
  Thorpe Rehabilitation Network. The work hardening component
  includes physical conditioning, functional capacity evaluation using the
  ErgoScience Physical Work Performance Evaluation, job simulation,
  psychoeducation for injury prevention and healthy living focusing on
  proper posture and body mechanics, safe lifting techniques, nutrition
  and exercise principles, driver evaluation and training, psychological
  services and vocational counselling. A wide range of activities is available to the client including aquatics, spinal stabilization, weight training,
  stress management, relaxation training and biofeedback. Physical agent
  modalities (PAMS) are used for symptom relief and include transcutaneous electrical nerve stimulation (TENS), interferential current, heat
  and cold applications, massage, ultrasound, traction, joint mobilization
  and iontophoresis. The typical client attends the programme for 2–4
  hours a day, 3–5 days per week for a period of 4–6 weeks. Occupational
  and physical therapists, psychologists and industrial rehabilitation
  specialists who have extensive industrial work experience staff the
  programme.

- *The Associated Rehabilitation Consultants of Canada, Ltd* (2002) is a multidisciplinary work hardening programme staffed by occupational and physical therapists, athletic trainers, chiropractors, physiatrists (physicians who specialize in physical medicine and rehabilitation) and sports medicine physicians. The occupational therapist does an on-site job analysis and develops a return-to-work programme in cooperation with the client, employer, physician and other health care practitioners.

- *The Central Rehabilitation Clinic in Newfoundland, Canada* (Central Rehab Inc, 2002) offers a work hardening programme that is similar to those described above. The professional personnel in the programme include a certified occupational therapist, fitness instructor, kinesiologist, physical education instructor and licensed practical nurse. Initial assessment of the client includes sitting and standing tolerances, mobility, strength for lifting, carrying and pulling and pushing objects, gross and fine motor coordination, head and neck postures, repetitive foot movements and hand function. Daily notes are kept on the client's attendance, promptness in completing tasks, pain verbalizations, body mechanics, initiative, compliance with the programme demands, safety adherence and ability to accept criticism. In preparation for discharge the client is evaluated in terms of potential for return to work. Recommendations for modifying the equipment and workstation are provided. Discharge is recommended when the client has achieved his or her goals and can tolerate at least five 8-hour days of job simulation while using proper body mechanics, or when the client has reached a plateau or is no longer able to benefit from the programme.

Other occupational rehabilitation or work hardening programmes throughout the world are similar to the ones described above. Most of them have a referral process, admission criteria, evaluation and assessment process, physical or work conditioning programme, stress management and pain management component, on-site job analysis, job simulation and return-to-work counselling. Each of these components is briefly described in the following paragraphs. (See Chapter 6 for an in-depth discussion of stress management.)

Referral and admission to an occupational rehabilitation programme

The overall philosophy of an occupational rehabilitation programme is to teach the client to be an active participant in the process of learning how to do a job in a safe and efficient manner. This philosophy guides the injured worker's acceptance into the rehabilitation programme. The injured worker can be referred by private insurance carriers, physicians, other healthcare providers, self-insured employers, Workers' Compensation Board and, in some cases, attorneys representing the client. Admission criteria vary between rehabilitation agencies, but all consider the client's potential to benefit from the programme during a 3–8-week intensive period of physical work and work hardening.

As part of the referral process, the therapist, interdisciplinary team and client establish client goals cooperatively. The client becomes an active participant in the rehabilitation process. The emphasis is on helping the client to focus on function and being able to accomplish work rather than to focus on the client's complaints. The client should perceive the process as a way of building their strength and personal resources to accomplish tasks. The client is taught to take an active part in controlling symptoms and developing problem-solving skills in order to improve the work environment. Communication between the client and the interdisciplinary team is essential for the rehabilitation process to work effectively. Problems (e.g. location of pain on the body, frequency, intensity and timing of pain, triggers for pain, inability to carry out specific job tasks, severe stress that interferes with ability to do job, musculoskeletal symptoms and limitations of muscle strength and range of motion) should be stated clearly by the client. The client should have an opportunity to list in priority order the problems that are most disabling or aggravating.

In the referral process the occupational therapist works with the client to operationalize the goals into a realistic framework. For example, if the client experiences upper extremity pain, the therapist can have the client pinpoint where the pain is coming from by using a pain drawing or pain analogue scale (e.g. McGill Pain Questionnaire; Melzak, 1987), and describe the type of sensation accompanying the pain (e.g. numbness or tingling). The occupational therapist should orient the client to the occupational rehabilitation process, identify the steps involved and the approximate time period for completing the process. During orientation it is important to establish rapport with the client and to gain the client's cooperation by emphasizing the therapeutic alliance of the client with the interdisciplinary team. Practical information should be explained to the client verbally, even if the information is available in a pamphlet. Several issues should be discussed in the orientation phase, such as expecting muscle soreness at the beginning of the programme; keeping the staff informed of any activity that is causing severe pain or interfering with function; avoiding caffeine and nicotine; the availability of ice packs, physical agent modalities and assistive devices; and emphasizing that daily attendance is required and that it is important to notify the staff if absences are anticipated (Demers, 1992).

Examples of evaluation of physical, psychological and vocational factors

In the evaluation process the interdisciplinary team identifies the client's vocational goals, obtains a comprehensive work history, evaluates the client's work aptitudes and skills, and assesses the client's motivation to return to work. In the process the team identifies personal stressors in the client's life as well as in the work environment and tries to gauge whether the client is magnifying symptoms in order to gain personally from the occupational injury or delay in returning to work. Symptom magnification (Matheson, 1989) has been used as the term to identify workers who consciously try to deceive the treatment team. Although it is rare, it should be considered in cases where there is an inconsistency on functional tests or in observing the client's behaviour in the waiting room as opposed to performing tasks in the clinic. The client who is consciously malingering should be differentiated from the client who feels despair and hopeless about his or her ability to improve and return to work and because of this performs at a depressed level.

Tests and assessment tools are used in the evaluation process to gain a complete understanding of the client's aptitudes, interests, functional capacities and the extent of the work injury. A diagnosis can be corroborated and the prognosis for returning to work can be evaluated based on the results of the evaluation. A test battery can be established that includes (a) aptitude tests such as the General Aptitude Test Battery (GATB) (US Department of Labor, 1985) or one of the Wechsler intelligence scales; (b) interest tests such as the Gordon Occupational Checklist II (GOCL) (Gordon, 1981); (c) fine motor dexterity measures such as the Purdue Pegboard (Tiffin, 1948); (d) functional capacity instruments such as the Baltimore Therapeutic Equipment Work Simulator (BTE Technologies, 2005); (e) stress inventories such as the Stress Management Questionnaire (Stein and Associates, 2003); (f) pain scales, such as a visual analogue scale where the client ranks the intensity of pain, or the McGill Pain Questionnaire (Melzack, 1987) where the client describes the type of pain and location on the body; (g) commercial work samples such as the VALPAR (VALPAR, 1999–2005); (h) personality tests, such as the Minnesota Multiphasic Personality Inventory (MMPI; Hathaway and McKinley, 1970); and (i) independent living measures such as the Functional Independence Measure (FIM) (Keith et al., 1987).

Work conditioning programme in muscle strengthening and stretching

Implementing a physical conditioning programme early in the rehabilitation process is essential to avoid muscle atrophy that can result from inactivity and immobility (Hansen, 1998). Musculoskeletal injury causes increased stiffness in the joints, a decline in physical fitness, demineralization of bone and loss of bone density and an inhibition of the healing process. The muscle-strengthening programme is usually carried out by the physical therapist and assisted by the occupational therapist. The physical conditioning programme should include exercises to increase muscle strengthening that are important in the worker's job tasks as well as flexibility, mobility, motor control and aerobic endurance (Hilson and Hatlestad, 1996). It is important to encourage the client to engage in a daily aerobic exercise such as walking, bicycling or swimming since it is known that regular aerobic exercise improves sleep, cardiovascular function, regulates emotional state and may control pain. The occupational therapist can work in cooperation with the physical therapist in establishing an exercise programme that is meaningful and purposeful to the client such as embedding the exercise goals into everyday occupation such as walking, biking, gardening and shopping.

The physical therapist designs a graded exercise programme based on the results of a functional capacity test and by identifying specific muscles and muscle groups that are weak (Hilson and Hatlestad, 1996). Isometric and active exercises with weights, and resisted exercise machines, isokinetic machines, theraband, gymnastic balls and simulated work are used to achieve muscle strengthening. Other exercises that are indicated for persons with low back pain because of occupational injuries include flexion exercises such as the Williams' flexion exercises (Hooper, 2003). The Williams' flexion exercises include a pelvic tilt where the individual moves the abdomen up with the back and knees bent. Other Williams' exercises include curling the body while moving the knees to the chest and partial sit-ups. The purpose of the Williams' exercise protocol is to stretch the back muscles and to increase the strength of the abdominal muscles. Physicians and physical therapists also prescribe back exercises for extension.

All exercise regimens should be individualized to the needs of the client and carefully monitored by the physical therapist or other health professional. The programme prescribed is based on the type of exercise (e.g. isometric or isotonic), the frequency of the exercise (e.g. every day), the duration (e.g. 30–45 minutes) and the intensity of the exercise (e.g. mild, moderate or intense). It should become incorporated into the client's everyday schedule and the client should keep a record of the exercise and its benefits.

Stress management

The selection of a stress management programme for the client with an occupationally related injury is vital. There is increasing evidence that psychosocial stressors play an independent role in causing musculoskeletal disorders (Warren, 2001). Warren proposed that 'psychosocial stressors may produce chronically elevated muscle tension, thus predisposing soft tissue to the effects of biomechanical stressors' (p. 229). Stress is a risk factor in the workplace that can cause job dissatisfaction, lowered self-esteem, alcohol and drug dependence, cardiovascular disorders, lowered productivity, increased risk for accidents and occupational disorders (Holt, 1993). The stress management programme should include the evaluation of work stressors, the symptoms of occupational stress and the various coping behaviours that the individual can use to reduce the stress. (See Chapter 6 for a more complete discussion of stress.)

Pain management

The primary symptom of most clients attending an occupational rehabilitation programme is pain. Low back pain is the principal cause of impairment in occupational injuries (Callahan, 1993). Pain is usually the first symptom that the worker complains of and it is probably the most debilitating of all symptoms. In incorporating a pain management programme into a comprehensive approach, it is critical to help the client understand the physiological mechanisms of pain and to differentiate acute from chronic pain. Pain in general is one of the most common reasons why workers seek medical assistance. The International Association for the Study of Pain (2005) defines pain as 'unpleasant sensory and emotional experiences arising from actual or potential tissue damage' (Pain Terms, para 1).

Peripheral pain receptors are found in all parts of the body, such as the skin, foot pads, muscles, ligaments, fascia (fibrous tissue that covers, connects and separates muscles), joint capsules, periosteum (fibrous tissue covering bones) and the walls of blood vessels. Pain stimulates the sympathetic nervous system, which in turn can increase the pain by producing peripheral vasoconstriction. Pain increases heart rate, blood pressure and demand for oxygen consumption. Pain can interfere with one's sleep patterns and by so doing can reduce daily activity and affect work behaviour. The vicious cycle of pain creates inactivity, fatigue and muscle weakness and this can generate further pain.

On the one hand, acute pain has a self-limiting course and is associated with damage to tissue in the body that has pain receptors. Acute pain acts like a barometer in the body alerting the individual to the presence of an injury. Musculoskeletal injury is perhaps the most common cause of acute pain. The treatment for acute musculoskeletal pain can be described in the acronym 'PRICE': *protect* the body part with, for example, the use of a sling and first aid, *rest* the limb or extremity, *ice* applied to the affected area, *compression*, such as the use of an ace bandage, and *elevation* of the extremity to prevent swelling.

On the other hand, chronic pain continues after acute damage to the tissue. It is common in low back pain, fibromyalgia, osteoarthritis, carpal tunnel syndrome and other upper extremity disorders that are caused by cumulative trauma or repetitive motion. Chronic pain can cause the individual to reduce their activity, become frustrated and depressed, change their lifestyle, lose motivation for work while becoming less productive, and cause friction with family members and co-workers. In general, chronic pain can create a negative attitude towards health. If left untreated, chronic pain can affect cognition by reducing concentration, restricting problem-solving memory and impairing decision-making. On an emotional level, chronic pain can create a feeling of helplessness or a fear of engaging in activities.

The primary treatment of chronic pain in an occupational rehabilitation programme is to raise the pain threshold of the individual through behavioural approaches. These approaches include active participation of the client in biofeedback, relaxation therapies, yoga, Feldenkrais Method, T'ai-Chi, prescribed therapeutic exercises, diversionary occupations such as arts and crafts, board games and other activities that are purposeful and meaningful to the client. Passive approaches include hypnotherapy, acupuncture, massage, mobilization and chiropractic. Physical agent modalities (PAMs) that are effective in chronic pain include heat, cold packs, traction, transcutaneous electrical nerve stimulation (TENS), hydrotherapy, ultrasound, diathermy and fluidotherapy. Medications used in treating chronic pain include analgesics, anxiolytics to decrease the anxiety attached to pain, sedatives-hypnotics to help induce sleep and anti-depressants (McCormack, 2003).

Job simulation

Job simulation can be carried out in a clinic setting where the occupational therapist recreates the major components of a job and evaluates the worker's abilities to perform job-related tasks. The therapist tries to recreate a realistic work atmosphere where the client is responsible for coming to work on time and in keeping all appointments. The worker progresses in the designated job tasks until both the worker and the therapist feel that the worker is ready to return to his or her former job. This process of gradually preparing the worker to return to the job is part of the work hardening process. During this time 'the worker can experiment and practice different techniques, increase loads and learn the safest and most energy efficient way to complete job tasks' (Tramposh, 1996, p. 315).

The client starts the work hardening programme at a level that is comfortable and progresses to the point where gains have been optimized. Demers (1992) states, 'The goal of the programme is to begin at a safe level, and then progress beyond that level as the client makes gains' (p. 55). The client may be able to perform partially the job tasks in the beginning of the work hardening process. The therapist measures the client's performance abilities continuously so as to inform the client of his or her progress. The use of job-simulated activities increases the client's motivation as well as increasing the client's muscle strength, range of motion, dexterity, endurance, coordination and ergonomically correct posture while completing the job tasks. Feedback is provided by the therapist regarding how the client lifts materials, reaches for objects, handles heavy objects and performs activities at the simulated workstation. The work hardening process gives the therapist the opportunity to teach the client the benefits of ergonomics, exercise and stress management. Simulated workstations can range from a cab of a truck, assembly plant, computer workstation to a packing plant news-stand and restaurant.

On-site job analysis

The on-site job analysis is a systematic evaluation of the worker and the work environment. It is a key component in the occupational rehabilitation process and the work hardening programme. It is usually carried out by an occupational therapist who has knowledge of the occupational description of the job, the equipment and tools used on the job, and the factors on the job that potentially can put a worker at risk for job injury (Key, 1996).

Discharge criteria

During the rehabilitation process, the worker may not be able to complete the programme successfully. This may occur if the client is not compliant with the programme policies. For example, the worker may have habitual poor attendance, seem to be malingering in order to justify an insurance claim, or appear not to be motivated to return to work. The client may be discharged if it is apparent to the interdisciplinary team that further medical or psychological services are necessary before the client is ready for a rigorous programme of rehabilitation. The client may also be discharged at the point where improvement has plateaued and the client has reached the maximum benefit from the programme. The most successful criterion for discharge is the client's readiness to return to work (Power, 2000).

Return to work

Vocational counselling regarding return to work considers the following possibilities: (a) return worker to his or her former job with the same employer; (b) place the worker in a related job at the same company if the worker is unable to do the job because of residual effects of the work disability, or if the worker is at risk for further injury; (c) explore the possibility of the worker being in a similar job with a different employer; or (d) explore the possibility of a new job with the worker and the need for further job training. The return to work phase of the occupational rehabilitation process is in essence the outcome measure. It is the primary goal of the client and rehabilitation team.

Follow-up

It is essential to follow up on the worker's success on the job and to evaluate the worker's ability to apply what was learned in the rehabilitation programme to on-the-job tasks. Does the worker use good body mechanics when performing the job? Is the worker as productive after the injury as before the injury? Has the worker modified the workstation to eliminate major job risks? These are some of the questions that the occupational therapist would ask when doing a follow-up on-site job analysis.

A case example of an occupational rehabilitation programme in Sweden

The following description of a work programme in Sweden demonstrates the occupational rehabilitation model and how it is used with individuals with traumatic brain injury. Simulated work tasks for a teacher were developed by the occupational therapist (Söderback et al., 1993).

The client, a 50-year-old man with a subarachnoid haemorrhage in the middle cerebral artery, was referred to occupational therapy for assessment of cognitive function in connection with evaluation of his work ability. 'John' had been discharged from the hospital's neurological emergency ward. He lived with his wife in a house in a suburb. Their children were grown and had left home. His leisure interests revolved around his family and friends, playing tennis, skiing and being in the country. He was on medical leave from his job as a high school teacher and was not undergoing any other treatment or rehabilitation.

Phase 1: Result of functional and/or ability assessments. At his first visit to the occupational therapy department, John completed an overall cognitive functional ability assessment, an interest questionnaire and a test for assessing finger dexterity (i.e. VALPAR 201; fine finger dexterity). Results showed that he perceived problems with emotional and cognitive functions. He stated that he had problems with reading, writing, comprehending oral and written language, and understanding what he watched on television. He had difficulty following conversations when there were several people talking. John reported that he takes longer to accomplish everyday tasks. This was confirmed by the results of the Box and Block test (Mathiowetz et al., 1985a), where his score for the right hand was below average. John said that he often felt tired after completing a complex task, such as driving a car. He said his life has changed and he was not entirely satisfied with the situation. John's primary rehabilitation goal was to return to his former job as a teacher. The occupational therapist administered a cognitive functional assessment using the Allen Cognitive Level Test (Allen, 1985) and the Intellectual Household Assessment (Söderback, 1988). John performed the assessment tasks in leatherwork of the Allen Cognitive Test according to the requirements for level 4. This indicated that he had certain difficulties in following instructions. The results on the Intellectual Household Assessment indicated that John's problems consisted chiefly of poor attention. As a consequence, he found it difficult to remember instructions until the test administrator demonstrated the task. During the tests, he had difficulty planning, monitoring and performing two or more work items simultaneously. It was concluded from the assessments that John could benefit from systematic training for cognitive functioning.

Phase 2: Job analysis interview. The one-and-a-half-hour audiotaped interview took place at the occupational therapy department. John had worked full-time as a high school teacher in a municipal school with about 400 pupils (about 30 in each class). The teachers had a common room where each had a table for lesson preparation. John stated that most teachers prefer to do prepare lessons at home since it is generally impossible to work uninterrupted in the school. The Swedish Compulsory

School curriculum determines what pupils are to learn and what the contents of lessons should be. John considered that his job gave him academic freedom for his teaching style, but not for the academic content. He stated that teaching could be stressful. For example, colleagues did not have time to talk about the problems that arose. Despite this, John thought he had support from his colleagues since they all had similar problems. John taught German, English, history and religion. He had twenty-four 40-minute teaching hours a week, sometimes in two-hour lessons. The rest of his time at school involved preparation, staff meetings, contacts with pupils and parents, and specific duties which required about six hours a week.

When he was to return to work, John worried about misspelling words on the blackboard. This could lead to discipline problems with students because he might be perceived as a 'bad teacher'. John was also doubtful about his ability to teach history and religion because these subjects require longer and more careful preparation than preparing to teach a second language.

Worksite visit. The workplace visit took the form of participatory observation by the occupational therapist at John's school. The visit lasted two hours and was videotaped. As a guide for analysis of the observations, the 'descriptive question matrix' (Spradley, 1980) was used.

The first observation took place in the pupils' common room. This large room was two stories high. It had a conical glass roof, brick walls, tiled floor and balconies along the walls. There were metal lockers along the walls. The goal of the teacher on duty was to maintain order and discipline and to solve conflicts. During the videotaped visit, 52 pupils passed in front of the camera, but there were actually 200 in the room. There was talking, shouting, stamping and the banging of locker doors. Pupils walked about, sat, chatted in groups, jostled each other and argued. In one group, the supervising teacher had to intervene to settle a conflict.

The other documented event took place in one of the school's classrooms. The observer was at the back of the room. The blackboard was on the opposite wall, with a lectern, overhead projector and other teaching material in front of it. Between the lectern and the observer were 30 desks arranged in rows. To the left was a window running the length of the wall and to the right, a door and bulletin board. The teacher had to teach, maintain order and help the students learn the German language. The documented event was 25 minutes of a German lesson. Apart from the observer, those present were a male colleague of John's and 18 compulsory school pupils. The teacher asked the pupils questions in German, then all read aloud with the teacher. The pupils were asked to read the German text to themselves and the teacher went round the room answering questions. He used the overhead projector to explain points of grammar. After giving brief general information, he asked questions. He corrected one pupil and then wrote on the board. The pupils were to translate Swedish sentences into German. While the pupils worked quietly on their translation, the teacher continued writing on the blackboard. Then the pupils reported their translations and the teacher wrote the answers on the board. Teacher and students read aloud together, then each pupil read a paragraph aloud. Then they were asked one by one to translate from the text just read into Swedish. When the lesson was over the pupils got up and left the classroom talking loudly. Many feelings were expressed during the lesson, chiefly happiness when they were successful and irritation when they were having difficulty.

Summary. The teacher's work tasks consisted of teaching, keeping discipline in the classroom, and supervising pupils during breaks. The teaching task included asking questions, encouraging, reading aloud, listening, understanding, informing, explaining, writing and talking. These work tasks make demands chiefly on the cognitive, verbal and logical functions. This means that the teacher must communicate all the time, take in several simultaneous actions and activities, and make decisions as to when teacher resources are needed. The teacher must also be able to perform these work tasks when there is a high level of noise among many people, and when several things are happening at once.

Considering the impairments and disability described under phase 1, the occupational therapist judged that John could not, at that time, perform these work tasks in a manner satisfactory to those involved. At John's request and in discussion with the Head Teacher and a representative of the health unit, it was decided that work training would be carried out according to a combination of phases 3 and 4. The two colleagues who had taken over John's teaching while he was absent would be brought in as support and contact persons.

Phase 3: Evaluation of work ability and work training with simulated work tasks. The work training was introduced with two treatment sessions of simulated tasks at the occupational therapy department. John's simulated tasks were in the form of planning and preparing lessons. Intellectual Function Training was carried on with the aim of improving his attention span so that communicative ability and simultaneous action improved. The effect was to be evaluated after six months using the Intellectual Housework Assessment (Söderback, 1988). This work training continued once a week, in parallel with work training in a 'real' environment.

Phase 4: Work training measures at previous place of work. John underwent work training at his previous workplace for 20 hours a week. The work was modified so that John was not a duty teacher and was concerned only with language teaching. For eight lessons a week, John was involved with a colleague who had the main responsibility for teaching. John *taught* one lesson a week on his own. The main goal of the work hardening programme was for John to be involved the following term in 12 lessons a week, six of which he was to teach on his own.

Follow-up workplace visit. The follow-up workplace visit took place during a lesson in the same manner as the introductory visit. At the follow-up visit, within 15 minutes, John misspelled four words on the blackboard, and hesitated four times before writing on the blackboard and twice before speaking to the class. He thought these actions occurred too often and was afraid they might lead to disciplinary problems with the students. John also expressed his inadequacy at not being able to complete his lesson. On the basis of the problems described and in consultation with John, subgoals were formulated for the next two weeks' work training to reduce the number of misspellings and to prepare the lesson more carefully by writing out and rehearsing the lecture.

Phase 5: Evaluation of outcome
The subgoals were evaluated by using the Goal Attainment Scaling Instrument (GAS) (Kiresuck et al., 1994) as a self-assessment after each lesson. At the occupational therapist's follow-up visit, John was observed teaching a lesson again. The therapist's assessment using the GAS was compared with John's self-assessment and results showed a high correlation.

After eight weeks, discussion with his colleagues and others showed that John's programme according to the new Swedish work programme guidelines was successful and that he was performing his duties in a manner that is satisfactory to all concerned. The programme was expected to continue for 32 more weeks, in order to accommodate for the length of time required to recover from brain damage.

(Söderback et al., 1993, pp. 42–45)

Job analysis

Job analysis is defined as the gathering, evaluating and recording of accurate, objective and complete data regarding a specific job. The process of analysing a job includes (a) what the worker does in terms of activities or function; (b) how the work is performed (methods, techniques or processes involved and the work devices used); (c) the results of the work; (d) worker characteristics (skills, knowledge, adaptations needed to accomplish the work task); and (e) environmental and organizational factors needed to accomplish the task.

Background on job analysis

The earliest concept of a job analysis started with the work of Bernadino Ramazzini (1633–1744). Ramazzini, who is considered the originator of occupational medicine, studied the relationship between occupations and disease (Hunter, 1978). In his studies, he was interested in examining those components of the job that were hazardous or were contributing factors to the onset of occupational disease. He used observation of the worker's tasks in his 'job analysis'. Through detailed observation he analysed the hazards of jobs that were common in Italy during the seventeenth and eighteenth centuries. These included the work of chemists, potters, tinsmiths, glass workers, cleaners of cesspits, farmers, stonemasons, tanners and other workers. Ramazzini was very thorough in identifying the risk factors among workers and observing the causes of disease, and thus was able to recommend health and safety precautions to prevent injury and disease. Recommendations included rest intervals, adequate ventilation, exercise, change of position during work tasks, adjustment of the temperature in the workplace, use of mouth rinses for workers exposed to toxic chemicals, personal cleanliness and protective clothing (Hunter, 1978).

The process of examining the hazards of jobs by Ramazzini led to the field of occupational medicine and job analysis. However, it wasn't until the twentieth century that job analysis was done in a scientific and systematic way. Frank and Lillian Gilbreth (1921) used time-and-motion analysis for studying job tasks done by workers. Micro-motion studies and a timing device to obtain a record of the worker's movements in performing a task were used.

> However, to make the process uniform, between practitioners, they needed a method of categorizing the types of motions. The method would also have to be a system that could easily apply to all types of activities and yet still allow identification of what the Gilbreths viewed as unnecessary or fatigue producing motions.
>
> (Ferguson, 2000, para 6)

The various motions in the classification system, called 'therbligs' (Gilbreth spelled backwards), include 18 different motions. They were identified both by a symbol/icon and by a colour. The 18 motions include search ⌀, find ⌀, select →, grasp ∩, hold ∩, transport loaded ◡, transport empty ◡, position 9, assemble #, use ∪, disassemble #, inspect ◊, pre-position ◊, release load ⌀, unavoidable delay ⌒, avoidable delay ◡, plan β and rest ᴸ (Ferguson, 2000). Therbligs were used as shorthand to take notes and compile charts on the worker's movements during a specific task. '[B]y examining the charts, one could determine which Therbligs were taking too long or which could be eliminated by rearranging the work. They could also identify periods of delay caused be either the tool/part layout' (Ferguson, 2000, para 7).

As a result of the initial observations of Ramazzini and the time-and-motion studies of the Gilbreths, job analysis became the core for all vocational assessment and occupational rehabilitation programmes. Job analysis is an essential component of vocational evaluation and is used in the following ways:

- *Initial selection, screening, recruitment and placement* of workers ranging in positions that include both unskilled and skilled workers. Job analysis is used when advertising employment opportunities to acquaint the potential worker with the tasks involved. In the initial screening process, a job analysis helps the interviewer to ask appropriate questions to determine the interviewee's qualifications and relevant experiences, and to answer questions regarding the job.
- *Better utilization* of workers in determining physical demands of job factors in promoting workers and suggesting job changes to accommodate individuals with disabilities. First, a job analysis identifies the activity level and muscle strength needed to perform a specific task. Second, it is used to evaluate the worker's quality of performance as a basis for promotion. Third, job modifications and accommodations are identified through a job analysis to enable a worker with a disability to carry out the task.
- *Job restructuring* to make better use of the available workforce especially in jobs that are hard to fill. When there is a shortage of workers for specific jobs, the results of a job analysis can be used for retraining workers to expand their skills and perform new tasks.
- *Vocational counselling* to provide job information and educational requirements to counsellors to help clients make sound decisions regarding occupational choice. The results of the job analysis combined with occupational information enable the counsellor to suggest possible occupations.
- *Preparation* for further education and training of clients by identifying the content and time required for entry into a job. The job analysis identifies the entry skill level, education and experience necessary to perform a job.
- *Developing standards* for objective evaluations of a worker's on-the-job performance. The results of the job analysis can identify production norms for specific aspects of a job. These production norms can be used to develop standards that are approved by both employee unions and management and also determine promotions.
- *Improving health and safety* of the worker by identifying the risk factors on the job and attempting to find methods to reduce them. This may be the most important purpose of the job analysis, as it is used by OSHA in setting standards for heath and safety in the workplace.

Components of a job

The ergonomist performs a job analysis in order to select the most suitable or capable person for a specific job. The task is to match the skills, aptitudes and experience of the worker with the job description. The job analyst breaks down the job components into the smallest *elements* and identifies their sequence. The components include both cognitive processes (e.g. thinking, planning, organizing, attending) and physical motions (e.g. sitting, packing, moving, lifting). For example, the automobile assembly worker who puts together a car bench does the following: (a) selects the appropriate cushion and seat cover; (b) pulls the seat cover over the cushion; (c) installs the car rings to attach to the seat; (d) carries the assembled cushion to the car; and (e) installs it. The elements combine to make *tasks* that are goal-directed work activities, such as driving or installing a cushion in a car seat. These tasks are part of a worker's identified *position*, such as a truck driver or automobile car cushion installer for a specific firm. The position entails the total work assignments or tasks of a single worker in a specific job. Positions vary even under the same job title. In theory, there is a unique position for every worker in the country. In other words, there are as many positions as there are workers. Although many individuals share the same position title, such as truck driver, the actual work performed varies according to the how the specific worker performs the job.

The job is a group of positions that share the same occupational title. Each job has a unique description originally based on the *Dictionary of Occupational Titles* (US Department of Labor, Employment and Training Administration, 1991a) and is subdivided into more specific job titles (e.g. truck drivers, heavy; truck drivers, light; truck drivers, helpers). Current descriptions come from the O*NET™ OnLine (available at http://online. onetcenter.org).

The *Dictionary of Occupational Titles* organized worker functions under three headings: DATA, PEOPLE and THINGS. DATA worker functions consist of synthesizing, coordinating, analysing, compiling, computing, copying and comparing data. The worker *synthesizes* data by developing and creating knowledge (e.g. artist, writer, humourist, stage director, composer or researcher). A worker *organizes* data when employed as a manager, director of an industrial plant or organizes an advertising campaign. Analysing DATA requires the worker to make decisions (e.g. loan applications, evaluation of malfunctioning electrical systems or engines). *Compiling* data entails amassing data into usable formats, such as inputting data for computer files, maintaining inventory of goods, and interviewing individuals for employment using set criteria. *Computing* data relates to jobs involving computation of data (e.g. calculating costs of products and services, determines telephone charges). Individuals engaged in *copying* data are transcribing data from one record into another format (e.g. typing form letters on a computer, recording gas or electric meter readings). Individuals *comparing* data are involved in evaluating two or more data sets based on given criteria (e.g. editing texts, examining cars for scratches and dents, inspecting products using written standards or guidelines).

PEOPLE worker functions include mentoring, negotiating, instructing-consulting, supervising, diverting, persuading, speaking-signalling, serving and taking instructions-helping. In these worker functions, the individual's position and jobs depend on interacting with other people. *Mentoring* activities are carried out by counsellors or therapists, while mediators, referees and labour arbitrators are involved in *negotiating*. Teachers, allied health therapists or job coaches may implement *instruction and consultation*. *Supervisors* are usually managers or administrators who are responsible for directing and evaluating workers in various environments. *Diverting* activities are done by individuals who are performers (e.g. musicians, actors, public speakers, professional athletes). Politicians, attorneys and lobbyists are involved in the task of *persuasion*. Those involved in *speaking and signalling* include an intermediary who is giving directions or relaying information (e.g. stockbroker, dispatcher or radio operator). The role of *servers-assistants* is carried out by sales associates, airline stewardesses and stewards, or childcare workers. Workers in jobs that entail *taking instructions and helping* are in positions as aides, such as a Certified Nursing Assistant.

THINGS are tangible, inanimate objects, substances and materials; machines, tools and equipment; products as distinguished from human beings, substances or materials; and machines, tools, equipment, work aids and products. A thing is tangible and has shape, form and other physical characteristics. The categories of things include setting up, precision working, controlling, driving-operating, operating-manipulating, tending, feeding-off-bearing and handling. Example of *setting up* includes preparing machines and equipment for use and repairing them when necessary. *Precision working* is operating objects under specified standards and guidelines with tools that require calibration. *Controlling* involves operating the machines where there are dials or valves that control temperature, pressure or flow of liquids. *Driving-operating* involves the use of judgement in determining speed and direction of complex machines. *Operating-manipulating* requires motor coordination and manual dexterity to operate equipment. *Tending* involves using minimal judgements to start, stop and observe machines by using switches. *Feeding-off-bearing* includes feeding materials into a machine (e.g. conveyer belt), or removing materials from a machine (e.g. taking laundry out of machines). *Handling* tasks use the body, tools or special devices to load, move or carry objects. For example, a person may load and use a hand-truck.

In reality many jobs consist of an integration of data, people and things, and a multiplicity of tasks. For example, a receptionist is involved in answering the phone (data), responding to questions from the general public (people), taking messages (data and people), taking direction from a supervisor (data) and using a computer (things). In doing a job analysis it is important for the evaluator to describe the actual job. They should not try to fit the person into the job category, but to understand those components of the job that entail data, people and things. An example of analysing the components of a job (truck driver) is shown in Figure 5.1.

Components of Job

	Definition	Examples of each component
JOB	Group of positions sharing the same occupational title. These are defined by the *Dictionary of Occupational Titles*.	TRUCK DRIVER, HEAVY (any industry) 905.663-014: drive trucks or vans with a capacity of at least 26,000 Gross Vehicle Weight
POSITION	Tasks of a single worker in a specific job	Truck driver for a specific firm
TASKS	Goal-directed job-related activities	Long distance driving, handling materials, taking invoices, loading and unloading, vehicle inspection
ELEMENTS	Most basic movement or cognitive process that underlies the job tasks. Elements combined make up the task.	Cognitive • *Attending* • *Decision-making* • *Evaluating* Physical motions • *Sitting* • *Lifting* • *Upper extremity movements*

Figure 5.1 Job analysis for a truck driver. The components of the job include the elements, position, tasks and job description. Notice that the smallest components are the elements, and each of the other components builds on this.

Job skills

After determining the components of the job the evaluator assesses the skills necessary for a worker to complete the job tasks. The tasks comprising a job could range from unskilled to highly skilled. For example, when working on a computer the individual could be proficient in typing but not familiar with using filing systems in a word processing program. The degree of skill to perform a task will depend on the training and education necessary to preparing for the job and the experience necessary to being proficient. The vocational evaluator doing a job analysis should be familiar with the degree of skill necessary in performing the job. Other factors considered in the skills required for a job include (a) physical demands (e.g. lifting, standing and hand strength); (b) mental factors (e.g. decision-making, calculations, evaluating performances); (c) stress factors (e.g. meeting deadlines, functioning at a fast pace); (d) skill in using tools and equipment (e.g. computers, copy machines, drill press); (e) ability to work in environmental extremes (e.g. refrigerated environments, outside work in hot climates); and (f) ability to adapt to a hazardous environment (e.g. using protective clothing, respirator, ear muffs or goggles).

The client's self-perception of his or her skills to do the job is one of the most important predictive factors for returning to work after an occupational injury (Söderback, 2001). The worker assesses his or her feelings towards the job, the type of work performed, equity of pay, opportunities for promotion, supervision available and interactions with co-workers which comprise the worker's job satisfaction (Smith et al., 1996).

Functional capacity assessment (FCA) and work tasks

Functional capacity assessment (FCA), also referred to as functional capacity evaluation (FCE), is used to measure the worker's 'ability to perform a number of job-related functions such as lifting, lowering, pushing, pulling and carrying weights, climbing ladders and stairs, sitting, standing, bending, stooping, crouching, kneeling, crawling and grasping' (Key, 1996, p. 220). An FCA is prescribed when a worker has incurred a work-related injury and there is a question whether the worker has the physical capacity to perform the job. The results of the FCA will be able to identify the worker's physical abilities as compared with the physical demands of the job.

There are a number of standard evaluation programmes used in performance testing and published by occupational and physical therapists that evaluate the client's physical capacities (e.g. Hart et al., 1993; King et al., 1998; Matheson et al., 1996). Examples of FCAs include the Isernhagen Work System (Isernhagen 1988; Reneman et al., 2004); Key Functional Assessment (Key, 1996); The Physical Work Performance Evaluation (ERGOscience) (Lechner et al., 1991); Baltimore Therapeutic Equipment (BTE Technologies, 2005); Matheson Functional Capacity Assessment, (Matheson et al., 2002; and the Joule Functional Capacity System (Christopherson and Ruprecht, 1999). An FCA, in general, measures those whole body movements that are required for performing a specific job, such as a painting, plumbing, or carpentry.

The Smith Physical Capacities Evaluation (SPCE) (Smith and Baxter-Petralia, 1992) is based on 20 physical demands of activity as identified in the *Dictionary of Occupational Titles* (DOT) (US Department of Labor, Employment and Training Administration, 1991a). These functions include the ability to lift, carry, push, pull, balance, climb, stoop, kneel, crouch, crawl, run, jump, see, hear, recline, talk, grasp, reach, sit and stand. For each of these functions, a simulated activity administered by an occupational or physical therapist is presented to the client in a rehabilitation clinic. Equipment for the test includes stairs, ladder, ramps, boxes, pails, wheelbarrows, blocks and a dynamometer. The stated purpose of the SPCE is to evaluate the client's current level of functioning in physical capacities. Norms are used in each of the 20 areas and scored as 'able', 'impaired' or 'unable' to perform the task. The DOT is used as a reference manual in determining whether the task is required in the job.

In conjunction with the SPCE is the Baxter Physical Capacities Evaluation (BPCE) (Baxter-Pretralia and Smith, 1992), which is used with clients who have sustained upper extremity injuries. Five levels of work are identified (1) sedentary – lifting up to 10 pounds; (2) light – up to 20 pounds; (3) medium – up to 50 pounds; (4) heavy – up to 100 pounds; and (5) very heavy – lifing over 100 pounds. The BPCE is divided into (a) *biomechanical tests* (muscle strength, range of motion, pinch strength, isometric grip strength, dynamic grip strength); (b) *sensibility tests* (static two-point discrimination, moving two-point discrimination, light touch/deep pressure localization); (c) coordination tests (e.g. Purdue Pegboard (Tiffin, 1948), Nine Hole Peg Test (Mathiowetz et al., 1985b), Jebsen-Taylor Hand Function (Jebsen et al., 1969)); and (f) endurance tests, such as selected VALPAR tests (VALPAR, 1999–2005).

Assessment of work tasks

Another approach to evaluating an individual's ability to work is to examine the client's cognitive skills, and the social and cultural aspects of a job. In *Off to Work: A Vocational Curriculum for Individuals with Neurological Impairment*, Wehman and Sherron (1995) list work tasks that are rated according to their importance in the job and whether they can be accommodated with assistive devices or placement of furniture. The evaluation of the client's ability to do the job also includes academic areas, such as reading, writing, mathematics, oral and written communication skills, and the ability to learn. Social and cultural aspects of the job are also important, and include interactions with co-workers, dependence on other workers to complete the job, worker attitudes towards the work, male/female ratio and ethnic diversity. The client's ability to work in special environmental conditions (e.g. exposure to outside weather, temperature extremes, high noise levels, exposure to noxious fumes and dust, poor ventilation and extreme vibration) are considered. Floor type, lighting and size of work area can affect the client's placement in a job. For some clients, especially those using wheelchair accessibility to the workplace, consideration should be given to parking facilities for vans, ramps to building, lifts that accommodate a wheelchair, and space around work areas, water fountains, telephones and rest rooms (Wehman and Sherron, 1995).

Work samples

A work sample is defined as 'a well-defined work activity involving tasks, materials and tools which are identical or similar to those in actual job or cluster of jobs' (Dowd, 1993, p. 32). Work samples are used to assess a person's vocational aptitude(s) and interests, worker characteristics/abilities and/or vocational interests (Dowd, 1993). In general, work samples are designed to test if an individual has the ability to perform the actual work on a job as compared to the job description and skills required to do a specific job. The *Dictionary of Occupational Titles* (US Department of Labor, Employment and Training Administration, 1991a), *Occupational Outlook Handbook* (Bureau of Labor Statistics, US Department of Labor, 2004–2005) and *Revised Handbook for Analyzing Jobs* (US Department of Labor, Employment and Training Administration, 1991b) are useful starting points in designing a work sample or selecting a published work sample.

Power (2000) contrasts actual work samples that are taken directly from the worker's job and simulated work samples that are developed by occupational therapists or vocational evaluators in rehabilitation centres or vocational programmes. There are also commercial work sample systems, sometimes referred to as aptitude tests, or vocational evaluation systems such as the VALPAR and Micro-Tower (Brown et al., 1994). Most work samples have been developed for jobs with a strong physical component (Power, 2000). The work sample assesses (a) an individual's vocational aptitude and physical capacities; (b) cognitive abilities; (c) occupational interests; and (d) worker characteristics (e.g. attitudes towards a job, ability to receive supervision and cooperate with co-workers and capacity to work under specific environmental conditions). In designing a work sample, (a) the purposes should be clearly stated; (b) the materials and layout of materials needed in the assessment should be described; and (c) instructions for administering the work sample and directions for scoring should be in a test manual. For example, the work sample might require the client to assemble small parts while working on a conveyor belt using small tools such as pliers and screwdriver in a confined work space. It is important to be familiar with established norms for interpreting scores. Norms are derived from the actual scores of typical workers performing the given task while on the job. Production standards established by industry guidelines can also be used in setting norms (Power, 2000). Work samples can be used with other assessment tools, such as (a) observation of worker performance, and (b) interviews with the worker to gauge his or her vocational interests and motivation to perform the job.

Work samples can be categorized as a single trait or cluster of traits. A *single trait work sample* is used to measure one factor that may be the most important aspect of the job or a key component of a job. Examples can include manual dexterity, eye–hand coordination or gross motor skills. Aptitude tests such as the *Crawford Small Parts Dexterity Test* (Crawford and Crawford, 1975), *Pennsylvania Bimanual Work Sample* (Roberts, 1969), *Purdue Pegboard* (Tiffin, 1948) and *Hand Tool Dexterity Test* (Bennett, 1946) are considered single trait work samples since they measure the single characteristic or trait that is the key element for the job. A *cluster trait work sample* is used for assessing a number of traits inherent in a group of related jobs, such as upper extremity function, ability to work with small tools, fatigue tolerance and hand dexterity. For example, the evaluation of a truck driver's ability to work would include the cluster work sample of the skill of driving, strength in lifting packages, range of motion and ability to log inventories.

The work sample can be further classified as a *simulated* or an *actual* job sample. The work sample can be carried out on site (actual work sample), or developed by an occupational therapist (simulated work sample), or it can be a commercial vocational evaluation system.

A *simulated work sample* is devised by an occupational therapist or vocational evaluator, or commercially purchased. The work sample recreates the main components of the work tasks at a decreased intensity by eliminating some of the task repetition in the job. The therapist works with the client in improving the client's functional level while protecting the client's injured area. The client uses the work simulation experience as an opportunity to practise work strategies to decrease the risk of work injury. During the work simulation process the client is motivated to increase the intensity of the work output until reaching work standards for full-time employment.

Power (2000) describes the process in developing a simulated work sample in-house:

- An on-site job analysis and description of the important characteristics of the job. The job analysis should include physical demands and potential job modifications while being sensitive to the needs of workers with disabilities.
- An examination of job descriptions in ONET™ OnLine (http://online. onetcenter.org) or *Dictionary of Occupational Titles* (US Department of Labor, Employment and Training Administration, 1991a) to be sure that all elements are included.
- Interviews with the employer and employees to obtain further insight into the positive characteristics of the worker typically performing the job.
- Identification of the tools, equipment and materials used in performing the job.
- Determination of the education, training and experience necessary in performing the job. This information is available in the *Occupational Outlook Handbook* (Bureau of Labor Statistics, US Department of Labor, 2004–2005).
- Establishment of normative data to perform each aspect of the job. This is sometimes known as production goals.
- Carrying out research for the simulated work sample to determine reliability and validity of the work sample.

- Performing a field test to determine the feasibility and practicality of the work sample.
- Re-testing the reliability and validity of the work sample.

Vocational interests

Vocational interest inventories have received much attention from psychologists and counsellors since the turn of twentieth century. How does a client's interests relate to a job analysis? In determining whether a client will experience job satisfaction or be bored by a job, it is important to examine the client's vocational interests. A client will be more productive and have fewer absences from the job if he or she enjoys his or her work and if the interests match the job description. Use of vocational interest inventories during a rehabilitation process facilitates decisions about relevant occupational categories or occupations for clients who do not have employment or who could not resume previous work.

Commercial work evaluation (CWE) sample systems

Brown et al. (1994) have described several commercial work evaluation (CWE) systems that can be helpful to the occupational therapist or vocational evaluator. Commercial work evaluation systems are multi-cluster job samples that systematically and objectively evaluate an individual's ability to work. They were developed and designed to assess the work-related abilities of individuals in a controlled test situation. Objective methods to administer, score and report results are included. Reliability, validity and norms are provided in a test manual.

The work evaluation systems consist of job-related tasks, tools and materials that are commonly encountered in a number of jobs. For example, items are included to test ability to read an advertisement in a newspaper, make changes, read blueprints and sort mail. Other CWEs such as the VALPAR (Valpar International Corporation, 1993) include performance tests with such items as testing the individual's ability to place nuts on bolts inside a box. The factors measured include manual dexterity, eye–hand coordination, clerical abilities and upper extremity range of motion.

The MICRO-TOWER work evaluation system is recognized as the first commercially published CWE (see Brown et al., 1994; or Power, 2000). The MICRO-TOWER is an acronym for Testing, Orientation and Work Evaluation in Rehabilitation. It was developed at the Institute for the Crippled and Disabled in New York City in the 1930s. Currently there are a number of other commercially available vocational evaluation systems used widely in rehabilitation centres throughout the world. A description of these systems is listed in Stein and Cutler (2000).

Ergonomic job analysis

The primary purpose of the ergonomic job analysis is to identify risk factors in the workplace and to design solutions that reduce the potential for injury and disease. Keyserling (personal communication, 1997) listed the major reasons for an ergonomic job analysis in an industrial setting. They are as follows:

- Improve industrial production by considering the equipment, tools and work methods. The ergonomist, with the help of industrial engineers, introduces new methods and redesigns tools and equipment to increase efficiency. This is especially important in a global economy where competition drives companies to reduce costs while maintaining the quality of the product.
- Establish compensation and earnings by looking at work standards, education, skills and training required for the job. The results of the job analysis set wage rates by identifying the pay for piecework or hourly wages.
- Determine staff requirements for a job. For example, the job analysis could identify the number of workers usually required to perform a task or job in an industrial plant, such as placing an engine into a car chassis.
- Document knowledge and skills and responsibility required to perform a job by establishing worker standards that identify measurable outcomes.
- Identify risk factors in the workplace that may expose the worker to injury and disease. These risk factors could be related to inadequate lighting, excessive noise, overexertion, prolonged standing on concrete floors, slippery surfaces, ulnar and radial wrist deviations, reaching over head for extended time, lifting heavy objects, awkward positions, local contact stresses, vibration, temperature extremes, repetitive motion or exposure to toxic chemicals.
- Design ergonomic strategies to prevent injuries and hazards in the workplace. The solutions for eliminating risks can be formal or informal instruction classes for the employee on good ergonomic practices, such as (a) proper lifting; (b) scheduling warm-up exercise programmes and stretching muscles in the workplace; (c) scheduling periods for rest breaks; (d) using fatigue mats for individuals who stand for prolonged periods; (e) acclimatizing worker to extreme temperatures in a gradual manner; (f) recommending protective clothing, eye goggles, ear protection and insulated boots; or (g) improving lighting to eliminate glare in the workplace and improving the type of illumination needed for a proper job.
- Introduce engineering solutions to prevent injuries. These solutions involve changing equipment, designing tools and furniture and correcting the workstation.

- Develop detailed instruction sheets or videos to orient a new worker to a job task and to develop a sequence or job ladder function that the worker is expected to accomplish during a specified period. For example, the job analysis would identify the complexity of the job and the months or years of experience usually needed to become proficient in carrying out the job. These data could be applied in examining the quantity and quality of performance on the job that is expected over a period of time. It can serve as the basis for worker evaluation and promotion.
- Evaluate the effect of interventions on the reduction of work injuries. The job analysis can be used as an ongoing activity to achieve improvements in production and the reduction of work injuries.
- Consider special placement of worker with a disability by taking into account the job demands and the capacities of the worker.
- Identify legal and governmental requirements for establishing management–union agreements and OSHA (or relevant body's) standards.
- Research the epidemiology of occupational diseases and ways to measure outcome of intervention.

In carrying out an on-site ergonomic job analysis the following questions are suggested:

1 What is the title of the job?
2 What is the job description?
3 What are the physical characteristics of the worker (e.g. height and weight)?
4 What education or training did the worker have that is directly related to the job?
5 How long has the worker been on this specific job?
6 How many other workers perform this exact job?
7 What is the physical location of the job in relation to the whole industrial plant?
8 Can the work site be sketched on graph paper?
9 What is the shift start time and finish?
10 When are breaks scheduled?
11 What is the total time expended on the job?
12 How does the worker describe the job?
13 What are the worker functions as observed in the on-site visit?
14 What are the major skills performed by the worker?
15 Does the worker rotate job tasks?
16 What are the most common tools, devices or equipment used?
17 What are the goods or services produced?
18 Are there typical worker characteristics that are related to performing the job?
19 What are the physical demands of job? Examples include:
    - lifting objects from the floor
    - twisting and bending the body in performing tasks

- forceful exertions in using tools such as a pneumatic gun
- awkward posture in performing tasks or using equipment
- presence of vibration
- required to work in extreme temperature
- repetitive motions
- prolonged standing
- visual strain
- noise and toxic fumes in work environment

20 What are the cognitive requirements?
21 Are there educational or certification requirements?
22 What components of the job are psychologically stressful?
23 What are factors in the job that can lead to possible errors or failure?
24 Are there safety or health hazards on the job that have been observed or identified by the worker?
25 What is the nature of the worker's authority or responsibility in completing the job?
26 How is the worker supervised?
27 Does the worker have opportunities for in-service training to upgrade performance?
28 How is the worker evaluated for rises and promotion?

Vocational assessment

Vocational assessment is a comprehensive interdisciplinary process that comprises gathering and analysing information over a period of time. Interviews, observation, and real or simulated work tasks are used to assess the individual's education, work history, physical, mental and emotional function, capacity for work, work tolerance and work limitations. The object of the assessment is to provide insight into vocational potential (Dowd, 1993).

Söderback et al. (2000) developed a criterion-referenced multidimensional model for vocational assessment (CMVA). The model contains a description of the actual work requirements represented by the *DOT* (Dictionary of Occupational Titles) job description (US Department of Labor, Employment and Training Administration, 1991a), the worker's ability to complete the task as measured by the appropriate VALPAR components (VALPAR International Corporation, 1999–2005), the interpersonal dimension, represented by the Life Value Questionnaire (Montgomery and Johansson, 1988), and the psychosocial work environment represented by the support variable of the demand-control-support model (Karasek and Theorell, 1990). The CMVA vocational assessment model is designed to identify the client's work potential for a specified job and to identify workers who are at risk for being absent because of illness (Söderback et al., 2000).

Analysis of occupations for preventing work-related injuries

What are the vulnerabilities of specific jobs? If we know the vulnerabilities of a job can we set up prevention strategies to reduce or eliminate these vulnerabilities so as to reduce injuries on the job? These questions were asked by the teacher (FS) in a course on ergonomics at the University of South Dakota. As an assignment the students were asked to examine an occupation with which they are most familiar, such as having been employed in this occupation or knowing about the occupation from a family member or friend. The students were given the assignment of describing the most important job tasks of that occupation, identifying the major risks for accidents and injuries in the occupation and then problem-solving by coming up with strategies or job modifications to prevent injuries related to the occupation. The job tasks and solutions (Table 5.1) were based on the students' limited experience so that the exercise can be interpreted as a work in progress. It is important now for the reader to critically examine the occupations and use it as an exercise for problem solving. Can the reader come up with an additional occupation and outline the job tasks, vulnerabilities and prevention strategies?

Table 5.1 Analysis of occupations for preventing work-related injuries

Occupation	Job Tasks	Vulnerabilities	Prevention
Meat Cutter	• Cutting meat from the bone with a boning knife	• Laceration of hand/finger	• Keep knives sharp so 'sawing' action is decreased
	• Lifting heavy bundles of meat	• Lower back injury	• Wear an elasticized back brace
	• Walking from freezer to cutting table	• Fall	• Install grate in floor to allow droppings to fall through
	• Sawing large cuts of meat into specific cuts	• Awkward hand position	• Use a pistol-handled knife
	• Arranging meat in freezer area	• Extended exposure to cold temperature	• Wear insulated gloves
Veterinarian	• Suturing a wound	• Being stepped on, kicked or bitten	• Put animals in crushes. Assistant can coax and hold animal with a rope
			• Vet is educated and continually aware of how to approach animals

Table 5.1 Analysis of occupations for preventing work-related injuries (continued)

Occupation	Job Tasks	Vulnerabilities	Prevention
Veterinarian (contd)	• Removing a bandage	• Cutting oneself with a Scalpel or scissors	• Wearing leather gloves (with cut-outs so as not to reduce finger dexterity) • Vet is educated and continually aware of safe-cutting procedures
	• Mixing or applying topical medicine	• Skin irritation from chemicals	• Wearing protective clothing
	• Lifting heavy equipment or animals	• Back injury	• Use of proper body mechanics, use of an exercise, stretching and strengthening programme to keep body endurable, limber, and strong
	• Use of hot water or heated surgical instruments for surgery or sanitation	• Burns	• Be aware of high-risk temperatures, use protective gloves or hot pads, wait a specified amount of time for instruments to cool after sanitation before putting them away
	• Working outside in extreme cold weather	• Frostbite	• Wear appropriate clothing, work indoors whenever possible (even if it only provides a wind-block, but no heater) • Leave truck running and work in shifts (e.g. ten minutes of work time and three minutes of warm-up time) • Carry a portable heater
Truck driver with flatbed trailer	• Driving long hours	• Visual strain • Back strain	• Frequent breaks, clean windows to prevent glare, bug shield to keep windshield clean
	• Moving in and out of cab and sleeper	• Stretching of upper body • Fatigue	• Steps appropriate size, grab bars, sit-in or walk-in sleeper (rather than crawl-in sleeper)

Table 5.1 Analysis of occupations for preventing work-related injuries (continued)

Occupation	Job Tasks	Vulnerabilities	Prevention
Truck driver with flatbed trailer (contd)	• Tying a load down onto flatbed	• Back strain	• Secure straps, chains and binders while standing on flatbed or on platform so closer to trailer height
	• Sitting long hours		• Periodic stops, stretching exercises, short walks, drive truck on shorter routes
	• Putting side boards onto flatbed, covering loads with tarpaulin		• Use hinged side boards which lay on flatbed to prevent lifting and moving individual boards; rather than flatbed, pull an enclosed van so tarpaulin is not required to cover cargo
Cosmetician	• Cutting hair	• Finger and hand cramping • Frequent ulnar deviation • Repetitive hand motions	• Stretching exercises • Bend the scissors, not the hand • Use adaptive scissors where hand is allowed to wrap around the handle • Make the grip the proper size and shape for the individual • Spring load scissors so that they open automatically • Possibly wear a splint at night to take pressure off of the median nerve • Schedule appointments with breaks in between
	• Using chemicals for perms or dyes	• Skin becomes red, dry, chapped or sore • Possible allergic reaction	• Wear gloves during chemical treatments • Use a cortisone lotion on skin as needed
	• Frequent standing	• Back pain • Neck and shoulder stiffness • Foot pain	• Wear shoes with adequate support • Stretch frequently to loosen the back, neck and shoulders • Maintain UE strength through exercise

Table 5.1 Analysis of occupations for preventing work-related injuries (continued)

Occupation	Job Tasks	Vulnerabilities	Prevention
Cash Grain Farmer	• Fixing machinery	• Extremities getting caught in machinery may cause damage or amputation • Upper extremity problems with muscles, joints, or nerves	• Wear heavy clothing and work boots • No loose clothing • Turn machinery off and wait for it to completely stop before working on it
	• Stress and fatigue from working long hours and lack of sleep during planting or harvest time • Heavy lifting • Driving tractor in the elements • Mixing and pouring chemicals	• Reaction time and increased chance of injury • Loss of concentration • Back injury • Sunburn • Chemical burns	• Take regular breaks for eating and resting • Trade off drivers • Strengthening exercises for lower back • Education on proper lifting techniques • Apply sunscreen • Put a cab, canopy, or shield to the tractor • Wear a hat • Wear a mask • Wear gloves • Wear goggles • Follow instructions • Keep water and first aid kit near by • Wear boots • Wear an apron
Auto-body Painter	• Using a power sander to sand metal car parts (e.g. doors, sills, etc.) • Spraying paint onto cars	• Cumulative trauma disorder • Injury to eyes from debris • Hearing impairment • Respiratory problems	• Use a vibration damp-ening device on sander • Use proper posture (ladder/platform helpful to sand roofs) • Eliminate excessive twisting • Neutralize wrist • Modify handle so excessive grip force is not necessary • Wear goggles/eye protective wear • Wear mask/ventilator • Redesign trigger or handle on paint gun so that less force is required to grip

Table 5.1 Analysis of occupations for preventing work-related injuries (continued)

Occupation	Job Tasks	Vulnerabilities	Prevention
Auto-body painter (contd)	• Lifting heavy car parts	• Back injury	• Teach proper postures and biomechanics to avoid excessive twisting • Have a second person help lift
	• Using screwdriver to disassemble car parts and reassemble	• Carpal tunnel syndrome	• Use an adjustable power screwdriver; for manual screwdrivers, make sure handle is long enough and built up; grooved handles may improve torque (but they must fit the individual)
Livestock Production/ Pork	• Lifting buckets of feed to dump in bins • Carrying buckets of grain	• Fumes from grain dust fill lungs • Back strain • Shoulder strain	• Carry load closer to body, near waist. Arms extended at side with elbows bent slightly, not locked • Use a long stick to push and stir load when jammed • Wear a face mask, cover mouth
	• Grinding feed • Using a drying bin for harvested grain	• Extremely loud noise can damage hearing • Amputations of limb in grinder • Getting cut or stuck by needle	• Wear earplugs • Lifting fewer buckets at a time/decrease weight of load. Keep a lordosis curve in back, bend at the knees and lift with the legs
	• Vaccinating for disease and administering antibiotics		• Wear heavy gloves; have someone else hold the pig steady
HVAC & Refrigeration Technician (HVAC = Heating, ventilation, and air conditioning)	• Lifting/carrying compressors and large panels for assembling walk-in freezers	• Back strain/injury	• Education on proper lifting techniques (possibly back school) • Getting assistance when lifting heavy objects • Use of automated materials to lift/carry materials • Back brace wear • Begin day with exercise session to warm up muscles

Table 5.1 Analysis of occupations for preventing work-related injuries (continued)

Occupation	Job Tasks	Vulnerabilities	Prevention
HVAC & Refrigeration Technician (contd)	• Repair of compressors for refrigeration/freezers (source of loud noise)	• Hearing loss	• Use of ear plugs or ear muffs when in noisy areas • Wear protective gloves
	• Soldering of copper pipes and fittings together	• Burns	• Education on proper use of soldering torch • Slowing down to prevent injuries made in haste (e.g., touching pipes before they have had time to cool)
	• Repairing electrical wiring on refrigeration/freezing units (could have condensation/ice on) • Providing electrical wiring for air conditioning units	• Electrical shock	• Ensure that hands are dry when working with wiring • Slowing down to prevent accidental contact with wiring
	• Climbing ladders to install/repair air conditioning units, furnaces, etc. on the roofs of businesses	• Falls from ladders	• Slow down and be cautious when climbing ladder • When descending, worker should get on ladder prior to grabbing tools/equipment • Carry fewer items at a time while on ladder • Ensure that the ladder is straight and on an even surface • Ensure that bungy strap is secure around ladder and to building • Use ladder with a wider base

Anthropometric considerations in ergonomic solutions

Anthropometry, the science of measuring the human body (Pheasant, 1986), is an integral part of the day-to-day practice in industrial ergonomics and occupational safety (Keyserling, personal communication, 1994). Pheasant (1986) divides anthropometry into static and dynamic measurement. Static anthropometry is the measurement of the lengths, breadths and depths of the human body while standing or sitting. It includes total height, such as stature, segmental heights, such as eye height (i.e. the distance from the floor to the eye when standing) and elbow height (i.e. the distance from the floor to elbow while the individual is standing). Sitting measurements for eye heights, knee heights and shoulder to elbow length are other examples of static anthropometry. Dynamic anthropometry measurements consider the worker's reach and clearance of space in the work environment. Reach is measured by the worker's ability to reach objects, dials or controls while standing or sitting. The most efficient and healthy workspace is when the worker is comfortable when reaching for an object. If the worker extends their reach beyond a normal workspace for prolonged periods of time, it can create a risk of developing work injuries. Dynamic anthropometry also considers the dimension of clearance such as access and exits of passageways, crawling spaces and carrying objects between spaces.

Anthropometric measurements are used for the design of protective clothing and equipment, workstations and operating controls. Keyserling (personal communication, 1997) identified four basic types of anthropometric measurements: (1) whole body measurements of height, weight, and differences between males and females, used to determine dimensions of doorways for adequate head clearance, manhole diameters and overhead conveyor belts; (2) body landmark measurements of sitting eye height, and shoulder height used in ergonomic design guidelines (e.g. placing hand work at elbow height and designing the height of a bench); (3) body segment anthropometric measurements of arms, limb weights and distribution of mass within a body segments, useful in developing ergonomic guidelines for biomechanical strength and kinematic reach models; and (4) functional measurements such as range of motion (e.g. reaching for an object on an assembly-line, control dials or tools).

Anthropometry is of fundamental importance in the match between the human and the machine, such as the truck driver and the truck, or the computer operator and the computer. Anthropometry creates the scientific body of data that are applied to designing environments and tools that are ergonomically sound. How can the concepts of anthropometry be practically applied to ergonomics? If we define ergonomics as fitting the environment to the individual, then it is critical to understand the physical characteristics of the human so that workstations, tools, equipment, temperature and noise variables can be adapted to the individual. If workstations do not consider body size variability, then occupational disorders can occur. For example, Botha and Bridger (1998) examined the relationship between operational problems in the work environment of nurses and musculoskeletal pain. They found that back pain was caused by inadequate space and poorly designed equipment, especially for lifting. They concluded that body size variability can affect the onset of occupational injuries.

Guidelines for lifting and measurement for muscle torque (Kingma et al., 2001) are an important aspect of dynamic anthropometry (Pheasant, 1986). Dynamic anthropometry is important in designing aircraft cockpits and car dashboards, as well as analysing the assembly workers' reach. Clearance is an important concept in designing workspaces where the worker is in motion, such as in using tunnels and catwalks. In considering the normal characteristics most researchers separate out gender and age. It is known that as we age, physical capacities tend to decline. Samson et al. (2000), in a cross-sectional study of 74 healthy women and 81 healthy men aged 20–90 years, discovered that individuals over 55 years had lower values for muscle strength, hand grip and functional mobility in tasks such as walking than individuals aged 20–55 years. This information has important implications for those individuals who continue working after the age of 55.

Anthropometry utilizes the statistical concept of the normal curve in creating ergonomically healthy environments. For example, knowing that the average adult male is five feet nine inches tall enables the design engineer to design furniture and chairs to fit the average male. The normal curve assumes that 68 per cent of males will be plus or minus one standard deviation from the average value. If we know that one standard deviation for height for males equals approximately three inches, then we can assume that males between five feet six and six feet tall will be within minus one to plus one standard deviation units from the mean value of five feet nine inches. A chair that is comfortable for males from five feet six to six feet will accommodate approximately 68 per cent of the adult male population. Now if the design engineer can create a chair that is adjustable to persons who are two or three standard deviations from the mean of five feet nine then the chair can accommodate 98–99 per cent of the population, if it can be adjusted to fit males who are five feet to six feet six. The data from anthropometry can be used to design healthy ergonomic environments to fit the human characteristics. Tables for static anthropometric data are widely available in the literature (e.g. Pheasant, 1986) and on-line (http://www.iuna.net/survey_pdf/ tables41_423.pdf).

There is an increasing demand for anthropometric data for designing machinery and protective equipment to prevent occupational injuries (Hsiao et al., 2002). Stumpf et al. (2001), in a discussion of the anthropometric data of the design a work chair, stated that 'People on the edges of the "normal" distribution curve for any dimension may not be well served by work chairs designed for people at the center of the curve' (p. 1). In recommending a chair that fits smaller and larger people as well as the average person, they designed three different chairs to accommodate each sector of the population. This approach varies from the ergonomic designer who considers the chair to be adjustable and therefore designed to fit 98 per cent of the population (minus three standard deviations from the mean to plus three standard deviations from the mean).

The other factor to consider in applying anthropometric data is to consider the physical characteristic differences among occupational groups. Hsiao et al. (2002), in a large-scale study of over 32,000 workers, found that firefighters, police and security guards were taller and heavier than employees in other occupations. Agricultural workers such as migrant workers were significantly shorter in stature but had thicker wrists. This study illustrates the importance of applying local anthropometric norms in considering workstation design.

Anthropometric data can create constraints on the design of workstations, tools and equipment. For example, 'the height of a chair must not be greater than the vertical distance from the sole of the foot to the crook of the knee' (Pheasant, 1986, p. 18). The criteria for judging the adequacy of ergonomic equipment are the standards for measuring comfort, safety, efficiency and aesthetics. Constraints and criteria are basic concepts in applying anthropometric data to ergonomic design.

Guiding questions

When an occupational therapist is hired as a consultant to devise a plan to reduce the risk for injuries on the job, the following questions are appropriate to consider:

1 What are the ergonomic hazards on the job?
2 How is the job described by the workers and employer?
3 What are the ergonomic strategies required to reduce the risk of injuries on the job?
4 How many injuries currently occur on the job?
5 Are injuries in this plant more extensive than injuries in similar plants?
6 How much is the average cost for injuries in this plant?
7 How much is the average worker's compensation award for each work-related injury?
8 What are the presumed causes of the injuries on the job?
9 What are the nature and extent of the injuries?
10 How can a job analysis be applied in this plant?

Summary

Human beings usually define their lives by what they do in an occupation. Work is a key component of life. It creates meaning for an individual and fills an individual's time. In this chapter the authors have attempted to place work in the context of an occupational therapist's key roles in the prevention of work injuries and in assisting a worker with a disability to adjust to a work environment. Occupational injuries affect millions of workers and the costs are enormous. The major injuries that occupational therapists will encounter in the workplace, such as low back pain and carpal tunnel syndrome, are related to repetitive motion and cumulative trauma. The primary interventions in the workplace include a daily exercise programme, stress management, physical agent modalities, rest breaks, equipment modification, job rotation, wellness programmes, biofeedback, lifting devices, musculoskeletal education and organizational control methods that include pacing of the work on an assembly-line. There are many other interventions in the workplace that are specific to a work setting and result from the cooperative efforts of the worker, management and health care professionals to generate solutions. Job analysis, functional capacity assessment, anthropometry and work samples are the tools that occupational therapists use in the work setting to design occupational rehabilitation programmes.

Review questions

1 How is work defined in relationship to ergonomics?
2 What does an occupational therapist need to know about the theory and sociology of work to help an individual with a disability to return to work or to prevent work injuries?
3 What are the major musculoskeletal injuries that occupational therapists will encounter in the workplace?
4 What is the epidemiology of work-related injuries and what are the approximate costs to the employer and society at large?
5 What are the occupational interventions that are applied in the workplace?
6 What are the occupational health and environmental measures that corporations use in preventing and intervening in work-related injuries?
7 What are the major components of the occupational rehabilitation process?
8 How does work hardening enable an individual to return to work?
9 How does an occupational therapist select a test battery that is appropriate in an individual case?
10 What should the occupational therapist know about the National Institutes of Occupational Safety and Health (NIOSH) and Occupational Safety and Health Administration (OSHA) or related bodies?
11 What are the purposes of a functional capacity assessment?
12 What details should the occupational therapist know about an ergonomic job analysis and work samples?
13 Define anthropometry and discuss how it is used in ergonomics?

References

Allen, C. (1985). Occupational Therapy for Psychiatric Diseases: Measurement and Management of Cognitive Disabilities. Boston: Little, Brown.

American Occupational Therapy Association (1986). Work hardening guidelines. American Journal of Occupational Therapy, 40, 841–843.

Anannontsak, A. and Puapan, P. (1996). Effects of working postures on low back pain. Journal of Human Ergology, 25, 65–72.

Anderson, N. (1964). Dimensions of Work: The Sociology of a Work Culture. New York: David McKay.

Associated Rehabilitation Consultants of Canada, Ltd (2002) AARC clinic services – Work hardening programme. Retrieved 12 March 2005, http://www.arccmanitoba.com/ClinicServices/ARCCWorkHardeningPgm.html

Barnum, M., Mastey R.D., Weiss, A.P. and Akelman E. (1996). Radial tunnel syndrome. Hand Clinics, 12, 679–689.

Baxter-Petralia, P. and Smith, S.L. (1992). Baxter Physical Capacities Evaluation (BPCE). Baltimore: Chess Publications.

Beissner, K.L., Saunders, R.L. and McManis, B.G. (1996). Factors related to successful work hardening outcomes. Physical Therapy, 76(11), 1188–1201.

Bennett, G.K. (1946). Hand Tool Dexterity Test. San Antonio, TX: The Psychological Corporation.

Bernard, B.P. (Ed.) (1997). Musculoskeletal disorders (MSDs) and workplace factors. A critical review of epidemiological evidence for work-related musculoskeletal disorders in the neck, upper extremity, and low back (2nd edn). (DHHS (NIOSH) Publication No. 97-141.) Cincinnati, OH: National Institute of Occupational Safety and Health. Available at http://www.cdc.gov/ niosh/97-141pd.html

Birger M., Sha'anani R. and Pavlotzki F. (1997). Biofeedback treatment of Raynaud's disease. Harefuah, 133, 362–364, 414.

Botha, W.E. and Bridger, R.S. (1998). Anthropometric variability, equipment usability and musculoskeletal pain in a group of nurses in the Western Cape. Applied Ergonomics, 6, 481–490.

Brewer, C.C. and Storms, B.S. (1993). The final phase of rehabilitation: work hardening. Orthopaedic Nursing, 12, 9–16.

Brown, C.D., McDaniel, R.S., Couch R.H. and McClanahan, M. (1994). Vocational Evaluation Systems and Software. A Consumer´s Guide. Menomonie, WI: The Materials Development Center.

BTE Technologies (2005). Baltimore Therapeutic Equipment Work Simulator (BTE). Retrieved 12 March 2005, http://www.btetech.com/

Burdorf, A., Naaktgeboren, B. and de Groot, H.C. (1993). Occupational risk factors for low back pain among sedentary workers. Journal of Occupational Medicine, 35, 1213–1220.

Bureau of Labor Statistics, US Department of Labor (BLS) (2004a). Injuries, illnesses and fatalities home page. Retrieved 4 March 2005, http://www.bls.gov/iif/home.htm#tables

Bureau of Labor Statistics, US Department of Labor (BLS) (2004b). Lost-worktime injuries and illnesses: Characteristics and resulting days away from work, 2002. Retrieved 21 March 2005, http://www.bls.gov/news.release/pdf/osh2.pdf

Bureau of Labor Statistics, US Department of Labor (BLS) (2004c) Table 3: Repetitive motion by selected worker and case characteristics – 2002. Retrieved 5 March 2005, http://www.bls.gov/iif/oshwc/osh/case/ostb1258.pdf

Bureau of Labor Statistics, US Department of Labor (2004–2005). Occupational outlook handbook [Online]. Available at http://www.bls.gov/oco/

Burt, C.M. (2001). Work evaluation and work hardening. Occupational therapy: practice skills for physical dysfunction. In L.W. Pedretti and M.B. Early (Eds), Occupational Therapy. Practice Skills for Physical Dysfunction (5th edn; pp. 226–236). St. Louis: Mosby.

Buschbacher R.M. (1999). Median nerve motor conduction to the abductor pollicis brevis. American Journal of Physical Medicine Rehabilitation, 78, 1–8.

Callahan, D.K. (1993). Work hardening for a client with low back pain. American Journal of Occupational Therapy, 47, 645–649.

Center for Disease Control [CDC], Division of Media Relations (1997). Facts about occupational injuries [Fact Sheet]. Retrieved 5 March 2005, http://www.cdc.gov/niosh/injury/traumacause.html

Central Rehab Inc (2002). Central rehab, Newfoundland, work hardening. Retrieved 12 March 2005, http://www.centralrehab.com/Work_Hardening.htm

Chan, C.C.H., Li, C.W.P., Hung, L. and Lam, P.C.W. (2000). A standardized clinical series for work-related lateral epicondylitis. Journal of Occupational Rehabilitation, 10, 143–152.

Christopherson, B.B. and Ruprecht, M.E. (1999). Joule by Valpar: Introduction and Preliminary Report of Joule Effectiveness and Client Satisfaction. Tucson: Valpar International Corporation.

Cockburn, J.T., Thomas, F.N. and Cockburn, O.J. (1997). Solution-focused therapy and psychosocial adjustment to orthopedic rehabilitation in a work hardening programme. Journal of Occupational Rehabilitation, 7, 97–106.

Collins, J.W., Wolf, L., Bell, J. and Evanoff, B. (2004). An evaluation of a 'best practices' musculoskeletal injury prevention programme in nursing homes. Injury Prevention, 10, 206–211.

Commission on Accreditation of Rehabilitation Facilities (CARF) (2005). Retrieved 12 March 2005, http://www.carf.org/default.aspx

Community Memorial Hospital (nd). Work hardening programme. Retrieved 10 March 2005, http://www.communitymemorial.com/clinicalservices/Work_Hardening_programme.htm

Cooper, B.A. and Stewart, D. (1997). The effect of a transfer device in the homes of elderly women. Vertical Pole. Physical and Occupational Therapy in Geriatrics, 15, 61–77.

Cooper, J.E., Tate, R. and Yassi, A. (1997). Work hardening in an early return to work programme for nurses with injury. Work: A Journal of Prevention, Assessment and Rehabilitation, 8, 149–156.

Crawford, J.E. and Crawford, D.M. (1975). The Crawford Small Parts Dexterity Test. San Antonio, TX: The Psychological Corporation.

De Grazia, S. (1964) Of Time, Work, and Leisure. Garden City, New York: Anchor.

Dekker, S.W.A. and Nyce, J.M. (2004). How can ergonomics influence design? Moving from research findings to future systems. Ergonomics, 47, 1624–1639.

Demers, L.M. (1992). Work Hardening: A Practical Guide. Stoneham, MA: Butterworth-Heinemann.

De Smet, L. (2002). Median and ulnar nerve compression at the wrist caused by anomalous muscles. Acta Orthopaedica Belgica, 68, 431–438.

Deyo, R.A. (1998). Low-back pain. Scientific American, 153, 48–53.

Docherty, N. and Rummel D. (Producers) (2003). Frontline: A dangerous business: Costs of occupational injuries and illnesses. FRONTLINE/WGBH Educational Foundation. Washington, DC: Public Broadcasting Service. Retrieved 4 March 2005, http://www.pbs.org/wgbh/pages/frontline/shows/workplace/etc/cost.html

Dowd, L. (1993). Glossary of Terminology for Vocational Assessment, Evaluation and Work Adjustment. Menomonie, WI: Material Development Center, Stout Vocational Rehabilitation Institute.

Erikson, E.H. (1963). Childhood and Society (2nd edn). New York: W.W. Norton.

Ferguson, D. (2000). Therbligs: The keys to simplifying work. The Gilbreth Network. Retrieved 12 March 2005, http://gilbrethnetwork.tripod.com/therbligs.html

Feuerstein, M., Callan-Harris, S., Hickey, P., Dyer, D., Armbruster, W. and Carosella, A.-M. (1993). Multidisciplinary rehabilitation of chronic work-related upper extremity disorders'long-term effects. Journal of Occupational Medicine, 35, 396–403.

Freedman, R.R. (1989). Quantitative measurements of finger blood flow during behavioural treatments for Raynaud's disease. The Society for Psychophysiological Research, 26, 437–441.

Frost, H., Lamb, S. E., and Shackleton, C. H. (2000). A functional restoration programme for chronic low back pain. Physiotherapy, 86, 285–293.

Gerardi, S.M. (1999). Part I. Work hardening for warriors: Occupational therapy for combat stress casualties. Work. A Journal of Prevention Assessment and Rehabilitation, 13, 185–195.

Gilbreth, F. and Gilbreth, L. (1921). Time and Motion Studies as Fundamental Factors in Planning and Control. New Jersey: The Mountainside Press.

Greenberg, S.N. and Bello, R.P. (1997). Working stiff: Case study reveals benefits of work hardening for motivated workers. Rehabilitation Management: The Interdisciplinary Journal of Rehabilitation, 10, 80, 82–83.

Guerriero, R.C., Rajwani, M., Gray, E., Platnick, H., Da Re, R. and Dodsworth, P. (1999). A retrospective study of the effectiveness of physical rehabilitation of low back pain patients in a multidisciplinary setting. Journal of the Canadian Chiropractic Association, 43, 89–103.

Gyllenhammar, P.G. (2002). Cheferna har ansvaret (The bosses have the responsibility). Daily News, 8 September, p. 2. (In Swedish.)

Habes, D.J. (1996). Upper extremity cumulative trauma disorders: Current trends. In A. Bhattacharya and J.D. McGlothlin (Eds), Occupational Ergonomics, Theory and Applications (pp. 581–603). New York: Marcel Dekker.

Haider, C. (1996). Swedish working life fund case studies: Job rotation and new technique saved money for a restaurant kitchen. Retrieved 10 March 2005, http://www.arbetslivsinstitutet.se/alf/alfeng/alfeng2.htm

Hansen, M. (1998). Pathophysiology Foundations of Disease and Clinical Intervention. Philadelphia, PA: W.B. Saunders.

Hart, D.L., Isernhagen, S.J. and Matheson, L.N. (1993) Guidelines for functional capacity evaluation of people with medical conditions. Journal of Orthopaedic and Sports Physical Therapy, 18, 682–686.

Hartvigsen, J., Leboeuf-Yde, C., Lings S. and Corder, E.H. (2002). Does sitting at work cause low back pain? Ugeskr Laeger, 164, 759–761.

Hathaway, S. and McKinley, C. (1970). Minnesota Multiphasic Personality Inventory [MMPI]. Minneapolis: National Computer Systems.

Healy, B. and Comerouskik, J. (1999). Work hardening: Specialized health care for the injured worker. Inside Case Management, 5, 5–7.

Hedge, A. (2002). Lifting and back stress [electronic class notes]. Cornell University. Retrieved 5 March 2005, http://ergo.human.cornell.edu/studentdownloads/DEA325pdfs/Lifting.pdf

Hendrick, A. (1943). Work and the pleasure principle. Psychoanalytic Quarterly, 12, 311–329.

Hilson, J. and Hatlestad, S. (1996) Flexibility, mobility, strength and aerobic conditioning. In G. Key (Ed.), Industrial Therapy (pp. 295–314). St. Louis: Mosby.

Hodge J.C. and Bessette B. (1999). The incidence of sacroiliac joint disease in patients with low-back pain. Canadian Association of Radiologists Journal, 50, 321–323.

Holt, R.B. (1993). Occupational stress. In L. Goldberger and S. Breznitz (Eds), Handbook of Stress: Theoretical and Clinical Aspects (pp. 342–367). New York: The Free Press.

Hoogendoorn, W.E., Bongers, P.M., de Vet, H.C., Ariens, G.A., van Mechelen, W. and Bouter, L.M. (2002), High physical work load and low job satisfaction increase the risk of sickness absence due to low back pain: Results of prospective cohort study. Occupational Environmental Medicine, 59, 323–328.

Hooper, P. (2003). Whatever happened to Williams' flexion exercises? Retrieved 12 March 2005, http://www.chiroweb.com/archives/17/01/09.html

Hsiao, H., Long, D. and Snyder, K. (2002). Anthropometric differences among occupational groups. Ergonomics, 45, 136–152.

Hunter, D. (1978). The Diseases of Occupations (6th edn). London: Hodder and Stoughton.

Integris Health (2002). Integris Health: Specialties. Retrieved 10 March 2005, http://www.integris-health.com/INTEGRIS/en-US/Specialties/default.htm

International Association for the Study of Pain (2005). Pain terminology. Retrieved 12 March 2005, http://www.iasp-pain.org/terms-p.html#Pain

Isernhagen, S.J. (1988) Work Injury Management and Prevention. Rockville, MD: Aspen Publishers.

Jang, Y., Hwang, M. and Li, W. (1997). A work-oriented occupational therapy programmeme for individuals with physical disabilities. Occupational Therapy International, 4, 304–316.

Jebsen, R.H., Taylor, N., Treisman, R.B., Trotter, M.J. and Howard, L.A. (1969). An objective and standardized test of hand function. Archives of Physical Medicine and Rehabilitation, 50, 311–319.

Johnson, J.V., Hall, E.M. and Theorell, T. (1989). Combined effects of job strain and social isolation of cardiovascular disease morbidity in a random sample of the Swedish male working population. Journal of Work Environment Health, 15, 271–279.

Johnson, L.S., Archer-Hesse, G., Caron Powels, D.L. and Dowson, T.M. (2001). Work hardening: Outdated fad or effective intervention? Work. A Journal of Prevention Assessment and Rehabilitation, 16, 235–243.

Joy, J.M., Lowy, J. and Mansoor, J.K. (2001). Increased pain tolerance as an indicator of return to work in low-back injuries after work hardening. American Journal of Occupational Therapy, 55, 200–205.

Karasek, R. and Theorell, T. (1990) Healthy Work: Stress, Productivity, and the Reconstruction of Working Life. New York: Basic Books.

Kaufman M.W. and All, A.C. (1996). Raynaud's disease: Patient education as a primary nursing intervention. Journal Vascular Nursing, 14, 34–39.

Keith, R.A., Granger, C.V., Hamilton, B.B. and Sherwins, F.S. (1987). The functional independence measure. Advances in Clinical Rehabilitation, 1, 6–18.

Kerr, M.S., Frank, J.W. Shannon, H.S., Norman, R.W., Wells, R.P., Neumann, W.P. and Bombardier, C. (2001). Biomechanical and psychosocial risk factors for low back pain at work. American Journal of Public Health, 91, 1069–1075.

Key, G.L. (1996). Industrial Therapy. St. Louis: Mosby

King, P.M. (1993). Outcome analysis of work-hardening programmes. American Journal of Occupational Therapy, 47, 595–603.

King, P.M. (1992). Brief or new: Profiling the work-hardening therapist: Education and experience. American Journal of Occupational Therapy, 46, 847–849.

King, P.M., Tuckwell, N. and Barrett, T.E. (1998). A critical review of functional capacity evaluations. Physical Therapy, 78, 852–866.

Kingma, I. Baten, C.T., Dolan, P., Toussaint, H.M., van Dieen, J.H., de Looze, M.P. and Adams, M.A. (2001). Lumbar loading during lifting: A comparative study of three measurement techniques. Journal of Electromyographic Kinesiology, 11, 337–345.

Kiresuck, T., Smith, A. and Cardillo, J.E. (1994). Goal Attainment Scaling: Applications, Theory, and Measurement. London: Lawrence Erlbaum Associates.

Kohn, J. (1997) The Ergonomic Casebook: Real World Solutions. Boca Raton, FL: CRC Lewis.

Lacroix, C. (1995). Work hardening for sub-acute back injured workers: A new approach. Work. A Journal of Prevention Assessment and Rehabilitation, 5, 143-146.

Leboeuf-Yde, C. (2000). Body weight and low back pain. A systematic literature review of 56 journal articles reporting on 65 epidemiological studies. Spine, 25, 226–237.

Lechner, D.E. (1994). Work hardening and work conditioning interventions: Do they affect disability? Physical Therapy, 74, 471–493.

Lechner, D.E., Roth, D. and Straaton, K. (1991). Functional capacity evaluation in work disability. Work. A Journal of Prevention, Assessment and Rehabilitation, 1, 37–47.

Levangie, P.K. (1999). Association of low back pain with self-reported risk factors among patients seeking physical therapy services. Physical Therapy, 79, 757–766.

Lieber, S.J., Rudy, T.E. and Boston, J.R. (2000). Effects of body mechanics training on performance of repetitive lifting. The American Journal of Occupational Therapy, 54, 166–175.

Lilley, R., Feyer, A.M., Kirk, P. and Gander, P. (2002). A survey of forest workers in New Zealand. Do hours of work, rest, and recovery play a role in accidents and injury? Journal Safety Research, 33, 53–71.

Lings, S. and Leboeuf-Yde, C. (1998). Whole body vibrations and low back pain. Ugeskr Laeger, 160, 4298–4301.

Linton, S.J. and Buer, N. (1995). Working despite pain: Factors associated with work attendance versus dysfunction. International Journal of Behavioural Medicine, 2, 252–262.

Mahoney, F.I., Barthel, D.W. and Wade, D.T. (1992). Measurement in Neurological Rehabilitation. New York: Oxford University Press.

Malanga, G.A. (1997). The diagnosis and treatment of cervical radiculopathy. Medicine and Science in Sports Medicine, 29, 236–245.

Maslow, A.H. (1970). Motivation and Personality (2nd edn). New York: Harper and Row.

Matheson, L.N. (1989). Use of the BTE Work Simulator to screen for symptom magnification syndrome. Industrial Rehabilitation, 2, 15–17.

Matheson, L.N. and Brophy, R.G. (1997). Aggressive early intervention after occupational back injury: Some preliminary observations. Journal of Occupational Rehabilitation, 7, 107–117.

Matheson, L.N., Isernhagen, S.J. and Hart, A. (2002). Relationships among lifting ability, grip force, and return to work. Physical Therapy, 82, 249–256.

Matheson, L.N., Mooney, V., Grant, J., Leggett, S. and Kenny, K. (1996) Standardized evaluation of work capacity. Journal of Back and Musculoskeletal Rehabilitation, 6, 249–264.

Matheson L.N., Rogers, L.C., Kaskutas, V. and Dakos, M. (2002). Reliability and reactivity of three new functional assessment measures. Work. A Journal of Prevention, Assessment and Rehabilitation, 18, 41–50.

Mathiowetz, V., Volland, G., Kashman, N. and Weber, K. (1985a). Adult norms for the Box and Block Test of manual dexterity. American Journal of Occupational Therapy, 39, 386–391.

Mathiowetz, V., Weber K., Kashman, N. and Volland, G. (1985b). Adult norms for the Nine Hole Peg Test of finger dexterity. Occupational Therapy Journal of Research, 5, 24–38.

McClure, P. (2000). The degenerative cervical spine: Pathogenesis and rehabilitation concepts. Journal of Hand Therapy, 13, 163–174.

McCormack, G.L. (2003). Pain control. In J. Carlson (Ed.), Complementary Therapies and Wellness: Practical Essentials for Holistic Health Care (pp. 304–313). Upper Saddle River, NJ: Prentice Hall.

Medical Multimedia Group (1999–2005). Patient education cumulative trauma disorders TOC. [On-line]. Available at http://www.medicalmultimediagroup.com/pated/ctd.html

Melzak, R. (1987). The short-form of the McGill Pain Questionnaire. Pain, 30, 191–197.

Miranda, H., Viikari-Juntura E., Martikainen, R., Takala, E.P. and Riihimaki, H. (2002). Individual factors, occupational loading, and physical exercise as predictors of sciatic pain. Spine, 15, 1102–1109.

Montgomery, H. and Johansson, U.S. (1988). Life values: Their structure and relation to life situations. Göteborg: University of Goteborg, Department of Psychiatry.

MVP Physical Therapy Orthopedic and Sports Rehabilitation (nd). Physical therapy rehabilitation in the South Puget Sound Region of the Pacific Northwest. Retrieved 10 March 2005, http://www.mvppt.com/special_programmes_industrial_rehab.htm

National Institute of Occupational Safety and Health (NIOSH) (1997). Carpal tunnel syndrome. [Fact Sheet. Document #705001]. Retrieved 5 March 2005, http://www.cdc.gov/niosh/ctsfs.html

National Institute of Occupational Safety and Health (NIOSH) (1998). National occupational research agenda [NORA]: Low back disorders. Retrieved 5 March 2005, http://www.cdc.gov/niosh/nrlowbck.html#top

National Institutes of Health (NIH) (1997). Research on low back pain and common spinal disorders. (PA Number PA-97-058). NIH Guide, 26(16). Retrieved 5 March 2005, http://grants.nih.gov/grants/guide/pa-files/PA-97-058.html

Neff, W.S. (1985). Work and Human Behavior (3rd edn). New York: Aldine de Gruyter.

Niemeyer, L., Jacobs, K., Reynolds-Lynch, K., Bettencourt, C. and Lang, S. (1994). Work hardening: Past, present, and future – The work programmes special interest section national work-hardening outcome study. American Journal of Occupational Therapy, 48, 327–339.

Norris, R.N. (1996). Return to play after injury: Strategies to support a musician recovery. Work. A Journal of Prevention, Assessment and Rehabilitation, 7, 89–93.

Occupational Safety and Health Administration (OSHA) (nd). OSHA ergonomic solutions: Computer stations e-tools. Index for computer workstations. Retrieved 5 March 2005, http://www.osha.gov/SLTC/etools/computerworkstations/positions.html

O'Connor, D., Marshall, S. and Massy-Westropp, N. (2003). Non-surgical treatment (other than steroid injection) for carpal tunnel syndrome. Cochrane Database of Systematic Reviews 1:CD003219

Ogden-Niemeyer, L. and Jacobs, K. (1989). Work Hardening. State of the Art. Thorofare: SLACK.

Park H., Sprince N.L., Whitten P.S., Burmeister L.F. and Zwerling, C. (2001) Risk factors for back pain among male farmers: Analysis of Iowa farm family health and hazard surveillance study. American Journal of Industrial Medicine, 40, 646–654.

Pascarelli, E.F. and Hsu, Y.P. (2001). Understanding work-related upper extremity disorders: Clinical findings in 485 computer users, musicians, and others. Journal of Occupational Rehabilitation, 11, 1–21.

Pascarelli, E.F. and Quilter, D. (1992). Repetitive Strain Injuries: A Computer Users' Guide. New York: John Wiley.

Pheasant, S. (1986). Body Space. London: Taylor & Francis.

Pope, M.H. (1989). Risk indicators in low back pain. Annals of Medicine, 21, 387–392.

Pope, M.H., Goh, K.L. and Magnusson, M.L. (2002). Spine economics. Annual Review of Biomedical Engineering, 4, 49–68.

Power, P.W. (2000). A Guide to Vocational Assessment (3rd edn). Austin: ProEd.

Pransky, G., Benjamin, K., Hill-Fotouh, C., Fletcher, K.F., Himmelstein, J. and Katz, J.N. (2002). Work-related outcomes in occupational low back pain: A multidimensional analysis. Spine, 27, 864–870.

Quittan, M. (2002). Management of Back Pain. Disability and Rehabilitation, 24, 423–434.

Reneman, M.F., Brouwer, S., Meinema, A., Dijkstra, P.U., Geertzen, J.H. and Groothoff, J.W. (2004). Test–retest reliability of the Isernhagen Work Systems Functional Capacity Evaluation in healthy adults. Journal of Occupational Rehabilitation, 14, 295–305.

Robert, J.J., Blide, R.W., McWhorter, K. and Coursey, C. (1995). The effects of a work hardening programme on cardiovascular fitness and muscular strength. Spine, 20, 1187–1193.

Roberts, J.R. (1969). Pennsylvania Bimanual Work Sample. Circle Pines, MN: American Guidance Service.

Samson, M.M., Meeuwsen, I.B.A., Crowe, A., Dessens, J.A.G., Duursma, S.A. and Verhaar, H.J.J. (2000). Relationships between physical performance measures, age, height and body weight in healthy adults. Age and Aging, 29, 235–242.

Saunders, R. (1997). Work hardening: Getting the injured patient back to work: Psychosocial counseling and job simulation are key aspects. . . Eighth in a special series. Journal of Musculoskeletal Medicine, 14, 14–18.

Schultz, I.Z., Crook, J., Fraser, K. and Joy, P.W. (2000). Models of diagnosis and rehabilitation in musculoskeletal pain-related occupational disability. Journal of Occupational Rehabilitation, 10, 271–293.

Schwartz, M.S. and Kelly, M.F. (1995). Raynaud's Disease: Selected issues and considerations in using biofeedback therapies. In M.S. Schwartz and Associates, Biofeedback: A Practitioner's Guide (2nd edn; pp. 429–444). New York: Guilford.

Scully Palmer, C. (2000). Outcome study: An industrial rehabilitation programme. Work. A Journal of Prevention Assessment and Rehabilitation, 15, 21–23.

Smith S.L. and Baxter-Petralia, P. (1992). The Physical Capacities Evaluation: Its Use in Four Models of Clinical Practice. Baltimore: Chess.

Smith, P., Kendall, L. and Hulin, C. (1996). The Measurement of Satisfaction in Work and Retirement. Chicago,IL: Rand-McNally.

Söderback, I. (1988). A housework-based assessment of intellectual functions in patients with acquired brain damage. Development and evaluation of an occupational therapy method. Scandanavian Journal of Rehabilitation Medicine, 20, 57–69.

Söderback, I. (1999). Validation of the theory: Satisfaction with time delimited daily occupations. Work. A Journal of Prevention, Assessment and Rehabilitation, 12, 165–174.

Söderback, I. (2001). Klarar du jobbet? Undersökning av arbetsförmåga. [Do your job skills meet the job requirements? Scientific investigation of people's vocational capacity]. Svensk Rehabilitering, 2001, 23–25.

Söderback, I., Pekkanen, K., Ekholm, J. and Schüldt, K. (1993). Occupational therapy work training programmes for the brain-damaged individuals. A Swedish programme. Work. A Journal of Prevention, Assessment and Rehabilitation, 3, 37–47.

Söderback, I., Schult, M.-L. and Jacobs, K. (2000). A criterion-referenced multidimensional job-related model prediction capability to perform occupations among persons with chronic pain. Work. A Journal of Prevention, Assessment and Rehabilitation, 15, 25–39.

Spradley, J.P. (1980). Participant Observation. New York: Holt, Rineholt and Winston.

Staal, J.B., Hlobil, H., van Tulder, M.W., Koke, A.J., Smid, T. and van Mechelen, W. (2002). Return-to-work interventions for low back pain: A descriptive review of contents and concepts of working mechanisms. Sports Medicine, 32, 251–267.

Stein, F. (1968). Consistency of cognitive, interest personality variables with academic mastery. Unpublished doctoral dissertation, New York University, New York.

Stein, F. and Associates (2003). Stress Management Questionnaire: An Instrument for Self-regulating Stress. [Individual Version. CD-Rom]. New York: Thomson/ Delmar Learning.

Stein, F. and Cutler, S.K. (2000). Clinical Research in Occupational Therapy (4th edn). San Diego: Singular Publishing Group/Thomson Learning.

Stumpf, B., Chadwick, D. and Dowell, B. (2001) The Anthropometrics of Fit: Ergonomic Criteria for the Design of a New Work Chair. Zeeland, MI: Herman Miller.

Super, D.E. (1957). The Psychology of Careers. New York: Harper & Row.

Synnerholm, M., Karlsson, E. and Söderback, I. (1995). Stanna hemma eller gå till jobbet? Om skälen bakom kort sjukfrånvaro [Stay at home or go to work? Reasons for being on short-time sick list.] (In Swedish). [Report No. 1995:3]. Stockholm, Sweden: Östersund: Enheten för Socialförsäkringsfors-kning (Division of Social Insurance Research).

Talo, S., Rytokoski, U., Hamalainen, A. and Kallio, V. (1996). The biopsychosocial disease consequence model in rehabilitation: model development in the Finnish 'work hardening' programme for chronic pain. International Journal of Rehabilitation Research, 19, 93–109.

Tetro A.M. and Pichora D.R. (1996). Cubital tunnel syndrome and the painful upper extremity. Hand Clinics, 12, 665–677.

Tiffin, J. (1948). Purdue Pegboard. Rosemont, IL: London House.

Tramposh, A.K. (1996). Job simulation. In G. Key (Ed.), Industrial Therapy (pp. 315–341). St. Louis: Mosby.

US Department of Labor (1985). Manual for the USES General Aptitude Test Battery [GATB]. Reliability and comparability, Form C and D. Washington, DC: US Government Printing Office.

US Department of Labor, Employment and Training Administration (1972) Handbook for Analyzing Jobs. Manpower Administration, Washington, DC: Government Printing Office.

US Department of Labor, Employment and Training Administration (1991a). Dictionary of Occupational Titles (4th edn). Washington, DC: US Government Printing Office. Available at http://www.oalj.dol.gov/libdot.htm

US Department of Labor, Employment and Training Administration (1991b). The Revised Handbook for Analyzing Jobs. Indianapolis: JIST Works.

Valpar International Corporation (1993). Valpar Component Work Samples. Tucson, AZ: Valpar International Corporation.

VALPAR International Corporation (1999–2005). VALPAR Component Work Samples (VCWS). Tucson: VALPAR Inc. Retrieved 12 March 2005, http://www.valparint.com/

van Tulder, M.W. (2001). Treatment of low back pain: Myths and facts. Schmerz, 6, 499–503.

Voaklander, D.C., Beaulne, A.P. and Lessard, R.A. (1995). Factors related to outcome following a work hardening programme. Journal of Occupational Rehabilitation, 5, 72–85.

Warren, N. (2001). Work stress and musculoskeletal disorder etiology: The relative roles of psychosocial and physical risk factors. Work. A Journal of Prevention, Assessment and Rehabilitation, 17, 221–234.

Wehman, P. and Sherron, P. (1995). Off to Work: A Vocational Curriculum for Individuals with Neurological Impairment. Verona, WI: Attainment Co.

Weir, R. and Nielson, W.R. (2001). Interventions for disability management. Clinical Journal of Pain, 17, 128–132.

Wiegmann, S.M. and Berven, N.L. (1998). Health locus-of-control beliefs and improvement in physical functioning in a work-hardening, return-to-work programme. Rehabilitation Psychology, 43, 83–100.

Wilbourn, A.J. (1999). Thoracic outlet syndromes. Neurolologic Clinics, 17, 477–497.

Winniford, M.D, Jansen, D.E, Reynolds, G.A, Apprill, P., Black, W.H. and Hillis, L.D. (1987). Cigarette smoking-induced coronary vasoconstriction in atherosclerotic coronary artery disease and prevention by calcium antagonists and nitroglycerin. American Journal of Cardiology, 59, 203–207.

Wyman, D.O. (1999). Evaluating patients for return to work. American Family Physician, 59, 844–848.

Yip, Y. (2001). A study of work, stress, patient handling activities and the risk of low back pain. Journal of Advanced Nursing, 36, 794–804.

Zeller, J., Sturm, G. and Cruse, C.W. (1993). Patients with burns are successful in work hardening programmes. Journal of Burn Care and Rehabilitation, 14, 189–196.

CHAPTER 6

Occupational stress in the workplace

Contending with stressful situations in the workplace is a common occurrence for all health care providers. Stress has numerous devastating effects on the workplace environment, as well as upon individuals who become victims of stress. However, enhancing psychological hardiness may facilitate an individual's ability to deal with workplace stress. Psychological hardiness, a personality style consisting of commitment, control and challenge, encourages human survival and the enrichment of life through development.

Lambert et al., 2003, p. 181

Learning objectives

By the end of this chapter the learner will:

1 Understand the overall problem of occupational stress in the work environment.
2 Define occupational stress.
3 Understand the relationship between occupational stress and occupational injuries.
4 Identify potential factors in the workplace that can cause occupational stress.
5 Understand the relationship between occupational stress and the onset of disease.
6 Identify how workers can deal effectively with occupational stress.
7 Identify strategies to prevent occupational stress.
8 Design a stress management programme in the workplace.

Introduction to occupational stress

How many of the injuries and diseases experienced by workers are related to occupational stress? In a widely publicized large-scale national study in the USA, the Northwestern National Life Insurance Company in 1992, found that seven out of ten workers felt that job stress contributes to health disorders and interfered with their work output. Forty-six per cent of those surveyed indicated that their job was very stressful and many thought about leaving their jobs because of the stress on the job (Northwestern National Life Insurance Company, 1992). An abundance of research studies demonstrate a significant need to reduce stress in the workplace. Stress in general, and occupational stress in particular, is of epidemic proportions in the industrialized countries of the world. A study in Japan found that the percentage of employees with work-related stress increased dramatically from 1982 to 1992 (Shimizu et al., 1997).

Research on stress and its relationship to precipitating specific health disorders has increased since the early 1990s. For example, occupational stress can be a significant risk factor in contributing to low back pain (Feyer et al., 2000; Papageorgiou et al., 1997), cardiovascular disease (Belkic et al., 2004; Rozanski et al., 1999; Suurnakki et al., 1987), myocardial infarction (Hammar et al., 1998; Moller et al., 2005), mental health problems (Mino et al., 1999) and burn-out (Faragher et al., 2005), as well as contributing to violence in the workplace (Anderson, 2004; Firth-Cozens, 2000; Sharif, 2000) and lowering worker productivity (Holmes, 2001).

Papageorgiou et al. (1997), using a mail survey in which 4501 workers responded, found that dissatisfaction with work was associated with low back pain. Job dissatisfaction can result from occupational stress and has been shown to be a significant factor in worker absences and sick leave. Physical factors in the environment can also contribute to worker dissatisfaction and occupational stress. Woo et al. (1999) examined the relationship between stress and absenteeism and found that civil service workers were more likely to take medical leave when (a) lighting is poor; (b) temperatures are uncomfortable; (c) the workload is heavy; or (d) heightened psychological tension is present. When psychosocial stressors were intensified in the workplace, workers also tended to report more minor illnesses. In addition, Swaen et al. (2004) concluded that 'that high psychologic job demands, emotional demands, and conflicts with the supervisor and/or colleagues are risk factors for being injured in an occupational accident' (p. 521).

Occupational stress is a worldwide problem. According to a 2003 report from the Health and Safety Executive (HSE) by the Institute for Employment Studies (IES):

> The UK has one of the worst records in Europe for the return of employees to work after long-term illness, and over the last six years there has been a rapid increase in the numbers of people who report they are experiencing stress. The most recent figures from the HSE show that over half a million people said they were affected by stress at work and that 13.4 million working days were lost due to stress and related conditions. The average time taken off by workers as a result of stress is estimated at 29 days a year.
>
> Institute for Employment Studies, 2003, para 1

Further, the most stressful jobs in Britain as reported by the Health and Safety Executive (Smith et al., 2000) were management, teaching, nursing, security and road transport.

Definition of occupational stress

How is occupational stress defined? Occupational stress is the cumulative pressure in the workplace that causes psychophysiological symptoms and vulnerabilities to work injuries and disease (Stein and Cutler, 2001). In an earlier definition, Joseph LaDou (1980) defined occupational stress as 'the sum of the factors in the work environment that affect the psychological and physiologic homeostasis of the worker' (p. 197). In a more specific definition of stress, the University of Wales (nd) Health and Safety Committee defined 'work related stress as the "reaction people have to excessive demands or pressures, arising when people try to cope with tasks, responsibilities or other types of pressure connected with their jobs, but find difficulty, strain or worry in doing so"' (p. 1). Many similar definitions of occupational stress can be found in the literature. Essentially all the definitions implicate specific stressors in the work environment that trigger psychological and physiological symptoms or discomfort.

Stress in general may be interpreted on a continuum from 'eustress' to excessive stress. A moderate degree of stress can be positive and motivate the worker to be productive. Eustress, or mild stress, was initially identified by Selye (1974) as positive stress that can motivate an individual to perform or exert his or her best efforts. In these situations, stress acts as a motivating force, helping the individual to be productive and meet employer demands (e.g. meeting deadlines and production standards). Another example is the musician performing in a concert. In this case the musician is under pressure to perform at his or her best while demonstrating musical talent. On the other hand, excessive stress in the workplace can be experienced when unrealistic demands are made on the worker. In those situations, the worker may not feel competent to complete a task or may feel a lack of control in making decisions. There is a fine line between eustress perceived by the worker or employer as motivating and which results in increased productivity, and occupational stress that is debilitating to the worker and causes health problems, lower productivity, worker absences or vulnerability to job-related accidents.

Occupational stressors

Organizational causes of occupational stress

As well as creating illness and vulnerability for injury in the worker, excessive stress can lead to poor quality of products. McLean (1987) identified

five organizational issues in the workplace that can produce occupational stress and result in a company breakdown and low employee morale.
These interactional factors between the employer and the employee
demonstrate how organizational policies, downturns in the economy and
societal demands can increase worker stress:

1 *High demands and low control are often associated with higher
   levels of strain and distress.* The Demand, Control, Support Model
   proposed by Karasek and colleagues (Karasek, 1979; Karasek and
   Theorell, 1990; Karasek et al., 1998) examines the relationship
   between the worker and his or her environment and the interaction of
   job demands, decision-making and social support. Individuals in high-
   demand jobs who perceive themselves as having little control or
   support are considered to be at high risk of developing stress. This can
   occur, for example, in a hospital where nurses are expected to be
   responsible for patient care but are not given the authority to change
   the care plan when they think it is necessary. The nurse who is responsible for a patient's care usually carries out the orders from the
   physician, but often is not given the opportunity to provide suggestions for changing the patient's care plan. High demands are placed on
   the nurse in this situation while permitting only minimal control of the
   overall patient treatment plan. In another example, workers are given
   responsibilities for assembling parts of a product without allowing
   them to see the finished product or giving credit for the quality of the
   finished product. In this situation the worker feels alienated because of
   a lack of control over the finished product. On the other hand, situations where the workers' perceive themselves as having a high rate of
   job demands along with high decision-making may positively influence
   job motivation, new learning behaviours and coping patterns
   (Theorell, 1997).
2 *Stress is cumulative, additive and interactive.* The stress in the workplace can be unrelenting, especially when there is a shortage of workers.
   In such instances the employer may rely on fewer workers to carry a
   larger proportion of the workload. This is especially true in agencies
   and companies where there is a high turnover of workers and the
   remaining workers have to carry the heavy load. For example, in a city
   welfare office where social workers are assigned a formulated case
   load, the case load can be increased if a social worker leaves. The
   remaining workers have to carry the worker's load until a new social
   worker is hired. The stress in this type of situation is cumulative and
   becomes interactive when there are disputes between supervisors and
   employees. For example, during emergencies or periods of crises
   police or firefighters may be requested by city officials to work overtime. Conflicts may arise between management and personnel over the
   amount of time worked and the additional compensation for overtime.
   Stress is heightened during periods of turmoil. In another example,

during the 9/11 disaster in New York City the stress on the police and firefighters was extraordinary (Barry, 2002). Stress also increases in healthcare workers who enter the field expecting to spend most of their time helping patients. However, they become disillusioned when much of their time is spent in meetings and dealing with paperwork. The result is additional stress and burn-out (Griffin, 1992).

3 *The more a period of fear or uncertainty is prolonged, the greater the risk for psychosomatic illness and accidents.* During periods of high unemployment or economic downturns, many workers are fearful of being laid off from their jobs. This creates uncertainty and insecurity in the workers. This insecurity in turn can produce stressful reactions leading to illnesses. Employers can also create internal fears or uncertainty in workers when employees are fired or asked to resign without due explanation.

4 *One's fears are often greater than the eventual reality; planning from a 'worst-case scenario' can allow the individual and the organization to capitalize on their creative energy.* For example, the undue stress in an organization when there is a threat of bankruptcy can initially motivate personnel to become more efficient and cost-effective. However, the employers and employees know that if the company does not make positive changes, the company will fail and the employees will lose their jobs. The initial phases of the stress can be positive because the staff are motivated to find creative solutions. If the solutions do not result in positive change, the stress can be destructive and lead to panic among the workers.

5 *It is not the situation itself but the perception of the situation that determines one's response.* When a company is under investigation, such as in the Enron scandal in 2002 (Teather, 2003), rumours become rampant and the employees' uncertainty creates distrust and stress. In the Enron example the perception in the newspapers was that the company would fail and all the employees would lose their jobs. The reality was that the company remained in business and the employees indicted were the top administrators. Stress is heightened in organizations when there is change such as business mergers or administrative reorganization, and when the administrators do not readily share information with the staff.

As can be seen, organizational policies and unexpected events can cause occupational stress. However, there are positive strategies that companies can use to reduce or prevent job stress (McLean, 1987). They are:

• *The broader the sense of ownership of an organization's problems and responsibility for resolution, the more likely is a positive outcome.* For example, when employees are given the opportunity for input into company policies and work procedures, a more positive psychological environment is created for problem-solving and joint decision-making.

Collaborative efforts between management and unions result in 'win-win' situations such as 'Quality Circles'. Quality Circles are defined as 'a group of staff who meet regularly to discuss quality-related work problems so that they may examine and generate solutions to these' (Jarvis, nd, para 3). The concept of Quality Circles was first pioneered by the Japanese car manufacturer Honda as a way to increase worker input into the design and manufacture of the product. The concept of Quality Circles has been expanded to health care. In a related article Lee et al. (2000) reported the successful application of Quality Circles in improving job satisfaction, and reducing absenteeism and turnover among nurses.

- *Structured group sessions during times of change and crisis can have positive and long-term effects on both the individual participants and the work organization.* A good example of how organizations can respond to economic down-periods is the case of American automobile makers during the 1980s. During the 1960s and 1970s, Japanese-built automobiles gained an excellent reputation for quality and full efficiency among American buyers. This resulted in economic gains for Japanese automobile companies and dramatically declining sales and profits for American automobile manufacturers. The big three American automobile makers (Ford, General Motors and Chrysler) decided to make drastic changes to the way cars were produced. The reactions from management and workers were unanimous in changing the way business was done. Management brought in representatives from the United Auto Workers union to help change the attitudes of workers, to build trust among the workers and to begin thinking creatively about effective changes in the production methods. The result was that employees' attitudes became more positive, the quality of the automobile improved and sales increased. In this situation, employee stress, which had initially led to burn-out and caused sloppy work and poor quality control was changed by management and worker cooperation (UAW-Ford National Joint Committee on Health and Safety, 1996).

Occupational stressors

In a summary statement of the causes of occupational stress, the New South Wales (Australia) Public Employment Office (2003) identified the following factors in the work environment that increase the chances of stress:

- poor management of occupational health safety and rehabilitation
- poor work organization
- inadequate staffing levels
- excessive individual workload
- unsafe work practices

- excessive working hours
- unsafe systems of work
- poor working conditions
- occupational violence including sexual and other forms of work related harassment, victimization, bullying or aggressive behaviour at work (p. 2, #2).

Kahn (1987) classified occupational stressors into nine general categories; (1) job loss or threatened job loss, resulting in vulnerability to psychological depression; (2) specific occupations that are intrinsically vulnerable to stress by the nature of their work (e.g. firefighters, bus drivers, air traffic controllers, miners and police); (3) intrinsic properties of work tasks, such as prolonged manual handling and lifting, inputting data into a computer without rest breaks, or working on a tractor without protection from the sun; (4) role characteristics where the manager is continually making quick decisions under time demands; (5) adversarial interpersonal relationships causing continual conflict, such as workers in competition for the same job or irreconcilable personality differences; (6) lack of resources or proper equipment ignored by management and causing worker burn-out; (7) work schedules that are disruptive due to shift work or continuous demands for the worker to work overtime; (8) lack of organizational support, with workers' suggestions for improving the psychological climate of the corporation being ignored and no recognition being given to the workers for a job well done; and (9) organizations that create a 'type A' atmosphere and sharp competition between workers. All of these general factors contribute to a stressful work environment.

In a related study, Stein et al. (1999) identified specific types of stressors that trigger psycho-physiological symptoms. They are categorized as (a) *interpersonal* – for example, arguments with fellow workers; (b) *intrapersonal* – having feelings of inadequacy on the job; (c) *time demands* – too many deadlines and work demands without sufficient time; (d) *mechanical breakdown* – tools and equipment at work that fail and create further problems; (e) *performance demands* – inability to keep up with the employer's expectations; (f) *financial pressures* – salary or hourly wages do not meet current expenses and/or cost of living increases; (g) *illness* – work-related illness causes absenteeism, further exacerbating stress resulting in a vicious cycle of stress → illness → absenteeism → further stress → . . .; (h) *environmental disturbances* – characterized by excessive noise, congestion, poor lighting; and (i) *complex situations*, such as sexual harassment or racial, religious or ethnic discrimination. Each of these factors can increase the stress level on the job and cause physical and psychological symptoms. Both the employer and the worker benefit from the economic viability of a company; however, unless an adequate number of personnel are employed to do a job, the worker may be stretched thin and under continual pressure to be more productive. If extensive pressure is put on the worker, the result can be severe stress and burn-out. Standards established by the employer and governmental agencies can sometimes create an adversarial relationship between the employer and the worker, resulting in tension and added occupational stress. The most harmonious work environment is where the employer and employee reach a level where the work is challenging and the employer makes a profit.

Other factors related to occupational stress

The worker's lifestyle can also be a positive or negative factor in occupational stress. Stress that arises off the job such as in family conflicts, financial difficulties, problems with raising children and a lifestyle of inactivity can also affect the worker's job performance. These negative factors can be carried into the workplace and add to existing stress causing additional symptoms (Blom et al., 2003). On the other hand, positive control of one's lifestyle can aid the worker in coping with stress on the job.

Often it is difficult to separate out the stress originating in the family from occupational stress; however, the combination of personal problems and job stresses increase the likelihood of physical and emotional symptoms. An individual prone to drug and alcohol abuse is further at risk in developing job-related stress, especially when there is no direct intervention or counselling. Stress, as an aversive factor in the individual, can originate internally (e.g. feeling incapable of completing a job) or externally (e.g. too much to do in too little time).

The effect of stressors on the body

In general, the body reacts to extreme stressors by stimulating the production of adrenaline which increases heart rate, blood pressure, perspiration and muscle tone, while slowing down digestion as in a 'fight or flight' response (Cannon, 1939). Stress directly affects the autonomic nervous system, which is in a continual state of change. When an individual is under extreme pressure or stress the sympathetic nervous system mobilizes into action and stimulates the secretion of hormones and the release of neurotransmitters that produce strong responses and a heightened state of arousal as if it were under attack. Selye (1956) identified the physiological responses to stress as the General Adaptation Response (GAS) and stated, 'The G.A.S. consists of three stages: the alarm reaction, the stage of resistance, and the stage of exhaustion' (Selye, 1956, p. 64). While working with an animal model, Selye (1956) found that the pituitary and adrenal glands played an important role in the stress response by triggering the mechanisms that increased the body's arousal. If this response is too intense or prolonged it can lead to psychophysiological symptoms or adverse reactions. Severe stress can also impair one's thinking and disrupt cognitive processing such as in remembering and retrieving information (Sapolsky, 1998). Prolonged and severe stress has been well documented and shown to precipitate symptoms of depression (Day, 1998), coronary heart disease (Rozanski et al., 1999), inhibition of the immune system (Kemeny and Grunewald, 1999), stroke (Bowler, 2001), anxiety (Leonard and Song, 1996), gastrointestinal diseases (Collins, 2001), mental exhaustion (Faragher et al., 2005) and other illnesses and diseases.

Stress, a mind–body interaction, is a total response of the individual to cope with the everyday demands of living. In general, stress can be mild, moderate or severe. The ability to tolerate high amounts of stress is related to one's use of coping strategies and personal resources to manage stress. Some individuals with a high tolerance for stress can self-regulate their stress through coping activities such as exercise and meditation. Other individuals are more vulnerable to stress, where even mild stress may trigger psychophysiological symptoms. The ability to self-regulate stress has been defined as hardiness (Huang, 1995). An employee's ability to use coping strategies at work (e.g. his or her reactions to unfair treatment or to a personal conflict at the workplace) can be obtained by using a coping behaviour questionnaire (Schult, 2002). Stress management programmes that teach an individual relaxation techniques increase an individual's reliance on one's self.

Implementing stress management programmes in the workplace

Coping with stress in the workplace

In general, health and safety programmes and employee assistance programmes are the first lines of defence in reducing occupational stress. These programmes have been shown to be effective and can reduce or prevent employee absences, job burn-out and job-related accidents. An employer occupational health programme is an investment that is cost-effective for both the employer and the worker. Savings occur in worker's compensation awards, while increasing work production.

The active participation of the worker is vital in eliminating or reducing lifestyle risk factors. Compliance and motivation are key factors in the success of an occupational and safety programme. An occupational health programme typically includes exercise training, nutrition information, weight control, stress management, smoking cessation, and alcohol and drug counselling. Relaxation therapy, prescriptive exercise, biofeedback, meditation and visualization may also be included (Stein and Associates, 2003; Stein and Cutler, 2001; Stein and Nikolic, 1989; Stein and Smith, 1989). Management of occupational stress by an occupational therapist, psychologist or other health professional helps the worker to incorporate stress management techniques into everyday life (Stein, 2003).

When designing a stress management programme in the workplace, it is important for the therapist to consider the individual factors that can interfere with a worker's compliance. The primary principle of a stress management programme is to develop coping mechanisms for each individual based on one's lifestyle, interests and daily patterns of activity. A stress management instrument identifying stressors, symptoms and coping activities can be helpful in developing an individualized stress management programme (Stein and Associates, 2003).

Murphy (1996) critically reviewed 64 published studies on the effects of stress management programmes in the workplace. The investigator concluded that muscle relaxation, meditation, biofeedback and teaching of cognitive-behavioural skills were the most frequently used methods comprising stress management programmes in the workplace. In general, stress management in the workplace can positively affect the worker's physical and psychological health.

Strategies to implement an occupational stress management programme

Work-site stress management programmes have been shown to be effective in reducing health problems such as hypertension and depression, decreasing absenteeism and accidents and increasing job performance and job satisfaction. Ivancevich et al. (1990) found that stress management interventions in the workplace can be divided into three areas: individual, organizational and individual/organizational interface.

Individual stress management interventions include (a) techniques such as meditation, exercise, relaxation and cognitive approaches; (b) goal-setting to help the worker set realistic goals about promotion and advancement in the company; and (c) time management to enable the worker to be more efficient and reduce the pressure to produce.

Organizational interventions in the workplace include (a) organizational structure such as modifying responsibilities and the decision-making process in a company; (b) job redesign to reduce job stress; (c) selection and placement resulting in fitting the worker to a job compatible with skills and interests; and (d) improvement of working conditions and provision of in-service training and development, including upgrading the worker's skills and knowledge to keep abreast with new technology.

Interface interventions involve the cooperation of the employer, worker and union organization in developing intervention programmes acceptable to each party. *Job demands–person style fit* is organized to fit the worker to a job that best meets the need of the company. Ideally the worker's skills and education are used maximally so that the company benefits from the worker's expertise. *Participation preferences–practices* imply that the workers have input into the way the work is organized and the product manufactured. This may entail Quality Circles where workers discuss the most efficient way to manufacture a product so that the quality of the product increases and the costs are kept down. *Autonomy preferences–practices* allow the worker as much authority as possible in making decisions regarding individual workspaces and job descriptions. The worker's input into how the job is performed is respected and implemented by management. In many instances, the union will also reinforce the worker's recommendation for changes in the workplace or the introduction of new tools or equipment.

Improvement of co-worker relationships can be accomplished in the workplace by having workers work in teams in a cooperative way. Two ways to do this include teams of workers who develop camaraderie by assembling an entire product, or establishment of focus groups to discuss interpersonal relationships and creation of a positive work environment. Workers can be educated to be supportive of each other and help in times of family crisis or need. The policy of allowing workers to donate sick leave to a fellow worker is a tangible way that management and workers can cooperate positively and improve the relationship between co-workers.

Further, Ivancevich et al. (1990) identified outcomes that resulted from these interventions. Individual interventions were related to decreases in blood pressure, anxiety, depression, somatic complaints and enhanced quality of life. Organizational interventions increased worker productivity, and reduced employee turnover, absenteeism, accidents on the job and healthcare costs. Individual/organizational interface interventions increased job performance, job satisfaction and healthcare utilization while decreasing employee burn-out.

Designing a stress management programme in the workplace

The general principles or strategies for developing a stress management programme are given below:

- Devise a stress management programme in consultation with the worker that is congruent with the worker's lifestyle and interests. For example, identify from the worker the mechanisms or coping activities that the worker finds effective in controlling or managing stress.
- Help the worker incorporate these mechanisms into his or her everyday schedule. Have individuals describe their time spent in working, commuting, leisure, rest and sleeping. Emphasize the importance of eight hours of sleep, eight hours of work and eight hours of leisure and self-care in managing stress.
- Encourage the individual to schedule a stress management activity at the same time each day (e.g. right before breakfast, during a work break or before dinner). An important component of every stress management programme is teaching the client to learn how to relax.
- Educate the worker to the concept of scheduling an activity or exercise by being aware of the frequency (how many days a week), intensity (mild, moderate, intense) and duration of the activity (15, 30 or 45 minutes).

• Assist the worker to set up a schedule that is relevant, meaningful and appropriate for accomplishing goals, and that is achievable. Incorporating daily activities that reduce tension, enhance self-esteem and increase coping mechanisms are facilitated by using a stress management programme that is holistic.
• Ask the worker to compile a list of stressors that trigger symptoms of stress. Examples might include disagreements with fellow workers or the supervisor, unreasonable job demands or commuting long distances.
• Assist the worker to become aware of the symptoms of occupational stress (e.g. headaches, back pain, anxiety or insomnia).
• Have the worker keep a daily log of stress management activities (e.g. exercise, meditation, music), and identify how these mechanisms affect mood, energy level and overall feelings of health.
• Encourage the worker to employ stress management techniques in increments. For example, the worker might begin with five or ten minutes of restful sitting, eventually increasing this activity to a half hour.
• Help the worker identify a quiet unobtrusive environment to carry out the relaxation exercises.

Identifying the components of a stress management programme in the workplace

Risk counselling is one type of therapeutic intervention that can be used in the workplace (Maddocks, 2000). Risk counselling involves an interview with the worker to identify the sources of stress, symptoms and coping mechanisms in order to design an individualized stress management programme. The following questions, discussed with the worker, may be helpful when designing such a programme:

• *What are the job stressors, how severe are they and how frequently do they occur?* Job stressors can directly be experienced on the job such as an overload in work demands. The stressor can be mild, moderate or severe, and can occur hourly, daily or weekly. There are a number of tests that can be used in assessing stressors, including the Stress Management Questionnaire (SMQ) (Stein and Associates, 2003), the Stress Audit (Miller and Smith, 1994); and the StressMap (Essi Systems, 1991). The SMQ was first developed in 1986 as a paper-and-pencil test to help the client identify the symptoms in their life, stressors that trigger symptoms and the coping activities that manage stress. The SMQ is based on a client-centred model where the client develops their own stress management programme based on an evaluation of his or her ability to manage stress. An individual version of the SMQ has been developed where the therapist administers cards to the client to sort.

This version of the SMQ, The Sorting Out Stress Cards (Stein et al., 2003) has been tested successfully for reliability with 80 clients.

- *What are the personal stressors outside the work environment?* Personal stressors are experienced outside of the work environment, and may include death of a spouse, divorce, family problems, financial difficulties or social conflicts. In assessing personal stressors, The Survey of Recent Life Experiences (Kohn and Macdonald, 1992), The Social Readjustment Rating Scale (Holmes and Rahe, 1967) and The Life Value Questionnaire (Montgomery et al., 1996) are appropriate tools. The health professional should separate out those job stressors directly related to the job and personal stressors outside the job environment.

- *What are the symptoms of job stress, personal stress carried into the job and the interaction of these stressors?* Symptoms can be classified into (a) physical symptoms, such as headaches, back pain or stomach pain; (b) cognitive symptoms, such as difficulty concentrating or making decisions; (c) emotional symptoms, such as depression or anxiety; and (d) behavioural symptoms, such as insomnia or eating disorders.

- *What are the coping skills and personal resources used by the employee in dealing with stress?* How an individual responds to stress and the coping behaviours used can be either adaptive or maladaptive. Examples of maladaptive coping behaviour are smoking, over-consumption of alcohol, excessive eating, abusing others or obsessive gambling. On the other hand, positive behaviours include the use of a daily exercise programme, relaxation therapies, soliciting support from family members, friends and colleagues, listening to music and seeking personal counselling.

- *What is the lifestyle balance of the person experiencing stress?* Does the individual keep a balance of rest, work and leisure activities? The person with symptoms of occupational stress may have a long and arduous commute to and from work, may be working on a split shift that interferes with the circadian rhythm and sleep cycle, or may be moonlighting on a second job that deprives the individual of sufficient rest.

- *What is the plan to reduce the job stress, decrease the symptoms of stress and to increase the coping mechanisms in the person's life?* A plan should be devised in conjunction with the worker, and in some cases with the family, that is realistic, feasible and attainable.

- *What is the commitment of management and the employers to reduce occupational stress?* Any plan to reduce stress in the workplace should receive the approval of the employer and supervisors. Although the details of dealing individually with the worker should remain confidential, the employer should be informed of the general factors that contribute to occupational stress in the workplace and the therapeutic interventions that are recommended.

Stress management in the workplace

A stress management programme in the workplace can help workers to better deal with everyday hassles and gain control over stress-related health problems. Randolfi (1997) describes how a stress management centre 'can be situated within an employee assistance program, a work-site medical facility, or adjacent to a fitness facility' (p. 43). He recommends that the facility include a computer system with Internet access and stress assessment software, self-help instructional video, audio tapes and books, biofeedback equipment, reclining lounge chair, massage table, light-sound machines that create flashing lights and relaxing repetitive sounds, a stereo system with headphones and accompanying relaxation tapes, and a flotation room where the person can float on their back in a ten-inch solution of warm water (94 degrees) and Epsom salts. Randolfi also recommends that the healthcare professional who manages the stress management and relaxation centre at the worksite be a health educator with a graduate degree and special training in stress management and health promotion. An occupational therapist with an MA and special training in biofeedback and relaxation techniques would be an appropriate individual for this position.

The rest of this chapter covers those specific interventions in the workplace that are designed to reduce occupational stress. Some of this material is adapted from: Stein (2001); Stein and Associates (2003); Stein and Cutler (2001).

Relaxation therapy

Relaxation therapy is a broad term encompassing many techniques that include meditation, relaxation exercises, progressive relaxation, visualization, biofeedback, music and any other means to help the person relax. The two major programmes related to psychological variables that have generated the most research are meditation and the relaxation response. Taylor (1995), in a study of a behavioural stress-management programme that included progressive muscle relaxation, biofeedback, meditation and hypnosis with individuals who were HIV positive, found in a controlled study that the experimental group, compared with a no treatment group, showed significant improvement in decreasing anxiety and increasing self-esteem and positive mood. T-cell count also improved. The investigators concluded that a stress-management programme with a meditation component is effective in treating individuals with HIV infection.

Meditation

Meditation can be defined as a self-directed practice for relaxing the body and calming the mind. Essentially, meditation is a learned and practised skill where the individual tries to create a calm inner peace by remaining still, concentrating on pleasant thoughts and eliminating the worries of the day. As a relaxation therapy, it can (a) beneficially influence the individual's mood (Teasdale et al., 1995); (b) increase the secretion of endorphins, which in effect can decrease pain and increase pleasure (Elias and Wilson, 1995); (c) increase T-cell counts and by so doing increase the effectiveness of the immune system (Taylor, 1995); (d) decrease heart rate (Telles et al., 1995); (e) reduce anxiety (Miller et al., 1995); and (f) decrease blood pressure (Wenneberg et al., 1997).

Meditation is a self-discipline skill where individuals can train themselves to relax and learn how to concentrate on one thing at a time. The person meditating makes a concentrated effort to focus on a single thought – peace, for instance; or a physical experience, such as breathing; or a sound (repeating a word or mantra, such as Om, or a Sanskrit word, such as krim). The aim is to still the mind's busyness – its inclination to mull over the worries, demands and details of everyday life. Meditation is an ancient practice that has roots in religious traditions and silent prayer. It has been part of almost every religion in the Eastern and Western cultures such as Judaism, Christianity, Moslem, Sufism, Japanese Zen, Chinese Tao, Hinduism and Buddhism. It has been adapted by modern practitioners and incorporated into stress management and cognitive-behavioural treatment programmes (Benson, 1975, 1979; Carrington, 1993; Glueck and Stroebel, 1975; Smith, 1986).

The basic principles of all types of meditation are to sit comfortably in a quiet room, close one's eyes or focus on a specific point, use abdominal breathing, concentrate on an inner process or visualize a pleasant scene and repeat an encouraging phrase to oneself (mantra) such as 'alert mind, calm body' (Stroebel, 1982). One aspect of meditation is to focus one's attention on a visual object such as a spot on a wall so as to clear one's mind of preoccupying worries or fears. Meditation in this case is a type of displacement of thoughts and feelings that are negative, such as anxiety and depression by substituting a calming influence. Meditation can also be used as a way of releasing attitudes to allow one's mind to wander freely. When one focuses on a point or visual stimulus in a room such as an object or piece of furniture, the individual assumes a non-judgemental or neutral attitude.

The effect of meditation on biological processes
Meditation appears to have a profound influence on the autonomic nervous system by producing a calming effect. What is the connection between meditation and the autonomic nervous system? Meditation works as an opposite effect of stress because it calms the body by producing a parasympathetic response in the ANS. The effect is to lower the heart rate, blood pressure and oxygen consumption, increase temperature in the extremities, slow brain waves and decrease muscle tension.

However, not all of the parasympathetic responses are in synch with the relaxation response. The complexity of the autonomic nervous system and its relationship to stress versus relaxation is the focus of much current research. The empirical research does support the general concept that meditation as a relaxation therapy has a beneficial effect on the autonomic nervous system in reducing the symptoms of stress (Everly and Benson, 1989). It has also been suggested by animal studies that there is a relationship between chronic stress and the hypothalamic-pituitary axis (Keller et al., 1988). If meditation is effective, it must have an influence on the complex mechanism involving the hypothalamus, adrenal glands, neurotransmitters and hippocampus in reducing the stress reaction (McEwen and Mendelson, 1993). In a three-year follow-up study, Miller et al. (1995) re-examined 18 participants out of an original group of 22 patients with a diagnosis of anxiety disorders. The patients had taken part in an eight-week outpatient group stress reduction intervention based on meditation training. They used standardized tests such as the Beck Depression Scale (Beck et al., 1961) and the Hamilton Scale (Hamilton, 1967) to measure improvement. Miller et al. (1995) concluded that meditation can have a long-term beneficial effect on individuals diagnosed with anxiety disorders and depression.

In a study on stress reduction through meditation, Astin (1997) examined the effects of an eight-week treatment programme for volunteer patients who experienced chronic pain. In a controlled study comparing an experimental and randomized, no-treatment, control group of 14 participants in each group, the investigators found the following:

> The techniques of mindfulness meditation, with the emphasis on developing detached observation and awareness of the contents of consciousness, may represent a powerful cognitive behavioural coping strategy for transforming the ways in which we respond to life events. They may also have potential for relapse prevention in affective disorders.
>
> Astin, 1997, p. 97

Gelderloos, Walton, Orme-Johnson and Alexander (1991) reviewed 24 studies on transcendental meditation in the prevention and treatment of individuals with substance abuse. They found that all of the studies of transcendental meditation showed positive effects. The effects included long-range improvements in well-being, self-esteem and personal empowerment.

In general meditation is a useful technique for an individual to use to reduce occupational stress. There is a large body of research that supports its use as a therapeutic intervention. In teaching workers to use meditation it is important to emphasize the need to incorporate meditation into one's everyday schedule and to adapt the actual meditation protocol to the needs of the worker. It has to be a meaningful and purposeful activity to the person if it is to be successful.

The relaxation response

Herbert Benson (1975; 1979), a cardiologist, developed the relaxation response from transcendental meditation which he studied in India. As a cardiologist he was interested in non-pharmacological treatments of hypertension. Benson was also interested in applying a behavioural medicine approach that emphasized the mind–body connection. The relaxation response was conceptualized to be a generalized approach to stress reduction that depresses sympathetic arousal and decreases the body's 'fight and flight' reactions. Stein and Smith (1989) adapted the Benson Relaxation Response as a clinical intervention that can be applied in the work setting to reduce stress. Stein incorporated the Quieting Reflex (Stroebel, 1982) into the relaxation protocol. The protocol is based on four simple steps that can be done in about five to ten minutes. Visualization and breathing exercises can also be combined with the relaxation response. The protocol is described below:

- In a quiet undisturbed environment or room, the person should sit in an upright chair with his or her feet planted on the floor without crossing the legs. The hands should be placed in the lap.
- In this position the individual closes their eyes and creates a quiet relaxed inner state of being.
- In this relaxed state the person repeats the phrase 'alert mind, calm body' (Glueck and Stroebel, 1975). The person can also substitute a prayer if that makes the person feel secure.
- In the fourth step the person takes a passive attitude and allows the mind to focus on pleasant thoughts or enjoyable scenes such as being by a lake. Another way for the person to create a relaxed state is to visualize the warmth of the body.

Progressive relaxation

Progressive relaxation was developed by Edmund Jacobson (1929), a physician who believed that muscle relaxation exercises are helpful in decreasing a person's anxiety and tension. He felt that prolonged anxiety and tension produces physical symptoms such as headaches, back pain, gastrointestinal disorders and cardiovascular disturbances. As a family practitioner, Jacobson used progressive relaxation successfully in treating patients. He felt strongly that if patients can learn how to relax they can reduce the symptoms of stress.

In applying progressive relaxation the person learns how to focus on tensing and relaxing muscle groups of the body. In this way the person reduces the anxiety and muscle tension caused by stress. The premise behind progressive relaxation is that there is a mind–body connection that affects overall health. The individual can do the progressive relaxation exercise by sitting in a chair or lying on their back. The basic pattern is to tense a muscle group such as the arms for about five seconds and then to let go and relax for about twenty seconds. By tensing their muscles the person begins to consciously control body tension and feel the difference between tenseness and relaxation. The person is cautioned not to flex any muscle too tightly so as to avoid muscle pain. If the person is sitting in a chair the person should be in an ergonomically neutral position with feet planted on the floor, back straight and head upright. The person can gently massage parts of the body that seem especially tight such as the back of the neck. When the person feels ready for the exercise they should close their eyes and begin the exercise progressively starting from the muscle groups in the feet and ankles then to the legs and knees, up to the thighs and hips, buttocks, stomach, chest, hands and fists, arms, shoulders, neck and face. Relaxing music such as Pachelbel's *Canon in D* or other baroque music such as pieces by Bach can be used in the background to create a pleasant emotional state.

There have been a number of research studies evaluating the effectiveness of progressive relaxation as a clinical intervention. Webb, Smyth and Yarandi (2000) examined the effectiveness of progressive relaxation in the workplace in reducing blood pressure for African-American women. An experimental group of 22 women were taught progressive relaxation for seven muscle groups. They practised progressive relaxation at home using audiocassette tapes. A control group of 21 women practised at home for 30 minutes using only relaxation tapes but without being given instruction. Both groups were visited weekly at the worksite during the eight weeks of the study. Both groups improved in their blood pressure readings, but the experimental progressive relaxation group showed more significant reductions in psychological strain scores than the control group. The authors concluded that progressive relaxation is an effective intervention that can be used in the workplace for improving cardiovascular health.

Progressive relaxation has also been shown to be effective for reducing insomnia (Means et al., 2000), tension headaches (Blanchard et al., 1990) and chronic low back pain (Turner, 1982). In general, progressive relaxation is an effective intervention that can be incorporated into an occupational health programme in the workplace to reduce stress.

Exercise

It is well known that exercise is beneficial to all individuals (President's Council on Physical Fitness and Sports, 1996). However, the type of exercise, duration of time spent doing the exercise, intensity of the exercise such as mild, moderate and forceful and the frequency of doing the exercise will affect its success as part of a stress-management programme. The exercise programme established for a person must be meaningful and of interest to the person. In general, it is recommended that every person has at least one hour of exercise a day. This can be a combination of walking, working in the garden, bicycling or climbing stairs at work. Other individuals may prefer indoor exercises such as working with special equipment in a gymnasium or an onsite health facility. T'ai Chi and Qigong are also beneficial. The basic principle in using exercise as a therapeutic technique is to establish a daily pattern of exercise that is realistic and practical. In a work setting available exercise equipment is frequently unused, often because it is cumbersome. It is preferable to establish with the worker a realistic exercise programme that is feasible and easy to carry out.

In establishing such a programme the following steps are recommended:

- *Measure one's fitness.* Gauge the individual's fitness by referring the person for a general check-up. The first component to consider is the present level of physical fitness. The client should have a physical examination to rule out any limitations in exercising (e.g. negative cardiovascular state). Identify the client's resting heart rate. The average adult heart rate is 72 beats per minute. Establish the client's blood pressure in resting condition. The average blood pressure is 80:120, diastolic:systolic. An individual's degree of physical fitness is an indication of his or her ability to engage in physical exercise. Physical fitness is defined 'as the ability to carry out daily tasks with vigor and alertness, without undue fatigue, and with ample energy to enjoy leisure-time pursuits' (President's Council on Physical Fitness and Sports, 1996, p. 20). A stress test is probably the best method to gauge physical fitness. The result of a stress test indicates the person's capacity to perform physical activity. The test measures the metabolic outputs (METS) that an individual is able to produce without feeling pain or fatigue. It is a measure of the individual's ability to perform physical activities.
- *Aerobic activity.* Select an aerobic activity that is meaningful and purposeful for the worker. Aerobic exercise is defined as engaging in vigorous physical activity where oxygen is metabolized. Aerobic activities include walking, jogging, swimming and bicycling. Engaging in aerobic exercise increases one's physical fitness as well as reducing stress, anxiety and depression. The link between exercise and the reduction of stress has been examined by a number of investigators. Cotton (1990) stated, 'This evidence suggests that aerobically fit individuals are more resistant to the physiological and psychological effects of stress, and that aerobically fit individuals may recover more quickly from stress' (p. 171).
- *Relaxation exercise.* Select a relaxation exercise, such as T'ai-Chi, Qigong or yoga, that is acceptable to the worker. The exercises usually involve cognitive control where the participant moves his or her joints in slow circular movements, such as in T'ai-Chi, or uses breathing, posture and visualization, such as in yoga or Qigong.
- *Massage.* Recommend massage or bathing which can be used to relax muscles.

- *Existing exercise programme.* Obtain from the client the physical activities in which he or she participates. For example, the client may state that he or she walks two to three times a week, plays golf once a week and walks up three flights of stairs every day.
- *Physical expenditure of activity.* The therapist should determine the total calories expended by the person's total activities. See table of MET equivalents (McArdle et al., 2001).
- *Selection of new activities.* The client and the therapist together should develop a list of new activities to be considered. In the selection of this activity, consider the interest of the client, the purposefulness of the activity, the affordability of the activity, time availability for the activity and whether the activity can be undertaken throughout the entire year. Activities that are not tied to changes in the weather, availability or friends are best. For example, walking, cycling and calisthenics can occur both indoors and outdoors. Skiing, on the other hand, can only be done in the winter when there is snow, and tennis involves the availability of another person. Goal-setting is important when selecting the new activity. For example, the client may wish to reduce his or her resting heart rate, blood pressure, anxiety or depression, or weight. By setting goals, the client will, in general, be more compliant, especially if he or she sees results from the activity.
- *Consider social and emotional needs of the activity.* The worker is more apt to comply if the activity meets his or her social or emotional needs. For example, if the activity provides friendly group interaction, relaxation, skill development or mental stimulation, and the worker values these, motivation and compliance will increase.
- *Achievability.* The exercise should be able to be rated in terms of duration, frequency and intensity. For example, walking can be increased from 20 to 30 minutes per day, from three to five days a week, from slow to fast walking or in the number of steps. Additionally, the success of the activity may depend on the client's physical fitness status, his or her body composition, motor abilities and prior activity experiences. For example, asking a person to play tennis when he or she has difficulty tracking the ball or moving quickly ensures failure.
- *Incorporation of activity into one's schedule.* It is important to stress that the client must incorporate this activity into his or her daily or weekly schedule and keep a log of the times in which he or she performs the activity.
- *Compliance and motivation to adhere to the exercise programme.* The benefits of exercise on the cardiovascular system and the psychological well-being of the individual have been widely cited and advocated by the Surgeon General (President's Council on Physical Fitness and Sports, 1996) and by other individuals in the public health sector. In spite of this, few Americans exercise regularly.

At any given time about 40 per cent of Americans do not exercise during leisure time, another 40 per cent are active at levels probably too low and infrequent for fitness and health gains, while only 20 per cent exercise regularly and intensely enough (Stephens et al., 1985) to meet current guidelines for fitness (American College of Sports Medicine, 1986) or to reduce the risk for several chronic diseases and premature death (Dishman and Gettman, 1980; Paffenbarger et al., 1986; Powell et al., 1986). A client, therefore, needs to be motivated and to apply self-discipline in order to comply with the programme.

Biofeedback

Definition of biofeedback

The term biofeedback was officially defined at the first meeting of the Biofeedback Research Society in Santa Monica, California, in 1969 as 'any technique using instrumentation to give a person immediate and continuing signals in changes in a bodily function that he is not usually conscious of such as fluctuating blood pressure; brain wave activity or muscle tension. The individual is then able to use the information to learn how to control these functions which were in the past automatic and involuntary'. In a later publication, Schwartz and Associates defined biofeedback in the following way:

> As a process, applied biofeedback is: a group of therapeutic procedures that uses electronic or electromechanical instruments to accurately measure, process, and feed back, to persons and *their therapists* information with *educational* and reinforcing properties about their neuromuscular and autonomic activity, both normal and abnormal in the form of analogue or binary, auditory and/or visual feedback signals. Best achieved with a competent biofeedback professional, the objectives are to help persons develop greater awareness of, *confidence in*, and an *increase in* voluntary control over their physiological processes that are otherwise outside awareness and/or under less voluntary control by first controlling the external signal, and then with internal psychophysiological *cognitions*, and/or by engaging in and applying behaviours to prevent symptom onset, stop it, or reduce it soon after onset.
>
> Schwartz and Associates, 1995, p. 41

Autonomic nervous system and biofeedback

Biofeedback theory is based on the voluntary control of autonomic nervous system responses. The landmark study by Miller (1969) established the possibility that animals could learn to control visceral and glandular responses that were previously thought to be involuntary and autonomic. Although Miller's discovery at that time came as a surprise to many traditional scientists, there was empirical evidence that Indian yogis could voluntarily control blood pressure, pain, heart rate and respiratory rate by bringing the body into a relaxed, meditative state (Green et al., 1970). Under ordinary circumstances, the ANS functions at the subconscious level. It acts to regulate the ongoing, reflexively driven activity of smooth muscle, cardiac muscle and glands, and integrates visceral systems with one another and with somatic motor functions (Gilman and Newman, 1992). In general, when an individual is highly emotional or under severe stress, sympathetic responses of the autonomic nervous system dominate behaviour due to the increased epinephrine or adrenaline. When the flight-or-flight response is activated, there is a sudden, massive increase in metabolic rate; increased blood pressure, heart rate and increased blood flow to the heart, brain and muscles (Preston et al., 1994). Additionally, these responses include increased activity in the sweat glands, dilation of pupils and increased glucose for energy. The individual may experience 'goose bumps' on the skin. Digestion of food in the gastrointestinal system is interrupted. When the body is at rest or an individual is meditating, the parasympathetic responses dominate behaviour. These responses result in a slowed heart rate, decreased blood pressure, relaxed muscles, normal digestion of food and increased secretion of thin saliva.

Biofeedback as a cybernetic model

Biofeedback is also based on the principle of cybernetics (Wiener, 1948); that is, input–process–output. Input is the cognitive information that stimulates an internal physiological response. Process represents the internal emotional reactions and physiological changes. The output is the organism's behavioural responses. Information can arouse and change the organism's emotional and physiological state causing an action response. For example, knowing that you have an illness can produce physiological changes in the body. Biofeedback works like an information loop where physiological data are recorded and cognitively processed to reduce symptoms. Biofeedback as an intervention in the workplace to alleviate the effects of occupational stress can, in combination with relaxation therapy, be effective in reducing the symptoms of, for example, hypertension, headaches, back pain and gastrointestinal pain. Instruments are used in biofeedback to make the person aware of physiological functions such as heart rate, finger temperature, sweating and blood pressure. In general, biofeedback is a method to enable the person to become aware of internal physiological changes (Stoyva and Budzynski, 1993).

There are many research studies that demonstrate the strong correlation between our emotions and our physiological responses (Christie and Friedman, 2004). For example, when we are angry our blood pressure may rise. When we are anxious or fearful we may experience physiological changes such as rapid heartbeat, cold hands, tight muscles, sweating and hand tremors. All of these changes are unique to individuals with differences in the type and intensity of reactions. Some people are able to control their feelings and remain calm when confronted with danger while other people respond with intense physiological symptoms. Occupational stress is linked strongly to physiological symptoms and, if prolonged, can result in diseases such as hypertension. Thus, it is useful for many individuals who are at risk to learn how to use biofeedback. Biofeedback is a self-regulating activity that can be used in conjunction with meditation, relaxation response and progressive relation to reduce anxiety and tension in the workplace. There are common indicators of reactions to stress such as neck and back pain, stomach ache, headache, dry mouth, cold sweaty hands, hand or knee tremor, an urgency to urinate or stammering. The first step in self-regulating behaviour through biofeedback is to help the client become aware of the individual symptoms or behaviours that are associated with stress.

Biofeedback modalities

The biofeedback modalities most commonly used in clinical practice are the following:

- *Electromyography* (EMG) (Neblett et al., 2003) is used for relaxation training, reduction of tension headaches, muscle re-education, and, in conjunction with behaviour modification, desensitization of the patient to phobias. Van Galen, Muller, Meulenbroek and Van Gemmert (2002) demonstrated that stress and muscular tension as measured by the EMG are related and that stress can precipitate work-related upper extremity disorders. In EMG biofeedback, the patient first becomes aware of the state of muscle tension and then later develops control in relaxing specific muscle groupings. A common body site for EMG biofeedback for relaxation/training is the frontalis muscle located in the forehead. The individual uses auditory and visual output from the EMG to learn how to reduce muscle tension and thereby to increase relaxation. The electrical impulses from the muscle are transmitted by a transducer (surface electrode) to a signal amplifier that magnifies the impulse. A signal processor then transfers the impulse to a visual or auditory display, such as a numerical value in microvolts or an auditory beep. The individual becomes aware of sensations in the muscle and identifies whether the muscle is tense or relaxed. The individual then tries to produce a relaxed muscle state through conscious control such as through meditation. EMG biofeedback has been applied successfully with patients experiencing tension headaches (Philips, 1977), anxiety (Townsend et al., 1975), temporomandibular joint disorders (TMJ) (Turk et al., 1993), insomnia (Raskin et al., 1973), hyperactivity (Braud, 1978), asthma (Peper and Tibbitts, 1992), upper extremity dysfunction (Tries, 1989), incontinence (Tries, 1990) and schizophrenia (Acosta et al., 1978).
- *Skin temperature or thermal biofeedback*. The portable skin temperature biofeedback instrument is designed to measure and display changes in skin temperature from a selected body site (Gaarder and Montgomery,

1981). The thermometer usually is used to detect minute changes in skin temperature in the forefinger reflecting blood flow. The purpose of skin temperature biofeedback is to help the client consciously to be able to raise and lower finger temperature. Skin temperature biofeedback has been used successfully with Raynaud's disease, a condition in which there is inadequate blood flow in hands and feet causing cold extremities (Blanchard and Haynes, 1975; Rose and Carlson, 1987). Migraine headaches have also been the focus of skin temperature biofeedback (Blanchard et al., 1990; Johnson and Turin, 1975; Morrill and Blanchard, 1989). Children have been taught to increase their finger temperature as a conscious method to control tension headaches (Arndorfer and Allen, 2001). Therapists have also used thermal biofeedback with clients to reduce blood pressure (McGrady, 1994).

- *Electroencephalogram* (EEG). The EEG is a record of the electrical activity of the cerebral cortex. It is used routinely by neurologists to detect abnormal brain activity such as that present in brain lesions and epilepsy. The EEG can also be used to monitor the waveforms of the normal brain. EEG biofeedback training is used to teach the patient to produce alpha brain waves, which are associated with relaxation and meditation (Moore, 2000). Alpha EEG feedback has been used clinically with patients suffering from anxiety (Glueck and Stroebel, 1975; Stroebel, 1982), chronic pain (Melzack and Perry, 1975), drug addiction (Cohen et al., 1977; Trudeau, 2000), attention deficit hyperactivity disorders (Nash, 2000) and migraine headaches (Andreychuk and Skriver, 1975).
- *Galvanic skin response (GSR) feedback equipment.* 'The purpose of portable modular GSR feedback equipment is to detect and display changes in the skin resistance (or conductance) caused by changes in the subject's emotional state' (Gaarder and Montgomery, 1981, p. 202). The GSR can detect anxiety. Caprara, Eleazer, Barfield and Chavers (2003) found that a patient's dental anxiety can be successfully detected by using the GSR. On the other hand, decreases in the GSR are usually associated with increased relaxation. In recording GSR, surface electrodes are attached to the palmar side of two non-adjacent fingers. Arousal, or tension in the autonomic nervous system, causes an increase in the galvanic skin response. GSR biofeedback has also been used clinically to diminish phobias (Javel and Denholtz, 1975).

Other biofeedback instrumentation

- Electrocardiogram (ECG) is a recording of the electrical activity accompanying the muscular contraction of the heart.
- A blood pressure cuff is used to monitor systolic and diastolic blood pressure (sphygmomanometer).
- The pulse rate records heart rate and rhythm.
- A pneumograph is used to record respiratory rate.

Using biofeedback technology

Biofeedback is one of the most active research areas in behavioural medicine. It has attracted researchers because it presents a treatment model that links physiological changes with emotions. The methodology enables the clinician to work cooperatively with the client in reducing psychophysiological and behavioural symptoms. The clinician can tangibly document changes in the client's behaviour. The client is an active participant in the treatment process, which is one of the ultimate goals of holistic practice. The client takes responsibility for his or her health by learning to monitor and control physiological responses. Biofeedback is congruent with the treatment philosophy of occupational therapy that rests on the principles of encouraging independence and self-regulation in the client (Abildness, 1982; Stein and Cutler, 2001). The health professional can incorporate biofeedback technology in the workplace and the occupational rehabilitation programme (Schult et al., 1995) to counteract occupational stress.

In using biofeedback technology with clients, the health professional should have sufficient educational background in the following areas:

- *Psychophysiology*: an understanding of the relationship between brain function and sympathetic and parasympathetic autonomic nervous system responses.
- *Electromyography instrumentation*: psychophysics of muscle potential and equipment methodology, such as precise placing of surface electrodes and readings from equipment.
- *Cybernetic theory*: an understanding of the feedback loop, thermostatic mechanisms and homeostasis.
- *Behavioural therapy*: reinforcement schedules and operant conditioning.

Summary

Occupational stress can have a very detrimental effect on the worker. It can contribute to depression, anxiety, cardiovascular symptoms, muscle tension, absenteeism, vulnerability to work injuries and job burn-out. There are many approaches to stress management that the employer and worker can use in creating an environment to reduce stress. The first step is for the management team to recognize that excessive stress in the work environment can be a risk factor to numerous health problems and can decrease productivity and quality of work. The second step is to identify the physical and psychological stressors in the work environment. This includes both an organizational analysis of factors and stressors due to work demands. The third step is to implement changes in the organizational structure that can reduce stress and that are agreeable to both the employer and workers. The fourth step is to devise an individualized stress management programme that can include meditation, relaxation response, progressive relaxation, exercise and biofeedback. Aspects of these techniques can be presented to the worker in the workplace as part of an occupational health or injury-prevention programme.

Review questions

1 What is a definition of occupational stress?
2 What are occupational stressors in the environment?
3 What are general factors that lead to occupational stress?
4 What are the symptoms of occupational stress?
5 How can an individual cope with stress in the workplace?
6 What are strategies to prevent occupational stress in the work environment?
7 What are potential interventions in the workplace to reduce occupational stress?
8 What is the relationship between occupational stress and job burn-out?
9 How can an occupational therapist plan therapeutic interventions with an individual and on an organizational level to affect positive change?
10 How can exercise and relaxation therapies be applied to work settings?
11 How can biofeedback be used in a work setting to decrease occupational stress?

References

Abildness, A. (1982). Biofeedback Strategies. Rockville, MD: The American Occupational Therapy Association.

Acosta, F., Yamanoto, J. and Wilcox, S. (1978). Application of electromyographic feedback to the relaxations of schizophrenic, neurotic and tension headache patients. Journal of Consulting and Clinical Psychology, 46, 383–384.

American College of Sports Medicine (1986). Guidelines for Exercise Testing and Prescription (4th edn). Philadelphia, PA: Lea and Febiger.

Anderson, D.G. (2004). Workplace violence in long haul trucking: Occupational health nursing update. American Association of Occupational Health Nurses, 52, 23–27.

Andreychuk, T. and Skriver, C. (1975). Hypnosis and biofeedback in the treatment of migraine headache. International Journal of Clinical and Experimental Hypnosis, 23, 172–183.

Arndorfer R.E. and Allen K.D. (2001). Extending the efficacy of a thermal biofeedback treatment package to the management of tension-type headaches in children. Headache, 41, 183–192.

Astin, J.A. (1997). Stress reduction through mindfulness mediation. Effects on psychological symptomatology, sense of control, and spiritual experiences. Psychotherapy of Psychosomatics, 66, 97–106.

Barry, D. (2002, 15 December). The nation: Time and motion; What firefighters do the rest of the time. Week in Review Desk. New York Times, Section 4, p. 3, col. 1.

Beck, A., Ward, C., Mendelson, M., Mock, J. and Erbaugh, J. (1961). An inventory for measuring depression. Archives of General Psychiatry, 4, 546–571.

Belkic, K.L., Landsbergis, P.A., Schnall P.L. and Baker, D. (2004). Is job strain a major source of cardiovascular disease risk? Scandinavian Journal of Work and Environmental Health, 30, 85–128.

Benson, H. (1975). The Relaxation Response. New York: William Morrow.

Benson, H. (1979). The Mind/body Effect: How Behavioural Medicine can Show You the Way to Better Health. New York: Simon and Schuster.

Blanchard, E. and Haynes, M. (1975). Biofeedback treatment of a case of Raynaud's disease. Journal of Behaviour Therapy and Experimental Psychiatry, 6, 230–234.

Blanchard, E.B., Applebaum, K.A., Radnitz, C.L., Morill, B., Michultka, D., Kirsch, C.L., Guarnieri, P., Hillhouse, J., Evans, D.D., Jaccard, J. and Barron, K.D. (1990). A controlled evaluation of thermal biofeedback and thermal biofeedback with cognitive therapy in the treatment of vascular headache. Journal of Consulting and Clinical Psychology, 58, 216–224.

Blom, M., Janszky, I., Balog, P., Orth-Gomer, K. and Wamala, S.P. (2003). Social relations in women with coronary heart disease: the effects of work and marital stress. Journal of Cardiovascular Risk, 10, 201–206.

Bowler, D. (2001). 'It's all in your mind': The final common pathway. Work. A Journal of Prevention, Assessment and Rehabilitation, 17, 167–173.

Braud, L. (1978). The effects of frontalis EMG biofeedback and progressive relaxation upon hyperactivity and its behavioural concomitants. Biofeedback and Self-Regulation, 3, 69–89.

Cannon, W.B. (1939). The Wisdom of the Body. New York: W.W. Norton.

Caprara, H.J., Eleazer, P.D., Barfield, R.D. and Chavers, S. (2003) Objective measurement of patient's dental anxiety by galvanic skin reaction. Journal of Endodontics, 29, 493–496.

Carrington, P. (1993). Modern forms of meditation. In P. Lehrer and R.L. Woolfolk (Eds), Principles and Practice of Stress Management (2nd edn, pp. 139–168). New York: Guilford.

Christie, I.C. and Friedman, B.H. (2004). Autonomic specificity of discrete emotion and dimensions of affective space: A multivariate approach. International Journal of Psychophysiology, 51, 143–153.

Cohen, H.D., Graham, C., Fotopoulos, S.S. and Cook, M.R. (1977). A double-blind methodology for biofeedback research. Psychophysiology, 14, 603–608.

Collins, S. (2001). Stress and the gastrointestinal tract. IV. Modulation of intestinal inflammation by stress: Basic mechanisms and clinical relevance. American Journal of Physiology – Gastrointestinal and Liver Physiology, 280, 315–318.

Cotton, D.H.G. (1990). Stress Management: Integrated Approach to Therapy. New York: Brunner/Mazel.

Day, G. (1998). Stress prevention, not cure. Director, 52, 46.

Dishman, R.K. and Gettman, L.R. (1980). Psychobiological influences on exercise adherence. Journal of Sport Psychology, 2, 295–310.

Elias, A.N. and Wilson, A.F. (1995). Serum hormonal concentrations following transcendental meditation-potential role of gamma aminobutyric acid. Medical Hypotheses, 44, 287–291.

Essi Systems (1991). StressMap. San Francisco: Available from Essi Systems, Inc., 70 Otis St., San Francisco, CA, 94103 or http://www.essisystems.com/assessments/stressmap_index.php3.

Everly, G.S. and Benson, H. (1989). Disorders of arousal and the relaxation response: Speculations on the nature and treatment of stress-related diseases. International Journal of Psychosomatics, 36, 15–21.

Faragher, E.B., Cass, M. and Cooper, C.L. (2005). The relationship between job satisfaction and health: A meta-analysis. Occupational and Environmental Medicine, 62, 105–112

Feyer, A.M., Herbison, P., Williamson, A.M., de Silva, I., Mandryk, J., Hendrie, L. and Hely, M.D. (2000). The role of physical and psychological factors in occupational low back pain: A prospective cohort study. Occupational and Environmental Medicine, 57, 116–120.

Firth-Cozens, J. (2000). New stressors, new remedies. Occupational Medicine, 50, 199–201.

Gaarder, K. and Montgomery, P. (1981). Clinical Biofeedback: A Procedural Manual (2nd edn). Baltimore, MD: Williams and Wilkins.

Gelderloos, P., Walton, K.G., Orme-Johnson, D.W. and Alexander, C.N. (1991). Effectiveness of the Transcendental Meditation programme in preventing and treating substance abuse. International Journal of Addiction, 26, 293–325.

Gilman, S. and Newman, S.W. (1992). Manter and Gatz's Essentials of Clinical Neuroanatomy and Neurophysiology (8th edn). Philadelphia, PA: F.A. Davis.

Glueck, B. and Stroebel, C. (1975). Biofeedback and meditation in the treatment of psychiatric illness. Comprehensive Psychiatry, 16, 303–321.

Green, E., Green, A. and Walters, E. (1970). Voluntary control of internal states: psychological and physiological. Journal of Transpersonal Psychology, 2, 1–25.

Griffin, R.M. (1992). Controlling stress to attain career goals. Occupational Therapy Practice, 3, 39–44.

Hamilton, M. (1967). Development of a rating scale for primary depressive illness. British Journal of Social Clinical Psychology, 26, 99–103.

Hammar, N., Alfredsson, L. and Johnson, J.V. (1998). Job strain, social support at work, and incidence of myocardial infarction. Occupational and Environmental Medicine, 55, 548–553.

Holmes, S. (2001). Work-related stress: A brief review. Journal of the Royal Society of Health, 121, 230–235.

Holmes, T.H. and Rahe, R.H. (1967). Social readjustment rating scale. Journal of Psychosomatic Research, 11, 213–218.

Huang, C. (1995). Hardiness and stress: A critical review. Maternal-Child Nursing Journal, 23, 82–89.

Institute for Employment Studies (IES) (2003) How the UK's 'stressed' employees are getting back to work. Retrieved 19 February 2005, http://www.employment-studies.co.uk/press/0307.php

Ivancevich, J.M., Matteson, M.T., Freedman, S.M. and Phillips, J.S. (1990). Worksite stress management interventions. American Psychologist, 45, 252–261.

Jacobson, E. (1929). Progressive Relaxation. Chicago, IL: University of Chicago.

Jarvis, C. (nd). Business learning open archives: Kaizen and quality circles. Retrieved 15 February 2005, http://www.brunel.ac.uk/~bustcfj/bola/quality/circles.html.

Javel, A. and Denholtz, M. (1975). Audible GSR feedback and systematic desensitization: A case report. Behaviour Therapy, 6, 251–253.

Johnson, W. and Turin, A. (1975). Biofeedback treatment of migraine headache: A systematic case study. Behaviour Therapy, 6, 394–397.

Kahn, R.L. (1987). Work stress in the 1980s: Research and practice. In J.C. Quick, R.S. Bhagat, J.E. Dalton and J.D. Quick (Eds), Work Stress: Health Care Systems in the Workplace (pp. 311–320). New York: Praeger.

Karasek, R. (1979). Job demands, job decision latitude and mental strain: Implication for job redesign. Administration Science Quarterly, 24, 285–307.

Karasek, R., Brisson, C., Kawakami, N., Houtman, I., Bongers, P. and Amick, B. (1998). The Job Content Questionnaire (JCQ) An instrument for internationally comparative assessments of psychosocial job characteristics. Journal of Occupational Health Psychology, 3, 322–355.

Karasek, R. and Theorell, T. (1990). Healthy Work. Stress Productivity and the Reconstruction of Working Life. New York: Basic.

Keller, S.E., Schleifer, S.J., Liotta, A.S., Bond, R.N., Farhoody, N. and Stein, M. (1988). Stress induced alterations of immunity in hypophysectomized rats. Proceedings of the National Academy of Science, 85, 577–566.

Kemeny, M.E. and Grunewald, T.L. (1999). Psychoneuroimmunology. Seminars in Gastrointestinal Disease, 10, 20–29.

Kohn, P.M. and Macdonald, J.E. (1992). Survey of Recent Life Experiences [SRLE]. Journal of Behavioural Medicine, 15, 221–236.

LaDou, J. (1980). Occupational stress. In C. Zenz (Ed.), Developments in Occupational Medicine. Year Book (pp. 197–210). Chicago, IL: Medical Publishers.

Lambert, V.A., Lambert, C.E. and Yamase, H. (2003). Psychological hardiness, workplace stress and related stress reduction strategies. Nursing Health Science, 5, 181–184.

Lee, L.C., Yang, K.P. and Chen, T.Y. (2000). A quasi-experimental study on a quality circle programme in a Taiwanese hospital. International Journal of Quality Health Care, 5, 413–418.

Leonard, B. and Song, C. (1996). Stress and the immune system in the etiology of anxiety and depression. Pharmacology, Biochemistry and Behaviour, 54, 299–303.

McArdle, W.D., Katch F.I. and Katch, V.L.(2001). Exercise Physiology: Energy, Nutrition and Human Performance (5th edn). Philadelphia, PA: Lippincott, Williams and Wilkins.

McEwen, B.S. and Mendelson, S. (1993). Effects of stress on the neurochemistry and morphology of the brain: Counterregulation versus damage. In L. Goldberger and S. Breznitz (Eds), Handbook of Stress: Theoretical and Clinical Aspects (pp. 101–126). New York: Free Press.

McGrady, A.V. (1994). Effects of group relaxation training and thermal biofeedback on blood pressure and related psychophysiological variables in essential hypertension. Biofeedback and Self-Regulation, 19, 51–66.

McLean, A. (1987). Therapeutic stress interventions. In J.C. Quick, R.B. Bhagat, J. Dalton and J.D. Quick (Eds), Work Stress Health Care Systems in the Workplace (pp. 249–251). New York: Praeger.

Maddocks, M. (2000). Occupational health. Health Services Journal, 110, 26–27.

Means, M.K., Lichstein, K.L., Epperson, M.T. and Johnson, C.T. (2000). Behavioural Research Therapy, 38, 665–678.

Melzack, R. and Perry, C. (1975). Self-regulation of pain: The use of alpha-feedback and hypnotic training for the control of chronic pain. Experimental Neurology, 46, 452–469.

Miller, N. (1969). Learning of visceral and glandular responses. Science, 163, 434–445.

Miller, L.H. and Smith, A.D. (1994) Stress Audit. Brookline, MA: The Biobehavioural Institute.

Miller, J.J., Fletcher, K. and Kabat-Zinn, J. (1995). Three-year follow-up and clinical implications of a mindfulness meditation-based stress reduction intervention in the treatment of anxiety disorders. General Hospital Psychiatry, 17, 192–200.

Mino, Y., Shigemi, J., Tsuda, T., Yasuda, N. and Bebbington, P. (1999). Perceived job stress and mental health in precision machine workers of Japan: A 2 year cohort study. Occupational and Environmental Medicine, 56, 41–45.

Moller, J., Theorell, T., de-Faire, U., Ahlbom, A. and Hallqvist, J. (2005). Work related stressful life events and the risk of myocardial infarction. Case-control and case-crossover analyses within the Stockholm heart epidemiology programme (SHEEP). Journal of Epidemiology and Community Health, 59, 23–30.

Montgomery, H., Persson, L-O. and Rydén, A. (1996). Importance and attainment of life values among disabled and non-disabled people. Scandinavian Journal of Rehabilitation Medicine, 28, 233–240.

Moore, N.C. (2000). A review of EEG biofeedback treatment of anxiety disorders. Clinical Electroencephalography, 31, 1–6.

Morrill, B. and Blanchard, E.B. (1989). Two studies of the potential mechanisms of action in the thermal biofeedback treatment of vascular headache. Headache, 29, 169–176.

Murphy, L.R. (1996). Stress management in work settings: A critical review of the health effects. American Journal of Health Promotion, 11, 112–135.

Nash, J.K. (2000). Treatment of attention deficit hyperactivity disorder with neurotherapy. Clinical Electroencephalography, 31, 30–37.

Neblett, R., Mayer T.G. and Gatchel R.J. (2003). Theory and rationale for surface EMG-assisted stretching as an adjunct to chronic musculoskeletal pain rehabilitation. Applied Psychophysiology and Biofeedback, 28, 139–146.

New South Wales Public Employment Office (PEO) (2003) Policy on occupational stress and premier's department guidelines on occupational stress – Hazard identification and risk management strategy. Sydney, Australia: Public Service Association. Retrieved 19 February 2005, http://www.psa.labor.net.au/publications/files/StressPSAGov.pdf

Northwestern National Life Insurance Company (1992). Employee Burnout: Causes and Cures. A research report. Part 1: Employee stress levels. Part 2: Addressing stress in your organization. Minneapolis: NWNL Employee Benefits Division.

Paffenbarger, R.S., Hyde, R.T., Wing, A.L. and Hsieh, C.C. (1986). Physical activity, all-cause mortality, and longevity of college alumni. New England Journal of Medicine, 314, 605–613.

Papageorgiou, A.C., Macfarlane, G.J., Thomas, E., Croft, P.R., Jayson, M.I. and Silman, A.J. (1997). Psychological factors in the workplace – do they predict new episodes of low back pain? Evidence from the South Manchester Back Pain Study. Spine, 22, 1137–1142.

Peper, E. and Tibbitts, V. (1992). Fifteen-month follow-up with asthmatics utilizing EMG/Incentive Inspirometer feedback. Biofeedback and Self-Regulation, 17, 143–151.

Philips, C. (1977). The modification of tension headache pain using EMG biofeedback. Behaviour Research and Therapy, 15, 119–129.

Powell, K.E., Spain, K.G., Christenson, G.M. and Mollenkamp, M.P. (1986). The status of the 1990 objectives for physical fitness and exercise. Public Health Report, 101, 15–21.

President's Council on Physical Fitness and Sports (1996). Physical activity and health: A report of the Surgeon General. Pittsburg, PA: US Department of Health and Human Services, Centers for Disease Control and Prevention, National Center for Chronic Disease Prevention and Health Promotion. Retrieved 21 February 2005, http://www.cdc.gov/nccdphp/sgr/contents.htm

Preston, J., O'Neal, J.H. and Talaga, M.C. (1994). Handbook of Clinical Psychopharmacology for Therapists. Oakland, CA: New Harbinger.

Randolfi, E.A. (1997). Developing a stress management and relaxation center for the worksite. AWHP's Worksite Health, 4, 40–44.

Raskin, M., Johnson, G. and Rondestvedt, J.W. (1973). Chronic anxiety treated by feedback-induced muscle relaxation. Archives of General Psychiatry, 28, 263–267.

Rose, G.D. and Carlson, J.G. (1987). The behavioural treatment of Raynaud's disease: A review. Biofeedback and Self-Regulation, 12, 257–272.

Rozanski, A., Blumenthal, J.A. and Kaplan, J. (1999). Impact of psychological factors on the pathogenesis of cardiovascular disease and implications for therapy. Circulation, 99, 2192–2217.

Sapolsky, R.M. (1998). Why Zebras don't Get Ulcers: An Updated Guide in Stress, Stress-related Diseases, and Coping. New York: Freeman.

Schult, M.L. (2002). Multidimensional assessment of people with chronic pain. Unpublished doctoral dissertations, University of Uppsala, Sweden.

Schwartz, M. and Associates (1995). Biofeedback: A Practitioner's Guide (2nd edn). New York: Guilford.

Selye, H. (1956). The Stress of Life. New York: McGraw-Hill.

Selye, H. (1974). Stress without Distress. Philadelphia, PA: Lippincott.

Sharif, B.A. (2000). Understanding and managing job stress: A vital dimension of workplace violence prevention. International Electronic Journal of Health Education, 3, 107–116.

Shimizu, Y., Makino, S. and Takata, T. (1997). Employee stress status during the past decade (1982–1992) based on a nation-wide survey conducted by the Ministry of Labour in Japan. Industrial Health, 35, 441–450.

Smith, J.C. (1986). Meditation: A Sensible Guide to a Timeless Discipline. Champaign, IL: Research Press.

Smith, A., Brice, C., Collins, A., Matthews, V. and McNamara, R. (2000). The scale of occupational stress: A further analysis of the impact of demographic factors and type of job. [HSE Contract Research Report 265/2000]. Centre for Occupational and Health Psychology, School of Psychology, Cardiff University. Retrieved 19 February 2005, http://www.hse.gov.uk/research/crr_pdf/2000/ crr00311.pdf

Stein, F. (2001). Occupational stress, relaxation therapies, exercise and biofeedback. Work. A Journal of Prevention, Assessment and Rehabilitation, 17, 235–245.

Stein, F. (2003). Stress management. In J. Carlson (Ed.), Complementary Therapies and Wellness (pp. 295–303). Upper Saddle River, NJ: Prentice Hall.

Stein, F. and Associates (2003). Stress Management Questionnaire: An Instrument for Self-regulating Stress. [Individual Version. CD-Rom]. New York: Thomson/ Delmar Learning.

Stein, F. and Cutler, S.K. (2001). Psychosocial Occupational Therapy: A Holistic Approach (2nd edn). Albany: Delmar.

Stein, F. and Nikolic, S. (1989). Teaching stress management techniques to a schizophrenic patient. The American Journal of Occupational Therapy, 43, 162–169.

Stein, F. and Smith, J. (1989). Short-term stress management programme with acutely depressed in-patients. Canadian Journal of Occupational Therapy, 56, 185–192.

Stein, F., Bentley, D. and Natz, M. (1999). Computerized assessment: The Stress Management Questionnaire. In B.J. Hemphill-Pearson (Ed.), Assessments in Occupational Therapy Mental Health: An Integrative Approach (pp. 321–337). Thorofare, NJ: SLACK.

Stein, F., Grueschow, D., Hoffman, M., Taylor, S. and Tronbak, R. (2003). The sorting out stress cards – A version of the SMQ: A reliability study. Occupational Therapy in Mental Health, 19, 41–59.

Stephens, T., Jacobs, D.R. and White, C.C. (1985). A descriptive epidemiology of leisure-time physical activity. Public Health Reports, 100, 47–58.

Stroebel, C.F. (1982). QR: The Quieting Reflex. New York: G.P. Putnam.

Stoyva, J.M. and Budzynski, T.H. (1993). Biofeedback methods in the treatment of anxiety and stress disorders. In M. Lehrer and R.L. Woolfolk (Eds), Principles and Practice of Stress Management (2nd edn, pp. 263–300). New York: Free Press.

Suurnakki, T., Ilmarinen, J., Wagar, G., Jarvinen, E. and Landau, K. (1987). Municipal employees' cardiovascular diseases and occupational stress factors in Finland. International Archives of Occupational and Environmental Health, 59, 107–114.

Swaen, G.M., van Amelsvoort, L.P., Bultmann, U., Slangen J.J. and Kant, I.J. (2004). Psychosocial work characteristics as risk factors for being injured in an occupational accident. Journal of Occupational and Environmental Medicine, 46, 521–527.

Taylor, D.N. (1995). Effects of a behavioural stress-management programme on anxiety, mood, self-esteem, and T-cell count in HIV positive men. Psychological Reports, 76, 451–457.

Teasdale, J.D., Segal, Z. and Williams, J.M. (1995). How does cognitive therapy prevent depressive relapse and why should attentional control (mindfulness) training help? Behavioural Research Therapy, 33, 25–39.

Teather, D. (2003, 7 March). Enron scams fill 2,000 pages. The Guardian. Retrieved 15 February 2005, http://www.guardian.co.uk/enron/story/ 0,11337,909130,00.html

Telles, S., Nagarathna, R. and Nagendra, H.R. (1995). Autonomic changes during 'OM' meditation. Indian Journal of Physiological Pharmacology, 39, 418–420.

Theorell, T. (1997). How will future worklife influence health. Scandavian Journal of Work, Envionment, and Health, 23(suppl. 4), 16–22.

Townsend, R.E., House, J.F. and Addario, D. (1975). A comparison of biofeedback-medicated relaxation and group therapy in the treatment of chronic anxiety. American Journal of Psychiatry, 132, 598–601.

Tries, J. (1989). EMG feedback for the treatment of upper-extremity dysfunction: Can it be effective? Biofeedback and Self-Regulation, 14, 21–53.

Tries, J. (1990). The use of biofeedback in the treatment of incontinence due to head injury. Journal of Head Trauma Rehabilitation, 5, 91–100.

Trudeau, D.L. (2000). The treatment of addictive disorders by brain wave biofeedback: A review and suggestions for future research. Clinical Electroencephalogy, 31, 13–22.

Turk, D., Zaki, H. and Rudy, T.E. (1993). Effects of intraoral appliance and biofeedback/stress management alone and in combination in treating pain and depression in patients with temporomandibular disorders. Journal of Prosthetic Dentistry, 70, 158–164.

Turner, J.A. (1982). Comparison of group progressive relaxation training and cognitive-behavioural group therapy for low back pain. Journal of Consulting and Clinical Psychology, 50, 757–765.

UAW-Ford National Joint Committee on Health and Safety (1996). Fitting Jobs to People: Ergonomics Action Guide. Detroit, MI: UAW-Ford National Joint Committee on Health and Safety.

University of Wales (nd). Policy statement on occupational stress. Retrieved 15 February 2005, http://www.swan.ac.uk/personnel/policies_and_procedures/K7742c%20Policy%20Occ%20Stress.pdf

Van Galen, G.P., Muller, M.L., Meulenbroek, R.G. and Van Gemmert, A.W. (2002). Forearm EMG response activity during motor performance in individuals prone to increased stress reactivity. American Journal of Industrial Medicine, 41, 406–419.

Webb, M.S. Smyth, K.A. and Yarandi, H. (2000). A progressive relaxation intervention at the worksite for African-American women. Journal National Black Nurses Association, 11, 1–6.

Wenneberg, S.R., Schneider, R.H., Walton, K.G., MacLean, C.R., Levitsky, D.,K., Wallance, J.W., Mandarino, J.V., Rainforth, M.V. and Waziri, R. (1997). A controlled study of the effects of the Transcendental Meditation programme on cardiovascular reactivity and ambulatory blood pressure. International Journal of Neuroscience, 89, 14–28.

Wiener, N. (1948). Cybernetics or Control and Communication in the Animal and the Machine. New York: John Wiley.

Woo, M., Yap, A.K., Oh, T.G. and Long, F.Y. (1999). The relationship between stress and absenteeism. Singapore Medical Journal, 40, 590–595.

CHAPTER 7

The case study of an administrative secretary: Working at a computer station

For the control of physical risk factors, this process of early identification of symptoms, combined with a process to fix the job, is the basis of a successful ergonomic programme.

N. Warren, 2001, p. 231

Learning objectives

By the end of this chapter the learner will:

1 Understand the work dimensions of a secretary.
2 Become familiar with ONET™ OnLine and how it can be used to define the work of the secretary.
3 Apply clinical reasoning in problem solving this case.
4 Apply a job analysis to the secretarial position.
5 Describe and analyse a computer workstation in relation to ergonomic design.
6 Devise a feasible ergonomic plan to reduce musculoskeletal injury and occupational stress in an administrative secretary.
7 Apply concepts learned in Chapter 5 and Chapter 6 to the case.
8 Apply the University of Michigan's model, for an on-site job-analysis (Keyserling, personal communication, 9–11 June 1997).

Definitions and background information

The purpose of this chapter is to introduce the reader to a case study of an administrative secretary based on an actual situation. Some of the actual details were changed. The first author had the opportunity to work with this individual in a university setting with the assistance of graduate students. The position of a secretary was selected for analysis since secretaries represent one of the largest portions of our work society who are vulnerable to upper extremity disorders and computer-related disabilities.

The first task was to analyse the work requirements for a secretary as defined by the United States Department of Labor. A comparison can be made between the individual client's capability or capacity to perform a specific job and the requirements of the job. This type of information is available through the Occupational Information Network (ONET™ OnLine) (ONet Corstortium, 2005) available at http://online.onetcenter.org/. ONET™ OnLine is a comprehensive database covering occupational titles, work competencies, job requirements and resources. In addition the ONET™ OnLine has been used for job analyses (Whitmore, 1997).

The ONET™ OnLine, which classifies occupations using the Standard Occupational Classification (SOC) system, is used by US Federal Statistical Agencies to classify workers into occupational categories for the purpose of collecting, calculating and disseminating data. Workers are classified according to their occupational definition. Detailed job descriptions for all occupations are included in this database. For example, the code number 43-6011.00 is specific to Executive Secretaries and Administrative Assistants, the subject of this chapter.

The SOC system analyses each job from three perspectives: (a) *knowledge*: organized sets of principles and facts that apply to a general domain; (b) *skills*: developed capacities that facilitate learning and performance of activities; and (c) *abilities*: the enduring attributes that influence performance. Each perspective is analysed into smaller components, which are then rated by percentage according to the importance in performing the occupation. The closer the rating is to 100 per cent, the more important the component. Details about each component, as well as additional information regarding training requirements, tasks, work values, work activities, work contexts and interests, can be found in Table 7.1.

A client who requires career planning advice will find information in the *Occupational Outlook Handbook* (OOH) (Bureau of Labor Statistics, US Department of Labor, 2004–2005) available at http://www.bls.gov/OCO). This 'is a nationally recognized source of career information, designed to provide valuable assistance to individuals making decisions about their future work lives' (para 1). The OOH is revised regularly, and provides information about work requirements, conditions, training, earnings and expected job prospects.

The *Dictionary of Occupational Titles* (DOT) (US Department of Labor, Employment and Training Administration, 1991a), provides standard information for about 20,000 occupations. Each occupation has a specific code based on the requirements of the job. Although the information is not as current as the ONET™ OnLine, it remains available because 'it is a standard reference in several types of cases adjudicated by the Office of Administrative Law Judges, especially labor-related immigration cases' (Background, para 1). The US Department of Labor recommends the use of ONET OnLine to obtain the most current information about jobs.

Table 7.1 Summary of Executive Secretaries and Administrative Assistants ONET™ OnLine Classification 43-6011.00

Job description Persons in this job are expected to provide high-level administrative support. Tasks include conducting research, preparing statistical reports, handling requests for information and clerical tasks such as correspondence, arranging schedules, greeting visitors. They may also train and supervise clerical staff.

Examples of tasks

* Managing and maintaining executives' schedules.
* Preparing invoices, reports, memos, letters, financial statements or other documents, using appropriate software.
* Reading, analysing and distributing incoming memos, submissions and reports.
* File and retrieve corporate documents, records and reports.
* Greet visitors and determine whether they should be given access to specific individuals.
* Prepare responses to correspondence containing routine inquiries.
* Perform general office duties such as ordering supplies, maintaining records management systems and performing basic bookkeeping work.
* Prepare agendas and make arrangements for committee, board, and other meetings.

Knowledge	Skills	Abilities
Clerical	Active listening	Oral comprehension
English language	Reading comprehension	Written comprehension
Customer and personal services	Time management	Written expression
Computer and electronics	Speaking	Oral expression
Administration and management	Writing	Speech clarity
Critical thinking	Near vision	
Active learning	Problem sensitivity	
Coordination	Information ordering	
	Deductive reasoning	

Work activities	Work context	Work styles
Administrative activities	Telephone	Cooperation
Interacting with computers	Contact with others	Attention to detail
Getting information	Face-to-face discussions	Dependability
Communicating with supervisors,	Electronic mail	Integrity
peers or subordinates	Letters and memos	Concern for others
Organizing, planning and	Importance of being	Self-control
prioritizing work	exact or accurate	Stress tolerance
Establishing and maintaining	Work with work group	Adaptability/flexibility
interpersonal relationships	or team	Independence initiative
Communicating with persons	Structured versus	
	unstructured work	

Adapted from the Summary of Executive Secretaries and Administrative Assistants ONET™ OnLine Classification 43-6011.00, by Occupational Information Network (ONET™ OnLine), available at http://online.onetcenter.org/link/summary/43-6011.00.

Components of a typical work environment for an administrative secretary

A computer station is comprised of: (a) the work surface; the height of the desk; (b) the sight (dissolution) of the computer screen; (c) the keyboard; (d) the mouse; (e) the working chair with arm rests; (f) foot rests; and (g) and the placement of the computer screen, the keyboard in relation to the desk and the working chair (American Federation of Government Employees, 2003). Improper use of the computer and inappropriate working positioning at a computer workstation may result in computer-related musculoskeletal injury. Schmidt, Amick, Katz and Ellis (2002) concluded that computer usage for four or more hours without a rest break remains the greatest risk for upper extremity musculoskeletal disorders for workers. It is well known that work-related musculoskeletal disorders are caused by physical, individual and psychosocial factors (Novak, 2004). Physical risk factors include (a) repetitiveness; (b) high frequency of working movements; (c) awkward upper body postures; (d) excessive muscular force; and (e) lack of variation of the work tasks (Occupational Safety and Health Administration (OSHA), nd). Feuerstein, Shaw, Nichols and Huang (2004) concluded that psychosocial variables such as mood, coping skills, job control, job satisfaction, job stress and social support are implicated in work-related upper extremity disorders. They also identified work style, defined as the worker's approach to coping with job demands, as another psychosocial factor. All of these factors place the secretary at risk for musculoskeletal disorders.

The case of Mary

Part one: Background information

A departmental head of a sociology department in a university requested assistance from the occupational therapy department at the same university. The request concerned evaluation of the workstation of one of the departmental secretaries. The occupational therapist was to make recommendations for the purpose of reducing the risk for musculoskeletal trauma disorders and stress symptoms caused by the work. The process of evaluating the workstation and making ergonomic changes is based on a number of variables that are analogous to the steps in occupational rehabilitation. These variables include (a) evaluation of physical, psychological and vocational factors; (b) evaluation of work tasks: simulating work tasks and functional capacity evaluation (FCE); (c) on-site job analysis; (d) interventions, such as ergonomic change of the workstation, stress management, and a physical exercise and/or relaxation programme if indicated.

Description of the case

Mary is 51 years old and has worked as a university administrative secretary for 12 years. The work has changed over the years as there is increased time required to (a) complete tasks on the computer and (b) schedule appointments in the department. The chair of the department has changed frequently during the past four years, which has influenced Mary's work tasks. During the past six months, she has been complaining of neck and back pains and eye strain.

According to the ONET-SOC Classification, the job description for Executive Secretaries and Administrative Assistants (http://online.onet-center.org/link/summary/43-6011.00) includes the following tasks:

- Answer telephone and give information to callers, takes messages or transfer calls to appropriate individuals
- Open incoming mail and route mail to appropriate individuals
- Answer routine correspondence
- Compose and distribute meeting notes, correspondence and reports
- Schedule appointments
- Maintain calendar and coordinate conferences and meetings
- Take dictation in shorthand or by machine and transcribe information
- Locate and attach appropriate files to incoming correspondence requiring reply
- File correspondence and other records
- Make copies of correspondence and other printed matter
- Arrange travel schedules and reservations
- Greet and welcome visitors, determine nature of business and conduct visitors to employer or appropriate person
- Compile and maintain lists and records using typewriter or computer
- Record and type minutes of meetings using typewriter or computer
- Compile and type statistical reports using typewriter or computer
- Mail newsletters, promotional material and other information
- Order and dispense supplies
- Prepare and mail cheques
- Collect and disburse funds from cash account and keep records
- Provide customer services such as order placement and account information.

Mary's job description according to her employee at the university includes the following tasks:

- Greet visitors, prospective students and answer questions or requests for information
- Obtain information from student files, using a computer
- Screen visitors to the department and decide who needs appointments with faculty or administrators
- Keep track of department chair's calendar, including making appointments (using a computer program)

- Advise prospective students on materials needed for completing applications
- Answer telephone, provide information or direction, route calls, take messages
- Type memos and letters as directed from the departmental chair and distribute appropriately
- Maintain computer files
- Take minutes at departmental meetings, make corrections under the supervision of the chair, and distribute minutes and memos to departmental faculty and staff
- Sort and distribute mail to faculty and staff
- Assist with clerical duties with regard to recruitment of faculty
- Make travel arrangements for fleet vehicles, hotels, airline reservations, travel request information, registrations for conferences and reimbursement forms.

Initial evaluation

An initial evaluation by the first author included an interview with Mary regarding her job responsibilities, work schedule, attitudes towards her work and feelings towards her supervisors. The author then observed Mary for one hour while she carried out her job duties, interacted with faculty, students and visitors. She was observed regarding such things as how she changed her body position when working on the computer, answering the telephone and retrieving files. The next step was to complete an on-site job analysis.

The on-site job evaluation

An on-site job analysis adapted from the University of Michigan Ergonomic Job Analysis method (Keyserling, personal communication, 6–10 June 1997) was performed on Mary's workplace. Acknowledgement is given to occupational therapy graduate students at the university who contributed to this job analysis. As noted, some of the information has been changed to lend itself better to a case study analysis. The results are given below:

- *Worker information*: female, age 51, height 5' 2", 120 pounds, right-handed, two years of college, 31/2 years' experience on the job as secretary, married with one child
- *Job title*: Secretary to chair of sociology department in university.
- *Work schedule*: shift start time 8:00 am to shift end time 5:00 pm, break schedules: 15 minutes, 10:00 am and 3:30 pm, and one-hour lunch break. Total work time: 450 minutes ($7\frac{1}{2}$ hours), total rest time 90 minutes ($1\frac{1}{2}$ hours).
- *Placement of the workstation*: Mary's workstation is near the entrance to the departmental office, right through the double doors that connect the office from the second floor corridor. She is the first person that any visitor to the department encounters when entering the office.

- *Furniture at workstation*: Desk that holds 15" monitor, computer keyboard, video display terminal (monitor), telephone, adjustable chair, foot rest, file cabinets that are readily available, book cases and bulletin board.
- *Equipment*: (fixed items) at workstation: computer, printer, copy machine, fax machine.
- *Tools* (hand-held items used while performing job of secretary): phone, pens, computer mouse, stapler, paper clips, tape dispenser, scissors, hole punch.
- *Handled materials*: parts and other items at the workstation: paper, student files, reference books, university catalogues, printed material of rules and regulations for admissions, travel requests, budget and related items, envelopes, manila folders, floppy disks, CDs.
- *Environment*: overhead fluorescent lighting, south window which provides light and passive heat, thermostat set at 70 degrees, noise in area due to radios of faculty and staff, phone calls, voices of students and faculty, off-white paint on walls, grey counter with rounded edges, boxes, purse and cartons with files under desk and near desk, light from south windows contribute to glare on the computer monitor.
- *Personal protective equipment*: headset for phone, adjustable ergonomic chair.
- *Work methods*: The computer, telephone, copier, are her main tools used on the job to perform written and verbal communication.
- *Work behaviour*. Mary greets people who come into her office. She demonstrates a pleasant personality in her interactions with visitors, students, staff and faculty. She smiles easily and is a good conversationalist. She stated she likes her job. The basic requirements for the job include a high-school diploma, skills in using a personal computer, familiarity with using the Internet and communicating by e-mail and interest in upgrading computer skills by attending in-service courses at the university. She is responsible for keeping the chair of the department's appointment calendar using a handheld palm computer, filing and supervising work-study students. Mary reported that the continuous ringing of the telephone and deadlines for completing minutes and reports were the most stressful parts of her job. She is frequently interrupted by the telephone and by faculty requests for copying class material while working on a task. Mary mentions that she sometimes has difficulty resuming a task when she is interrupted. The environment, in general, is pleasant and there are many opportunities for 'chit-chat' with students and faculty, which helps to create a friendly atmosphere in the office; however, it is also distracting and interferes with her work. She realizes that the people distracting her are also part of her work tasks, such as stopping to answer the telephone or helping a student with some of the bureaucracy of the university. In general, she likes her job.

- *Required skills on the job*: attending to tasks for prolonged periods, communicating well with others verbally or written.
- *Occupational requirements for a secretary job* is defined according to the ONET™ OnLine classification system. (See Table 7.1.)

Part two: Significant research studies related to the case study

Economics

According to the Occupational Safety and Health Administration (OSHA) (2003), musculoskeletal disorders 'now account for one out of every three dollars spent on workers' compensation. It is estimated that employers spend $20 billion a year on direct costs for MSD-related workers' compensation, and up to five times that much for indirect costs, such as those associated with hiring and training replacement workers' (para 4). Annual disability costs for work-related musculoskeletal injures represent 8–15 per cent of a company's payroll (Williams and Westmorland, 2002). In 2000, the Center for Disease Control (CDC) reported that 'direct disability lost-time costs were $91,360 per 100 workers, total disability lost-time costs (including indirect costs) were $458,150 per 100 workers, and medical costs were $268,539 per 100 workers' (Work Loss Data Institute, 2002, para 1).

Epidemiology statistics and outcome

In a national survey, Palmer, Cooper, Walker-Bone, Syddall and Coggon (2001) investigated 1871 individuals (i.e. computer operators, data processors, clerks, administrators, secretaries and typists) who use computers on a daily basis. They found that pain in the wrist, hands and shoulders were commonly reported by the workers. In another study, 'OSHA estimates that work-related musculoskeletal disorders in the United States account for over 600,000 injuries and illnesses (34 percent of all lost workdays reported to the Bureau of Labor Statistics (BLS)). In addition to these monetary effects, MSDs often impose a substantial personal toll on affected workers who can no longer work or perform simple personal tasks like buttoning their clothes or brushing their hair' (Occupational Health and Safety Administration, 2003, para 3).

Review of the recent literature

The following list itemizes factors in the computer workstation that impact on cumulative trauma disorders:

- Balci and Aghazadeh (1998) demonstrated in a study of video display terminal (VDT) operators that persons using bifocal lenses had significantly higher rates of neck pain than person's who used single focal glasses. The person with bifocal lenses had to change the position of the head many times to accommodate for the proper lens. This may cause the individual to place the neck in an awkward position. They recommended that a single focal lens for reading and working on the computer be used in place of a bifocal lens.

- Matias et al. (1998) explored the causes of carpal tunnel syndrome with 100 female VDT operators. The investigators examined work duration, position of the trunk, wrist extension and ulnar deviation and anthropometric variables. Discriminant analysis and multiple regression revealed that the main variable in predicting risk for carpal tunnel syndrome was the increase of the daily work duration on the computer (from one to four hours). The other significant factor was poor posture while typing. The anthropometric make-up of the individual was not a significant factor in putting an individual at risk of developing carpal tunnel syndrome.
- Serina et al. (1999) measured the wrist and forearm postures and motions of the 25 participants who were typing on a computer. There was strong evidence from the study that awkward wrist joint motions can contribute to musculoskeletal disorders.
- Demure et al. (2000) examined the relationship between musculoskeletal discomfort and ergonomic characteristics of a video display terminal (VDT) using 273 participants. They found that neck and shoulder discomfort was associated with spending more than seven hours a day at the VDT, less than complete job control, few or no breaks and middle age (40–49). Wrist and hand pain was related to many of the same variables and, in addition, to low job satisfaction, poor keyboard position, use of adjustable computer furniture and poor layout of the workstation.
- Haufler et al. (2000) investigated job stress and upper extremity pain in 124 female office workers who presented with pain symptoms. The workers completed a questionnaire that examined work demands, perception of the work environment, work style, pain intensity and absenteeism. Their results indicated that heightened job stress and a tendency to be perfectionists affected the worker's upper extremity pain and decreased the quality of work. In other words, the workers were trying to meet high standards on the job under heavy pressure, but it produced negative results in terms of quality of work.
- Treaster and Marras (2000) assessed the effect of alternative keyboards on tendon travel (e.g. how much work the tendons have to perform). They concluded that biomechanical data are important in assessing the impact of alternative keyboards on risk factors for cumulative trauma disorders.
- Zecevic et al. (2000) found that a fixed alternative segmented design keyboard for computer typing was effective in keeping the wrist in a neutral position with the forearm in moderate pronation.
- Simoneau and Marklin (2001) examined the effect of computer keyboard slope and height on wrist extension. They found that the downward sloping of the computer keyboard is beneficial in preventing injury to the wrist.

- Laursen et al. (2002) assessed the effects of the use of computer equipment on mental and physical demands. Twelve female participants used a computer mouse and keyboard while an EMG recorded their forearm, shoulder and neck muscles. The authors concluded that the neck extensors showed increased muscular activities as the individuals increased their work on the mouse and keyboard. Moreover, psychosocial factors combined with heavy demands on doing computer work could cause neck pain.
- Williams and Westmorland (2002) described the essential components and evidence of workplace disability management programmes related to musculoskeletal injuries and provided recommendations for disability management in the prevention and reduction of disability. The literature suggests that employer participation, a supportive work climate and cooperation between involved people performing their work tasks improve and possibly reduce work injuries.
- Berner and Jacobs (2002) surveyed staff and faculty members (n = 108) in a college in Massachusetts to identify level of compliance with ergonomic programmes. Fifty-five participants responded to an Internet-based survey regarding Upper Extremity Cumulative Trauma disorders. All the respondents had varying job responsibilities involving computers and 60 per cent had exposure to ergonomics information about a computer workstation. However, only 10 per cent reported implementation of their knowledge about computer workstation ergonomics.
- Balci and Aghazadeh (2003) compared the work–rest schedules for VDT operators considering data entry and mental arithmetic tasks using ten male college students as participants. The methodology included a discomfort questionnaire and performance measures. Three work–rest schedules (i.e. 60-minute work/10-minute rest, 30-minute work/5-minute rest, and 15-minute work/micro-breaks) and two tasks (data entry and a mental arithmetic task) were used. 'The 15/micro schedule resulted in significantly lower discomfort in the neck, lower back, and chest than the other schedules for data entry task. The 30/5 schedule followed by 15/micro schedule resulted in the lowest eyestrain and blurred vision. Discomfort in the elbow and arm was the lowest with the 15/micro schedule for the mental arithmetic task. The 15/micro schedule resulted in the highest speed, accuracy and performance for both of the tasks, compared with the 60/10 and 30/5 schedules. The data entry task resulted in significantly increased speed, accuracy and performance, and lower shoulder and chest discomfort than the mental arithmetic task' (p. 455).
- Hjortskov et al. (2004) examined the effect of mental stress on heart rate and blood pressure during computer work. The participants were 12 women who had their heart beat and blood pressure monitored as they worked on computer activities. They found that short periods of rest over eight minutes can normalize heart rate and blood pressure.

- Lassen et al. (2004), in a study of 6943 computer operators, found that continuous mouse and keyboard work can cause elbow, wrist and hand pain. They gathered self-report and clinical data at baseline and after a one-year follow-up.

Intervention and prevention studies aimed at cumulative trauma disorders include the following:

- Robertson and O'Neill (2003) developed an office ergonomics training programme and workplace intervention to decrease work-related musculoskeletal disorders in office workers. Self-reported data showed that education on ergonomic principles and workplace adaptation are effective in preventing work-related injuries.
- Martin et al. (2003) conducted a pilot study with 16 full-time clerical and office workers at a small private college. They developed a work-injury prevention programme that involved individualized training of ergonomic principles. In a randomized control intervention study, they concluded from the data that a work-injury prevention programme was effective in decreasing low back pain from pre- to post-measure.
- van den Heuvel et al. (2003) found that a computer software program describing the need to take short breaks and perform physical exercises was effective in increasing productivity and decreasing physical complaints in computer workers.

The summary of the research literature on computer operators shows a strong relationship between daily use of the computer for more than seven hours and the risk of developing cumulative trauma disorders in the upper extremities. Factors associated with putting an individual at risk include psychological and physical variables. For example, occupational stress, job dissatisfaction, cognitive overload and perfectionistic workstyle are factors that should be considered in reducing the risk of work injury. Physical factors include the individual's sitting posture while typing, the use of the mouse, the use of alternative split keyboards, the slope of the keyboard, rest breaks, prescribed glasses for computer use and wrist position. Interventions using ergonomic principles were effective in preventing work-related injuries. In generating solutions to this case study, the student should consider both the psychological and physical factors.

Applying ergonomic principles

In doing an ergonomic job analysis for an administrative or executive secretary, the following questions are proposed:

Psychological

- *Job satisfaction*. Is the worker unhappy with the work? What are the parts of the job description that the worker enjoys? What are the tasks in the job that creates stress? Is the worker bored? Is the job challenging? Does the worker plan to leave the job within the near future or is the job a long-term goal?

- *Occupational stress.* Is there cognitive overload? Is the worker experiencing physical, emotional, cognitive or behavioural symptoms that are related to the job tasks? Does the worker feel that she or he is overworked and taken advantage of by the supervisor? Are there specific stressors on the job that are directly causing symptoms? Which coping behaviours does the worker use to reduce the effects of occupational stress? Can a stress management programme be helpful to reduce the job stress?
- *Fixed equipment.* Are the chair and workstation ergonomically designed? Are feet on floor while the person is using the computer? Is there a need for a footrest? Is there lumbar support? Are the arms at 90 degrees while typing? Are the wrists in neutral position? Is there a wrist rest? Are the knees and thighs at approximately 90 degrees? Are the neck and spine straight and not hunched over while working on the computer? Is the head straight with the eyes about 15–30 inches from the monitor? Is the monitor at a 15–25 degree angle lower than the head? Is the angle of the monitor slightly moved upwards? Is the height of the table adjusted to the viewer's comfort zone? Does the individual use bifocal glasses? Does the person strain his or her neck when using bifocals?
- *Adaptive or added equipment.* Does the worker need a glare filter? Should the worker have a plastic floor mat under the chair to ease movement? Is a document holder indicated? Should the worker consider a pullout keyboard under the desk to decrease elbow flexion and wrist extension? Should the worker consider a mouse rest to keep wrists in neutral position while working on the computer? Should the worker consider a headset for the telephone or shoulder rest to decrease pressure on the neck?

Ergonomic strategies

Are stretching exercises at the beginning of the workday a consideration? Should the worker consider a five-minute rest break after an hour of typing? Should the keyboard be rearranged to be on the left side of the desk for right-handed people to allow for easy access to pens and message pads? Can the worker rotate tasks daily and limit continuous keyboard typing to five hours a day? Should frequently used manuals be placed at convenient levels while less frequently used references and manuals be placed in a file?

Summary

The case study is presented to help the learner use clinical reasoning of an actual case of an administrative secretary in a university setting. The background information includes the occupational description of administrative secretarial duties and tasks. The description of administrative tasks from the worker's perspective is presented as well as related research on computer operators. In this case study, the learner is presented with the background data, a literature review relevant in generating solutions and review questions to arrive at tentative solutions. Of course, there are many possible solutions in solving any ergonomic problem. The reader is encouraged to 'brainstorm' while generating many solutions, discuss these solutions and then to select the best solutions, based on feasibility in implementing and recommendations, worker compliance, cost, acceptance to employer and employee and maintenance of the quality of the work. This chapter should help the learner to integrate and synthesize the information from the former chapters.

The ergonomic principles should be applied by the occupational therapist in a holistic manner and consider the need to work in a healthy environment free of occupational hazards (Larson and Ellexson, 2000). Workers in the twenty-first century are expected to work at a rapid pace to meet the competition in a global economy. These expectations should not compromise worker safety and health. The commitment to ergonomics by the employer, government, worker and ergonomic professional is ongoing in protecting the worker while being cost-effective by eliminating or reducing the enormous costs attached to work-related injuries.

Review questions for the case study

1   What are the typical job functions of an administrative secretary?
2   What are the vulnerabilities of secretaries to work injuries?
3   What are the specific work injuries caused by repetitive motion in the upper extremities?
4   How does occupational stress affect the secretary's work output?
5   How do awkward body positions affect the onset of upper extremity symptoms?
6   What are the factors that can cause visual strain?
7   What are some of the ergonomic solutions that can reduce occupational injuries in persons using a computer for most of the day?
8   How can the keyboard be adjusted to keep the wrists in a neutral position?
9   What is the best chair for maintaining an ergonomic position?
10 How can rest breaks be incorporated into the secretary's work schedule?
11 What adaptations can be made to reduce visual glare?
12 Will a daily hand and arm exercise programme be useful in preventing injury?

References

American Federation of Government Employees [AFL-CIO] (2003). Ergonomics. Retrieved 21 March 2005, http://www.afge.org//Index.cfm? Page=Ergonomics

Balci R. and Aghazadeh, F. (1998). Influence of VDT monitor positions on discomfort and performance of users with or without bifocal lenses. Journal of Human Ergology, 27, 62–69.

Balci R. and Aghazadeh, F. (2003).The effect of work-rest schedules and type of task on the discomfort and performance of VDT users. Ergonomics, 46, 455–465.

Berner, K. and Jacobs, K. (2002). The gap between exposure and implementation of computer workstation ergonomics in the workplace. Work. A Journal of Prevention, Assessment and Rehabilitation, 19, 193–199.

Bureau of Labor Statistics, US Department of Labor (2004). Lost-worktime injuries and illnesses: Characteristics and resulting time away from work, 2002. Retrieved 21 March 2005, http://stats.bls.gov/news. release/osh2.nr0.htm

Bureau of Labor Statistics, US Department of Labor (2004–2005). Occupational Outlook Handbook [Online]. Available at http://www.bls.gov/oco/

Demure, B., Luippold, R.S., Bigelow, C., Ali, D., Mundt, K.A. and Liese, B. (2000). Video display terminal workstation improvement programme: I. Baseline associations between musculoskeletal discomfort and ergonomic features of workstations. Journal of Occupational Environmental Medicine, 42, 783–791.

Feuerstein, M., Shaw, W.S., Nicholas, R.A. and Huang, G.D. (2004). From confounders to suspected risk factors: psychosocial factors and work-related upper extremity disorders. Journal of Electromyography Kinesiology, 14, 171–178.

Haufler A.J., Feuerstein M. and Huang G.D. (2000). Job stress, upper extremity pain and functional limitations in symptomatic computer users. American Journal of Industrial Medicine, 38, 507–515.

Hjortskov, N. Rissen, D., Blangsted, A.K., Fallentin, N., Lundberg, U. and Sogaard, K. (2004). The effect of mental stress on heart rate variability and blood pressure during computer work. [On-Line]. European Journal of Applied Physiology, 92, 84–89.

Job-Analysis Net work (nd). Job analysis internet guide. Retrieved 21 March 2005, http://www.job-analysis.net/

Larson, B.A. and Ellexson, M.T. (2000). Blueprint for ergonomics. Work. A Journal of Prevention, Assessment and Rehabilitation, 15, 107–112.

Lassen, C.F., Mikkelsen, S., Kryger, A.I., Brandt, L.P., Overgaard, E., Thomsen, J.F., Vilstrup, I. and Andersen, J.H. (2004) Elbow and wrist/hand symptoms among 6,943 computer operators: a 1 year follow-up study (the NUDATA study). American Journal of Industrial Medicine, 46, 521–533.

Laursen, B., Jensen, B.R., Garde, A.H. and Jorgensen, A.H. (2002). Effect of mental and physical demands on muscular activity during the use of a computer mouse and keyboard. Scandinavian Journal Work Environment and Health, 28, 211–213.

Matias, A.C., Salvendy, G. and Kuczek, T. (1998). Predictive models of carpal tunnel syndrome causation among VDT operators. Ergonomics, 41, 213–26.

Martin, S.A., Irvine, J.L., Fluharty, K. and Getty, C.M. (2003). A comprehensive work injury prevention programme with clerical and office workers: phase I. Work. A Journal of Prevention, Assessment and Rehabilitation, 21, 185–196.

Novak, C.B. (2004). Upper extremity work-related musculoskeletal disorders: A treatment perspective. Journal of Orthopedics, Sports and Physical Therapy, 34, 628–631.

Occupational Safety and Health Administration (OSHA) (nd) Ergonomics: Contributing conditions. Retrieved 21 March 2005, http://www.osha-slc.gov/SLTC/ergonomics/job_analysis.html

Occupational Safety and Health Administration (OSHA) (2003, November). Unified agenda No. 2222: Prevention of work-related musculoskeletal disorders. (RIN 1218-AB36). Retrieved 21 March 2005, http://www.osha.gov/pls/oshaweb/owadisp.show_document?p_table=UNIFIED_AGENDAandp_id=4530

ONet Consortium (2005). Occupational Information Network (ONET™ OnLine). Available from http://online.onetcenter.org/

Palmer K.T., Cooper, C., Walker-Bone K., Syddall, H. and Coggon, D. (2001). Use of keyboards and symptoms in the neck and arm: Evidence from a national survey. Occupational Medicine, 51, 392–395.

Robertson M.M. and O'Neill, M.J. (2003). Reducing musculoskeletal discomfit: effects of an office ergonomics workplace and training intervention. International Journal of Occupational Safety and Ergonomics, 9, 491–502.

Schmidt, L.L., Amick, B.C. Katz, J.N. and Ellis, B.B. (2002). Evaluation of an upper extremity student-role functioning scale using item response theory. Work. A Journal of Prevention, Assessment and Rehabilitation, 19, 105–116.

Serina, E.R., Tal, R. and Rempel, D. (1999). Wrist and forearm postures and motions during typing. Ergonomics, 42, 938–951.

Simoneau, G.G. and Marklin R.W. (2001). Effect of computer keyboard slope and height on wrist extension angle. Human Factors, 43, 287–298.

Treaster, D.E. and Marras, W.S. (2000). An assessment of alternate keyboards using finger motion, wrist motion and tendon travel. Clinical Biomechanics (Bristol, S. Glocs.), 15, 499–503.

US Department of Labor, Employment and Training Administration (1991a). Dictionary of Occupational Titles (4th edn). Washington, DC: US Government Printing Office. Available at http://www.oalj.dol.gov/libdot.htm

US Department of Labor, Employment and Training Administration (1991b). The Revised Handbook for Analyzing Jobs. Indianapolis: JIST Works.

van den Heuvel, S.G., de Looze, M.P., Hildebrandt V.H. and The, K.H. (2003). Effects of software programs stimulating regular breaks and exercises on work-related neck and upper-limb disorders. Scandinavian Journal of Work, Environment and Health, 29, 106–116.

Warren, N. (2001) Work stress and musculoskeletal disorder etiology: The relative roles of psychosocial and physical risk factors. Work. A Journal of Prevention, Assessment and Rehabilitation, 17, 221–234.

Whitmore, K.D. (1997). A review of the literature: Implementation and management of an on-site ergonomics program – The occupational therapist's role. Work. A Journal of Prevention, Assessment and Rehabilitation, 8, 121–130.

Williams, R.M. and Westmorland, M. (2002). Perspectives on workplace disability management: A review of the literature. Work. A Journal of Prevention, Assessment and Rehabilitation, 19, 87–93.

Work Loss Data Institute (2002). Disability lost-time costs exceed medical costs, according to new report from CDC data. Retrieved 21 March 2005, http://www.odg-disability.com/pr_repmdc.htm

Zecevic A., Miller D.I. and Harburn K. (2000). An evaluation of the ergonomics of three computer keyboards. Ergonomics, 43, 55–72.

CHAPTER 8

Using ergonomic principles to effect change in industry

The theme of alienation from work is widely used to describe the disengagement of self from the occupational role. As some of the personal accounts showed, workers tend to become frustrated by the lack of meaning in the tasks allotted to them and by the impersonality of their role in the work organizations.

S. Parker, 1972, p. 53

Learning objectives

At the end of the chapter, the learner will:

1 Examine in depth ergonomic case studies.
2 Apply problem-solving in actual case examples.
3 Identify on-the-job interventions to prevent work-related injuries.
4 Be able to analyse factors in an assembly-line job that can lead to upper extremity disorders.
5 Understand the components of an organizational research case study.
6 Be able to develop a research proposal in ergonomics.

Introduction

This chapter includes three case studies (1) the return to work case study, (2) the job analysis case study, and (3) the organizational research case study. The case studies, taken from the authors' experiences, have a shared goal; that is, injury prevention and the creation of safe work practices and productive environments. The occupational therapist, using sound ergonomic principles, can apply his or her skills in developing a comprehensive plan that utilizes physical, psychological and social approaches.

The first case study, return to work, examines a systems approach to disability management in a light manufacturing plant, using ergonomic principles along with functional testing. The second case study is centred on job analysis at an oil refinery. It demonstrates the process in identifying potential ergonomic stressors and the design of an on-the-job plan to prevent work-related injuries. The third case study presented is an organizational case study that demonstrates the importance of ergonomic interventions in preventing musculoskeletal injuries in a large assembly plant. It is based on an actual study that was undertaken in response to a call for research proposals with an international company.

The return to work case study (1)

An occupational health nurse employed in a light manufacturing plant received a corporate mandate to address increasing disability costs. This mandate included both workers' compensation- and non-workers' compensation-related cases, many of which had remained unresolved and were still outstanding after several years. No process existed to re-evaluate individuals on restrictions or those out on disability and subsequently there was little progress towards case resolution.

The company wanted a programme that would resolve outstanding cases and produce a model to deal with future cases in a more timely and cost-effective manner. An occupational therapist from a nearby clinic was contacted to work with the occupational health nurse in the programme design and implementation.

The process

The occupational health nurse and occupational therapist met and agreed on a programme framework. The programme would include a functional capacity evaluation and job-specific testing, ergonomic analysis and individualized return-to-work plans. The process needed to be non-discriminatory while addressing the individual concerns of each employee. The first step would require extensive job analysis. The analysis results would provide the necessary information to (a) identify and validate current job functions; (b) determine the actual or simulated work tasks of the work products to be used in functional testing; (c) identify areas for potential ergonomic modifications; and (d) develop ongoing education and prevention programmes. A standardized Functional Capacity Evaluation (FCE) would be given in combination with job-specific testing. The FCE would serve two purposes: (a) identify the worker's overall physical abilities in the event that he or she could not return to the original job; and (b) provide baseline information for the design of a return-to-work programme.

Before the programme began, the occupational therapist was asked to sign a confidentiality agreement with the company. To allow the programme to move forward, the employer authorized payment of the job analysis, FCE testing and four days of additional job-specific testing for each individual. If the outcome of the functional testing indicated the need for further intervention, the occupational therapist would secure reimbursement through the workers' compensation funder. The results of the ergonomic analysis and functional testing would provide documentation for requesting payment authorization. Once all the pieces were in place and authorization for payment secured, the programme would be initiated. Due to the number of cases to be addressed, the occupational health nurse determined when each employee would begin the programme.

To begin the job analysis process, a plant walk-through took place to increase the occupational therapist's understanding of the employer's product and work flow. Existing job descriptions were updated and validated. Ergonomic issues were identified. Work simulation tasks were developed from actual product and tools supplied by the employer. These tasks would be the basis for the job-specific testing. Employees, supervisors and the occupational health nurse came to the provider's clinic to validate the job-specific test items. Ergonomic modifications were considered when setting up the testing for each employee. Employees went through an FCE followed by three hours of job-specific testing on four consecutive days.

Return-to-work plan

Based on the results of the functional testing, a return-to-work plan was designed for each employee. If the problems identified in testing were due to worker strength, endurance, or poor technique, a work-conditioning programme was initiated. Ergonomic solutions were implemented on an individual basis. These solutions ranged from job restructuring, job rotation, job modification or reasonable accommodation, tool or equipment modification, or job redesign. For those employees whose physical abilities matched the critical job demands, restrictions were lifted and they returned to their pre-injury job status with no intervention required.

Outplacement was recommended for one employee, a female who worked in the production/inspection area. She had been receiving ongoing medical treatment for problems in her neck and left shoulder. The employee had been on restrictions for several years and was currently on short-term disability. She underwent an FCE followed by job-specific testing. Based on the results of the functional testing, discussion with the physician and the employee, and her work history, the company decided to pursue outplacement. The employee was hired by another company at slightly less than her current wage. The employer's short-term costs following the outplacement were 10 per cent greater than the savings realized. However, within two years' outplacement cost equalization was achieved, meaning no further costs for the employer. The employee was placed in a job that was better suited to her physically and psychological-ly and the employer achieved case closure through the outplacement process.

Summary comments

The health care system fails in the disability process when injured employ-ees are kept off work or in therapy longer than necessary (Lopez, 1998), when work restrictions are not based on functional abilities, or when providers attempt to make ergonomic recommendations without knowl-edge of the job. A thorough job analysis that includes the employer's and employees' perspectives of the job, observation of work techniques, objective measurements, identification of ergonomic stress factors and job-specific functional testing provide a solid basis for return-to-work programming.

Discussion questions

1 Why would a company require an occupational therapist to sign a con-fidential agreement?
2 What is the value of job-specific testing?
3 Why is it important to validate job descriptions and what is the role of the therapist in the process?
4 Why is a walk through the plant important when providing consulta-tion services to industry?
5 Why was it important to include both standardized FCE testing and job specific testing in the programme?
6 What considerations are important when developing the individualized return to work plan?
7 What role did the occupational therapist play in helping the employer make the decision on outplacement for one employee?

Job analysis case study (2)

A large petroleum company, with a strong focus on worker safety and health, identified an increase in injury claims at one of their refineries. On closer review it was determined that the highest incidence of injury occurred in the maintenance job with the next highest in the reformer operator job. Most of the injuries were muscle strains and muscle pulls and in the maintenance job included shoulder, hand and low back, while in the reformer job they were elbow and shoulder.

The company decided to retain the services of an occupational thera-pist to analyse the jobs and identify ergonomic stressors. The information from the occupational therapist's report would be used by the company as a framework for the development of an injury prevention programme, as well as for budget requests to justify ergonomic changes and programme development costs.

Workplace specifics

The oil refinery was located in the northern part of the United States of America. Products included gasoline, kerosene, heating oil, asphalt and commercial chemicals. The refinery had approximately 300 employees and operated 24 hours per day, 365 days per year. Work hours were Monday to Friday, 7:30 am to 4:30 pm with on-call rotation for weekends, holidays and emergencies. The only time the refinery closed was due to a breakdown or a scheduled turnaround.

The main part of the refinery was housed in one large outdoor complex several stories high. Within this complex was a series of buildings that housed important functions including administration, product monitoring, safety and maintenance. Blending tanks were located away from the main complex. Product was moved to and from these tanks and throughout the refinery by pipeline.

The ground surface of the refinery was cement and the structural stairs and walkways were made of metal grating. Caged, vertical stairways provided a means to access the different levels throughout the refinery.

Personal protective equipment included hard hats, chemical-resistant gloves, safety glasses, earplugs, fire-retardant outer clothing and steel-toed work shoes. Depending on what tasks were being done, additional protective gear and respiratory equipment was required in the units where chemicals used in the refining process were housed. Chemical-resistant gloves were worn at all times, due to the chemicals used in the refining process.

Job analysis process

The analysis would include four on-site visits. The occupational health nurse scheduled the visits and introduced the occupational therapist to the employees. The Industrial Hygienist explained the processes carried out at the refinery and discussed safety issues related to the different jobs. He arranged for access to pertinent areas of the refinery, and accompanied the consultant to all job sites. It is important to note that company policy required that anyone doing business at the refinery complete a five-day safety course before being given access to any part of the refinery without an escort. Since this consultation required four days on-site, it was decided the Industrial Hygienist would escort the occupational therapist.

The occupational therapist began the process by observing and asking questions of employees who performed each job. This step helped alleviate the initial reluctance of employees to participate in the process by establishing a trust relationship (Perry et al., 1997). Once this trust was established, the employees were extremely helpful in demonstrating tasks, assisting with measurements and answering questions.

The essential functions of the job were videotaped, measurements of specific critical demands were taken and ergonomic stress factors identified and recorded.

Description of the maintenance job

The maintenance job employees number 15. The mean age of the workers is 53–55 years. The maintenance job has the highest heights and the heaviest loads in the refinery. The maintenance workers are responsible for ongoing maintenance and repairing of multiple compressors, pumps, fans and other equipment required. Once equipment is taken apart, it is either worked on at the site or transported by pickup trucks or cranes to the maintenance shop for repairs or cleaning. General maintenance includes replacing valves, pipes, and old or worn parts. Valve jobs on compressors and fans are scheduled unless a breakdown occurs.

Ergonomic stress factors – maintenance

Forces and weights

A variety of hand and power tools are used to work on refinery equipment and parts. For example, air jacks weigh about 17.5 kg; impact wrenches, up to 19 kg. Wrenches range from standard size used mostly inside the maintenance shop, to 37.5 kg when used outside on the largest compressors. Forces to turn bolts range from a few pounds up to 42.5 kg. The forces can be affected by the amount of corrosion on the valves. Parts and equipment, such as valves and valve covers, range in weight from 12.5 kg to 35 kg. Mechanical assists are available to move heavier parts.

Frequency

Maintenance tasks are assigned on a priority basis. The time spent on each task depends on what needs to be done. Valve jobs are carried out on the larger compressors, on average, once every six months, and on smaller compressors, once every eight weeks. Other maintenance is done as needed on an ongoing basis. Emergency situations take precedence.

Hold time/rest time

Hold time for the tools is approximately 6–20 seconds. Rest time varies depending on the task. Employees often work in teams and share the task, allowing longer rest times.

Angle/twist/posture

Due to the location of the compressors, tanks, valves, fans and other equipment, awkward positions are frequently adopted to access the equipment and parts that require maintenance. As an example, accessing the fans for repair or replacement requires both low and high reaches.

The fans are located in the highest level of the refinery. Workers access the area by climbing up caged vertical stairs. They then use various tools and pulleys to loosen bolts and free equipment, and often are required to work in awkward positions. An employee has to crouch down to get at the valves in the metal grate flooring that operates the fans. The fans themselves are positioned about 2 m from the floor. When working in the chemical unit additional protective gear is required, including wearing a breathing tank and respirator.

Work time duration

The maintenance shift is a straight eight-hour day. Overtime is on an as needed basis. Employees have scheduled breaks and lunch.

Temperature

Due to the geographic location of the refinery, workers are exposed to both summer and winter weather extremes. Assembling, removing and replacing parts or equipment takes place outdoors. Workers climb different levels and work in man baskets at high levels. Gloves are worn all year round to protect employees from contact with chemicals.

Risk factor identification

The maintenance job reports the most injuries. Maintenance employees are seasoned workers who have put in many years in other jobs at the refinery. Because the job is full-time, with overtime only scheduled as needed, and does not involve shift work, the maintenance job was coveted. Getting a maintenance job is based on seniority.

Potential ergonomic stress factors – maintenance

- Newer equipment is more compact than the older equipment making it harder to access.
- Bolts could be frozen, requiring greater forces on the shoulder and upper extremity in order to remove them.
- Thick gloves are worn at all times.
- Certain areas of the refinery require additional equipment (e.g. oxygen tank and respirator).

Observation of the use of good ergonomic principles

- Mechanical assists are used whenever possible.
- Harnesses and other safety equipment are put on when necessary.
- Tool extenders and cheater bars are used on tools when possible.

Description of the reformer operator job

There are twelve reformer operators at this refinery. The mean age of the workers is 32 years. The reformer operators work 12-hour shifts. After working four 12-hour days, they rotate shifts. The rotation schedule changes on a monthly basis.

The reformer operator monitors pressures, temperatures and chemical balances in the tanks, draws samples of product from tanks and towers for testing, maintains temperatures and pressures at proper levels, and responds to situations indicating emergencies. The reformer area has the highest pressures (up to 900 psi) and temperatures (up to 900–1000 degrees Farenheit; 425–500 degrees Celsius) in the refinery. These temperatures and pressures are needed to produce high-octane gas.

Ergonomic stress factors – reformer operator

Force

Most of the valves are cylindrical and range in diameter from 3" to 18" (7.5–43 cm). Forces to turn the valves range from 5 to 85 pounds (approx. 2.3–40 kg). The larger valves require a cylindrical/power grasp and both hands to operate them. The smaller valves require a disc grip and one hand to open and close. Some of the smaller valves can be turned using the head of a wrench placed between the spokes of the valve. A few of the valves have a lever handle and require negligible force to operate.

The frequency for turning the valves varies:

• The valves that need to be opened and closed for approximately a half hour four times per day require 15–25 pound forces.
• The 10–18" diameter valves that require both hands to open and close and take 50–85 pounds of force are handled only a couple of times per day.

Repetition

It takes approximately 6–18 seconds to open and/or close a valve. Valves are opened to take samples, or to adjust pressures or temperature. The operator moves throughout the reformer area adjusting, opening and closing the valves as necessary. The time between turning valves varies from 1 to 5 minutes depending on what needs to be done to keep everything operating smoothly. Valves are turned most often when things are not running well.

Frequency

Operators work indoors observing a computer terminal to monitor pressures, temperatures and chemical balances in the reformer area. The operators patrol the reformer area every two hours. It takes approximately 30–45 minutes to complete required tasks. During this time the operator is visually checking gauges, taking samples and adjusting temperatures or pressures throughout the reformer. Valves were turned as often as every minute to once every five minutes.

Angles/twists/body mechanics

The valves, gauges, pipes, compressors and other equipment that must be checked by the operator are located at different heights and require a variety of postures and body positions to access. To reach specific sites in the reformer area, operators are required to walk, climb metal stairs, occasionally crouch, bend or squat to climb over or stand on pipes. When taking samples the operator carries a bucket or crate of bottles, which holds the samples. When full, the crate or bucket weighs 20–25 lb (10–12 kg).

Wrist posture

Wrist posture varies depending on the location of the valve. Valves are positioned several inches off the ground to eight feet or higher requiring a ladder to reach. Wrist flexion or extension and radial and ulnar deviation are required depending on the horizontal or vertical position and size of the valve. The smaller diameter valves are turned with one hand, or by using a pipe wrench.

Temperature

Employees are subject to the both summer and winter temperature extremes because of the geographic location of the refinery.

Safety

Employees go through extensive training on safety and operational procedures prior to becoming a reformer operator. Safety is promoted throughout the refinery. Day-to-day as well as emergency procedures are in place and frequent safety meetings are held to update and inform all employees of current procedures.

Potential ergonomic stressors – reformer area

- The design of certain areas requires operators to duck under pipes and conduits to access gauges.
- Corrosion on the valves increases forces required to turn them.
- Thick gloves are worn at all times.

Good ergonomic principles observed

- Filing down of the head of the wrench to use the tool to turn valves instead of the hand.
- Engineering changes in the cooling shack where chemicals are moved through pipes operated by a system of valves instead of being poured and dumped by hand.
- Safety procedures were in place and used by employees.

Summary

The assistance of the Occupational Health Nurse and Industrial Hygienists helped establish an environment for productive, efficient and timely work. The employees who provided assistance during the analysis process were vital to this project. They answered questions and were readily available to assist when asked.

Videotape and still pictures were included with the report as well as validation of the essential job functions and critical job demands for both the maintenance and reformer operator jobs. The videotape was not all-inclusive, but rather a representation of the critical tasks required in each area. Pictures supplemented the videotape. Ergonomic stress factors were identified for each job.

Considerations

As stated above, the average age of workers in the maintenance job was 53–55 years. The estimated annual growth of workers 55 years of age and older was 3.7 per cent between 1996 and 2006 (Czaja, 1999). As an occupational therapist working in industry, it is important to be aware of how the physiological and functional changes of aging can affect work performance (Bass-Haugen et al., 2005). In making suggestions for ergonomic changes, the population demographics of the workers should be considered.

Review questions

1 What ergonomic stress factors in the maintenance and reformer operator jobs could be related to the musculoskeletal injuries identified in the case study, especially with regard to the age of the workers?
2 How would climate affect individuals working in the refinery?
3 What is the effect of gloves on the grip required to open and close valves?
4 How would the additional personal protective equipment of a breathing apparatus and respirator affect the worker?
5 Was repetition an issue in the reformer operator's job and if yes, what were the health consequences?
6 What ergonomic principles would you use to address the awkward postures and positions required in both the reformer operator and maintenance jobs?

Organizational research case study (3)

An occupational therapy department in an academic institution was invited by an international food manufacturing company to develop a research proposal to prevent upper extremity injuries in workers who were at risk of developing hand and wrist injuries as they performed their work activities, specifically de-boning and cutting up chickens on a conveyor belt. The organizational research case study describes the process from the point of solicitation of a research proposal to programme development. The research proposal presented can serve as a model for developing an ergonomic research study in a factory setting. Some of the details of the case study were changed from the original in order to update the material and to leave out irrelevant details.

Components of the organizational research case study

The organizational research case study is presented with (a) an overview of the letter of request from the company; (b) proposal evaluation criteria; (c) clinical reasoning assignment; and (d) the draft of the proposal. In the letter of request for research proposals, the company indicated that it was seeking a research study that was comprehensive as well as feasible so that it could be used as a model for preventing injuries at a number of plants.

The objectives of the research proposal were as follows: (a) to examine the factors in the setting that predispose the workers to trauma disorders and muscle strains of the upper extremities and (b) to explore a variety of interventions to reduce these problems. The study was to have primarily a prevention orientation and to include contributions from the disciplines of physiology, industrial psychology, sociology and clinical medicine, as well as occupational therapy. A total of US$50,000 would be awarded for the study.

The principal investigator would be responsible for writing the research protocol, making sure to include preventative, adaptive and remedial components. The principal investigator would also be responsible for (a) making several site visits to the plants chosen for the study; (b) training and coordinating an occupational therapist near the plant site to supervise the interventions; (c) working with plant supervisors and officials; and (d) collecting and analysing objective and qualitative data. The principal investigator would work closely with a project coordinator from the company in implementing the research protocol. The project would be a cooperative arrangement between the investigator and the company.

In its letter of request for research proposals, the company attached: (1) proposal guidelines, (2) an evaluation synopsis from the company's department of ergonomics, (3) a videotape showing poultry workers 'on the job', and (4) a copyright agreement. Proposals were reviewed by a panel applying criteria including practicality, originality, simplicity and cost-effectiveness. This consulting panel from the company included representatives from corporate ergonomics, the Medical Department, the Institute for Health and Fitness and related divisions.

Videotape

The video sent to the principal investigator depicted workers in a factory setting where chickens are de-boned. The workers, who are standing on a wooden platform in front of a conveyer belt, have protective heavy clothing, latex gloves and boots. There is approximately 2 metres between each worker. The floor appears to be slippery from chicken fat. Because of the nature of the work, the temperature must be below normal room temperature, at about 55 degrees Fahrenheit (14–16 degrees Celsius). Overhead fluorescent lighting is used.

The steps involved in the work process include:

1 Unloading the chickens from a truck at the loading dock.
2 Placing the whole chickens on a hook attached to an overhead conveyer belt.
3 Using a sharp knife to take the chicken meat off the bones. The wrist movement consists of flexion and radial deviation, with supportive movements in the shoulder and forearm.
4 Separating the chicken parts on the conveyor belt.

Description of the workday

Each workday is eight hours, divided into three shifts. The first shift is from 6:30 am to 2:30 pm; the second shift, from 2:30 to 10:30 pm; and the night shift from 10:30 pm to 6:30 am. Two 15-minute rest breaks and a half-hour meal break are provided. Approximately, 35 per cent of the workers smoke during the rest break, while the others drink coffee and have snacks.

Evaluation criteria

The following proposal evaluation criteria were redesigned by the authors.

Applicants should be aware that the research design might be as important as the research type. It is important to remember that projects should be designed to achieve the maximum score possible. Applicants may wish to review the criteria in order to determine whether their proposal will be competitive.

The points identified are provided as a range from which the Evaluation Committee will determine a score.

Research design: 60%

Points will be awarded based on the research design. Consideration will be taken for practicality, innovation, simplicity and cost-effectiveness.

1 Quality of the proposal   25%
2 Soundness of intervention procedures   15%
3 Control of extraneous variables   10%
4 Cost-effectiveness   10%

Credentials of the principal investigator and the consultants: **25%**

Credentials will be judged on the experience and education of each person as delineated in the résumé and letters of recommendation from affiliated agencies.

Feasibility of the study: **15%**

Points will be awarded on the ability of the applicant to successfully complete a grant within the time period allotted. Points may be deducted for applicants whose previous grant performance is not consistent with the commitments made in their previously funded proposal. This may include failure to execute a contract, numerous contract extensions or poor grant performance.

Critical thinking assignment for the case study

The reader is presented with an actual proposal that was submitted to the company with slight revisions (see Appendices A–J at the end of this chapter, pp. 268–77).

The reader is now given the assignment to evaluate the request for a study, critique the proposal, update the references and design a new proposal.

Exploration of the problem

The exploration of the problem includes the variables (a) exercise, (b) ergonomics and (c) a stress-management programme as a means of preventing repetitive motion injuries.

Repetitive motion injuries to the upper extremities are the major cause of carpal tunnel syndrome and tendonitis in the workplace (Armstrong et al., 1986; Kao, 2003; Pflazer and McPhee, 1995; Silverstein et al., 1987). These injuries may result in lost time from work (Bloswick et al., 1998), hand surgery (Masear et al., 1986; McNally and Hales, 2003) and worker's compensation cases (Wellman et al., 2004). In previous literature, it has been estimated that 10–25 per cent of workers in industries that require considerable wrist flexion or extension, and elevation and internal rotation of the shoulder, will develop an upper extremity disorder (Armstrong et al., 1982; Hymovich and Lindholm, 1966; Punnett et al., 2004).

Why do certain individuals develop repetitive motion injuries while others exposed to the same work environment are injury-free? Are there predisposing factors or constitutional vulnerabilities present in the injury-prone? Can workers be screened to determine who will develop repetitive motion injuries? Are certain physical attributes such as grip strength, upper extremity range of motion, work capacity and general health related to the onset of repetitive motion injury? Can a profile be established for the injury-prone individual? Are there psychological or personality variables that are associated with repetitive motion injuries?

Investigators (Armstrong et al., 1982; Blair and Bear-Lehman, 1987; Finkel, 1985; Madeleine et al., 2003; Masear et al., 1986) who have explored the problem of repetitive motion injuries in meat, fish and poultry workers, conclude that further research is needed to objectively evaluate various methods to prevent injury. These researchers and others have identified the following measures as possible preventative interventions:

- Sharpen tools so as to decrease force in cutting meat.
- Use cotton gloves to absorb excess moisture.
- Pace boning where the speed on the assembly-line is fast in the beginning of the shift and slowed down toward the end of the shift.
- Rotate jobs (e.g. wings, breasts, legs and carcass de-boning rotated every two hours).
- Use wrist supports to prevent extremes of wrist flexion or extension.
- Engage in exercises which strengthen the wrist and/or increase, range of motion.
- Provide platforms for workers to stand on and raise or lower work tables to improve posture.
- Provide education to supervisors and workers on proper biomechanics and joint protection.
- Include stress management training so as to reduce muscle tightness that can make the worker vulnerable to joint injury.

Methods and procedures

Eighty subjects will be recruited for this study. Two groups will be established (i.e. the control or 'retrospective well adaptive' group) and the experimental group. Forty subjects (20 from each plant) will be identified as the retrospective group and meet the following criteria: (a) at least three years working full-time as a de-boner at the company; (b) no previous or present history of hand, arm or shoulder injury; (c) voluntary consent to be in the project. These forty subjects who make up the retrospective well adaptive group have demonstrated good adaptation skills and will serve as a resource or 'quality circle' for identifying methods to prevent repetitive motion injury. Questionnaire and group dynamics data will be collected from this group to explore two questions: (a) Why do some individuals adapt successfully to assembly-line work? and (b) What factors enable an individual to prevent repetitive motion injuries?

The second group of subjects (experimental group) will meet the following criteria: (a) between 18 and 35 years old; (b) at least six months on the job; (c) no previous history of hand, arm or shoulder injury; (d) full-time employment; (f) voluntary consent to be in the study. Forty subjects (20 from each plant) who meet the criteria for the experimental group will be included in the study. These subjects will be randomly assigned to four intervention groups which will cross over (rotate) during three periods of intervention:

1 Education for joint protection
2 Exercise
3 Ergonomics and job rotation
4 Stress management and biofeedback.

Stages of the study

A cross-over research design will be used in this study where each subject is their own control (Stein and Cutler, 2000). The study is designed for one year.

- Stage 1 – 15 March to 30 April. Preparation for study (ordering of equipment and tests); selection and administration of pre-tests to retrospective well adaptive group and experimental group.
- Stage 2 – 1 May to 31 January. In this phase of the study, three periods of intervention will be established at the two plants (1 May to 31 July, 1 August to 31 October, and 1 November to 31 January). The subjects at the two plants will have the opportunity to experience two treatment methods.
- Stage 3 – 1 February to 28 February. Post-test measures will be collected and results will be statistically analysed.

Diagram of research design

Stage 1: Preparation for study and pre-testing (1 March–30 April)
I Selection of subjects: All subjects will be asked to sign a consent form. The following data will be collected from all subjects in the study:

a Pre-test evaluation battery
   i Demographic/ergonomics questionnaire devised by the principal investigator (see Appendix C)
   ii Stress Management Questionnaire (Stein and Associates, 2003)
   iii The Quality of Well-Being Scale (Kaplan et al., 1997). This is an interviewer-administered questionnaire. The data include the person's function level along three scales: mobility, physical activity and social activity. Scores range from 0 to 1 indicating no symptoms.
   iv Grip-strength as measured by the Jamar dynamometer (Flood-Joy and Mathiowetz, 1987)
   v Pinch strength as measured by the Pinch gauge (Mathiowetz et al., 1984)
   vi Purdue Pegboard (Tiffin, 1948) (a test of finger manipulation and assembly ability).

  b Administer tests to:

   i Retrospective well adaptive group (40 subjects)
   ii Experimental group (40 subjects)

II Train supervisors at two poultry plants.

Stage 2: Intervention (1 May to 31 January)

	Period 1 1/5–31/7	Period 2 1/8–31/10	Period 3 1/11–31/1
Site I			
Group 1 (N = 10)	A	D	C
Group 2 (N = 10)	B	C	A
Site II			
Group 3 (N = 10)	C	B	D
Group 4 (N = 10)	D	A	B

Stage 3: Re-evaluation/post-test (1 February to 28 February)

I Schedule of re-evaluation:

   Period 1   31 July
   Period 2   31 October
   Period 3   31 January

II The experimental group will be re-evaluated (31 July, 31 October and 31 January) on the following tests

   i Self-evaluation (see Appendix E)
   ii Grip strength
   iii Pinch strength
   iv Evaluation of Stress Management Questionnaire (See Appendix D)

How the data will be secured

The pre-test data will be collected in two days at each plant. Tests and questionnaires will be administered in groups while the grip strength, pinch strength and Purdue Pegboard will be administered individually.

The research team (i.e. principal investigator and two occupational therapy consultants) will spend three days at each plant to secure subjects and administer group and individual tests. The research team will return to the poultry plants to educate supervisors and to initiate research interventions at the beginning and end of each treatment period.

How the data will be treated and interpreted

Results will include qualitative and quantitative data. Data will be analysed using descriptive and inferential statistics. Frequency distributions, histograms and statistical pies will be used to describe variables in the following:

- Demographic/ergonomics questionnaire (e.g. pace of work, job rotation, environmental factors, troublesome areas on job; see Appendix C)
- Index of Well-Being (Kaplan et al., 1997)
- Grip strength as measured by the Jamar dynamometer (Flood-Joy and Mathiowetz, 1987)
- Pinch strength as measured by the Pinch gauge (Mathiowetz et al., 1984)
- Purdue Pegboard (Tiffin, 1948)
- Stress Management Questionnaire (Stein and Associates, 2003)

Inferential statistics (analysis of variance (ANOVA)) will be used to compare differences between the groups and within the groups. Interval scale data (i.e. grip strength and pinch grasp) will be used in the analysis. Chi-square analysis will be used in analysing frequency differences between groups from the self-evaluation items.

The following research questions will be applied to the data collected:

- What percentages of the subjects have had previous injury or surgery to their arm, hand and shoulder?
- Is the pace of work too fast?
- Was the training period for the job adequate?
- Are there factors in the workstation that can be improved?
- What are the specific factors that cause job stress, such as pain, noise, fatigue, shift work, repetitive motions?
- What are the present symptoms of stress?
- What are the everyday stressors in the environment?
- What activities are used in managing stress?
- How does an individual successfully adjust to the job?
- What is the overall health of the subjects?
- What is the average grip strength and pincer grasp strength of the group?
- Are there significant differences between groups in finger manipulation and assembly ability?
- Are there significant differences between four interventions (i.e. ergonomics, exercise, stress management and education) in decreasing symptoms of repetitive motion injury?

The results of the analysis will be documented in a report. Specific recommendations for effective interventions to decrease occupational injuries will be included.

Experience of the investigators and job description

The principal investigator (PI) has published over 50 journal articles and a book on research design. The investigator has been the PI on three research grants from the federal government. He has had extensive experience in administration and budgeting. His areas of research interest are wide and include ergonomics, stress management and wellness.

Two of the occupational therapy consultants, who also are the co-investigators, were employed in an industrial medicine unit in a rehabilitation department of a hospital. They treated, on daily basis, patients with upper extremity work-related injuries such as carpal tunnel syndrome, tendonitis and DeQuervain's disorder.

The third occupational therapy consultant is a training specialist at New York University. She has had extensive experience as a hand therapist and has published widely in the areas of hand rehabilitation, carpal tunnel syndrome, functional capacity evaluations and the treatment of industrial hand injuries.

The job description for the principal investigator is as follows:

1 Coordinate goals of project with co-investigator and consultants
2 Develop research methodology for the research study
3 Carry out statistical analysis of results
4 Develop questionnaires for initial data collection and re-evaluation
5 Do on-site supervision of research project at both job sites
6 Supervise clerical support project
7 Prepare and monitor budget
8 Order tests, equipment and supplies for the study
9 Report and document results of study
10 Prepare research protocol for biofeedback and stress management.

The job description for the occupational therapy consultants is as follows:

1 Coordinate goals, purposes and research design with principal investigator
2 Develop research protocols for exercise, ergonomics/job rotation, joint protection education
3 Administer pre-tests
   a grip strength
   b pinch strength
   c questionnaires and tests
4 Administer outcome measure questionnaire and grip and pinch strength
5 Collect and organize research data to be analysed.

Proposed budget

The proposed budget includes $36,000 for PI and consultants' salaries, approximately $4000 for equipment and $10,000 for travel expenses.

Summary of case study

The purpose of this organizational research case study is to present an actual example of the application of an ergonomic approach to an industrial setting. This example also gives the reader the opportunity to problem-solve specific ergonomic solutions creatively in an actual case study.

Review questions

1   What are recent research findings in ergonomics that can be used in updating the proposal and designing new interventions?
2   Does the current research literature support the interventions identified in the proposal?
3   What are the primary questions from the referring agency and are the issues still relevant?
4   What are the potential cost benefits to the company and employees of this type of study?
5   What further information is needed about the workers' behaviour in designing new interventions and preventive measures?
6   What are the major ergonomic problems identified in the work setting?
7   How can the proposal have an interdisciplinary focus?
8   What background information regarding the work environment is needed to carry out the study?
9   Are there new research studies to guide the investigator in the development of an updated proposal?
10 Is the proposal presented realistic?
11 What changes would be recommended to strengthen the proposal?
12 Is the abstract complete?
13 Is the research proposal justified in terms of economic costs and prevention of work injuries?
14 How can the exploration of the problem be strengthened?
15 Are the interventions recommended viable?
16 How many participants should be included in a new study?
17 How many research groups should be identified? Should there be experimental and control groups?
18 What are the screening criteria for worker inclusion in the study?
19 How will the experimental and control groups be implemented?
20 How long should the study take place?
21 Is the informed consent form adequate?
22 Is the overall diagram of the research design clear to the reader? If not, how can it be improved?
23 What assessments should be used for measuring outcome?
24 How will pre-test data be compared statistically with post-test data?
25 What demographic data should be collected and what is the rationale for collecting these data?
26 What are the research hypotheses in the study?
27 What are the necessary levels of education and experience of the principal investigator for carrying out the study?
28 What consultants should be hired and why?

29 Are the job descriptions of the principal investigator and consultants adequate?

30 Is the proposed budget realistic and adequate? Update these figures for actual time.

Chapter summary

The occupational therapist's role in applying ergonomic principles to actual case studies in industry is presented. The reader is provided opportunities to problem solve solutions to these cases and to respond to questions that are posed. Solutions to ergonomic problems in industry should be based on research and clinical evidence. The reader is encouraged to examine the recent literature on the topics presented, such as repetitive motion injuries, carpal tunnel syndrome and other disabilities that are described in these case studies.

Appendix A: Abstract of proposal

Exercise, ergonomics and stress management programme to prevent repetitive motion injuries

The purpose of this study is to measure the effects of education for joint protection, exercise, ergonomics and job rotation, stress management and biofeedback on the prevention of repetitive motion injuries in workers employed in poultry processing plants of an international food manufacturing company. The research project is designed to explore intervention methods that can be incorporated readily into a factory environment. An innovative research design is proposed that systematically alternates treatment interventions while allowing the subject to be one's own control. Data will be analysed to determine individual differences in environmental controls fitting the needs of the workers (Morse, 1986; Pheasant, 1991).

The subjects for the study will come from two of the company's poultry plants. Forty subjects will be randomly selected from each plant. The evaluators will be experienced occupational therapists who are employed in an industrial medicine unit of a rehabilitation medicine department.

The experiment is designed for one year. The timeline is as follows: the first 45 days, the selection of subjects, pre-test evaluations, ergonomics design, purchase of equipment and supplies; the next 60 days, the first period experimental treatment; the next 60 days, the second experimental period; the next 60 days would see the third period experimental treatment; and the last 30 days would include the analysis of test data.

A cross-over research design is used in this study. Four treatment situations would be identified: (a) *Exercise*, using a seven-minute exercise and relaxation programme; (b) *Ergonomics and Job Rotation*, an approach used in industrial medicine; (c) *Stress Management and Biofeedback* – this includes heart-rate monitoring and the Relaxation Response (Benson, 1975); and (d) *Education*.

All subjects will be administered the following assessments: (a) demographic ergonomics questionnaire, including work history; (b) Stress Management Questionnaire (Stein and Associates, 2003); (c) grip strength (dynamometer) (Flood-Joy and Mathiowetz, 1987); (d) Quality of Well-Being Scale (Kaplan et al., 1997); and (e) self-report of the subject's qualitative evaluation of intervention.

Contents of the proposal

1 Exploration of the problem
2 Methods used
3 Diagram of research design
4 How data will be secured
5 How data will be treated and interpreted
6 Experience of investigators and job description

7 Proposed budget

8 Appendices

  i Appendix B: Informed consent form for participation in the prevention study

  ii Appendix C: Demographic/ergonomics questionnaire

  iii Appendix D: Evaluation of the Stress Management Questionnaire (Stein and Associates, 2003)

  iv Appendix E: Self-evaluation questionnaire

  v Appendix F: Upper extremity exercise protocol (Columbia Hospital Audiovisual Department, personal communication, 1985)

  vi Appendix G: Job rotation protocol

  vii Appendix H: Education protocol (supervisors and employees)

  viii Appendix I: Guidelines for intervention at the worksite

  ix Appendix J: Stress management protocol

Appendix B: Informed consent form for participation in prevention study

The purpose of this research is to study techniques that may help people to prevent on the job injuries to hand, arm and shoulder. Participation in this study is voluntary. If you agree to participate in this study, you will be randomly selected for one of four groups. All subjects will be asked to complete three questionnaires, be tested for manual dexterity, grip strength and pincer grasp. If you are selected for an experimental group, you will have the opportunity to take part in a ten-minute warm-up exercise, adapt your workstation, and practise stress management and biofeedback. You will also have the opportunity to evaluate your experience and you will be retested for grip and pinch strength.

The exercise is based on principles of relaxation. An analysis of your workstation will be undertaken to make the job best fit the person. The biofeedback device, which is as small as a hand calculator, records your heart rate by attaching a simple lead to your ear lobe. By taking part in this study, it may help you to prevent injuries to your hands, arms and shoulders. It may also help, in the future, individuals like yourself to prevent injuries on the job.

Your name will not be used in analysing the data or in reporting the results of the study. You are free to drop out of the study at any time without any penalty. All information collected from you up to that point will be destroyed if you so desire.

There are no known physical or psychological risks in participating in this research. If you decide not to take part in this study, it will not affect your job and your decision will not be shared with your employer.

CONSENT FOR PARTICIPATION IN PREVENTION STUDY
If you have any questions regarding the purpose of this study, please call the investigator at the School of Allied Health Professions. If you have any complaints about your participation in this study, please call or write to the Institutional Review Board for the Protection of Human Subjects. Although Dr Stein will ask your name, all complaints are kept in confidence.

I have received an explanation of the study and agree to participate.

_____   _____
Signature of participant   *Date*

This research project has been approved by the University Institutional Review Board for the Protection of Human Subjects.

Appendix C: Demographic/ergonomics questionnaire

Social Security Number_____   Today's Date_____

Date of Birth_____   Sex: Male__   Female__

Height_____ Weight_____

What job(s) did you have previously to this one?

1 Job title or description of job: _____
   Name and address of company: _____
   Dates of employment: _____

2 Job title or description of job: _____
   Name and address of company: _____
   Dates of employment: _____

3 Have you every experienced pain in:
   arm?   Yes___   No___
   hand?   Yes___   No___
   shoulder?   Yes___   No___

4 Have you ever had an injury or surgery to:
   arm?   Yes___   No___
   hand?   Yes___   No___
   shoulder   Yes___   No___

How long have you been working in the present job as a full- or part-time poultry plant worker? _____

Current job description _____

Slow or fast pace _____

Continuous number of hours in activity _____

Number and lengths of breaks during day _____

What type of training did you receive for this _____

Do you feel that any aspect of your work station can be changed to make it more comfortable?   Yes___ No___

If yes, how?_____

What type of protective clothing or gloves do you wear on the job? ____
_____

What recommendations do you have? _____
_____

Would you be interested in rotating your job with a related task?
Yes___ No___

If yes, how often would you want to rotate your job?

1 every 2 hours	Yes___	No___
1 every 4 hours	Yes___	No___
Daily	Yes___	No___
1 week	Yes___	No___
2 weeks	Yes___	No___
3 weeks	Yes___	No___

Do you feel the temperature in the plant is:

Too cold?	Yes___	No___
Too hot?	Yes___	No___
Just right?	Yes___	No___

Do you feel the lighting to do the job is:

Too bright?	Yes___	No___
Too dark?	Yes___	No___
Just right?	Yes___	No___

Do you feel you have enough room to do the job?   Yes___ No___

If you use a knife in trimming meat, is it adequate for its purpose?
Yes___ No___

If not, how can it be improved? _____

What factors in your job are the most difficult to handle?

1	Shift schedule (night)	Yes___	No___
2	Repetitive nature of work	Yes___	No___
3	Pain in wrist	Yes___	No___
4	Pain in hand	Yes___	No___
5	Pain to upper arm	Yes___	No___
6	Pain to elbow	Yes___	No___
7	Pain to shoulder	Yes___	No___
8	Psychological stress	Yes___	No___
9	Noise	Yes___	No___
10	Fatigue	Yes___	No___
11	Standing in one place	Yes___	No___
12	Numbness in the hand	Yes___	No___
13	Tingling (pins and needles) in the hand	Yes___	No___

Of the factors above, what are the three most troublesome areas?
1 _____
2 _____
3 _____

Appendix D: Evaluation of Stress Management Questionnaire (Stein and Associates, 2003)

We are interested in improving the usefulness and clarity of this questionnaire. Your feedback and responses will be helpful to us in revising the questionnaire.

Please circle Yes, No or Unsure.

1 Was the questionnaire too long?   401 Yes   402 No   403 Unsure

2 Were the directions clear?   404 Yes   405 No   406 Unsure

3 Did you find the questionnaire interesting?
407 Yes   408 No   409 Unsure

4 Did the list of items accurately reflect your feelings?
410 Yes   411 No   412 Unsure

5 Did the questionnaire help you to become more aware of the stressors in your everyday life?   413 Yes   414 No   415 Unsure

6 Did you identify from the questionnaire any new methods to manage stress?   416 Yes   417 No   418 Unsure

7 Do you feel you would benefit from an individualized stress management programme?   419 Yes   420 No   421 Unsure

8 When you are stressful do you use
alcohol?   500 Yes   501 No
drugs?   600 Yes   601 No
cigarettes?   700 Yes   701 No?

9 Are you currently being treated for a medical disorder?   800 Yes   801 No?

802 If yes, please list the condition(s) _____

_____

422 Sex _____   427 Marital Status _____

423 Year of Birth _____   428 Religion (Optional) _____

424 Occupation _____   429 Ethnic Group _____

425 Student Major _____   430 Today's Date _____

426 Level of Education _____

Appendix E: Self-evaluation questionnaire

1 Social Security Number Plus Code_____

2 Experience:
   _____ Education for joint protection
   _____ Exercise
   _____ Ergonomics and job rotation
   _____ Stress management and biofeedback

3 Plant site_____

4 Group_____

5 Today's date_____

Evaluation of effectiveness

On a scale from 1 to 5, did the experience improve your job in the following areas:

6 Made you feel less stressful?

1	2	3	4	5
Worse	Not at all	Same	Improved	Greatly improved

7 Made you feel less fatigued?

1	2	3	4	5
Worse	Not at all	Same	Improved	Greatly improved

8 Made the actions less painful?

1	2	3	4	5
Worse	Not at all	Same	Improved	Greatly improved

9 Increased your ability to do your job accurately?

1	2	3	4	5
Worse	Not at all	Same	Improved	Greatly improved

10 During the past three months, have you experienced the following:

a	Numbness in the hand during the night?	Y	N
b	Tingling in the hand?	Y	N
c	Difficulty grasping objects?	Y	N
d	Weakness in the hand?	Y	N
e	Weakness in the wrist?	Y	N
f	Pain in the wrist?	Y	N
g	Pain in the elbow?	Y	N
h	Pain in the shoulder?	Y	N

Appendix F: Upper extremity exercise protocol

Guidelines

1 Three times per shift

  a Before beginning work
  b At the first break (not at mealtime)
  c At the second break (not at mealtime)

2 Five repetitions of each exercise
3 Exercises are for ROM (or mobility)

Exercises

Exercise 1 (see Figure 8.1).

1 Flexion: Cross arms in front of face, with hands in fist.

  a shoulder flexion
  b shoulder adduction
  c shoulder external rotation
  d forearm supination
  e wrist flexion with radial deviation
  f finger flexion and adduction
  g thumb adduction

2 Extension: Opens hands and lowers arms out to the sides, with palms facing behind client.

  a shoulder extension
  b shoulder abduction
  c shoulder internal rotation
  d forearm pronation
  e wrist extension with ulnar deviation
  f finger extension and abduction
  g thumb radial abduction

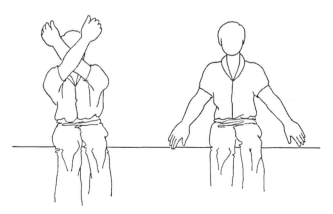

Figure 8.1
Exercise 1:
Proprioceptive neuro-
muscular facilitation
(PNF): Bilateral flexion
and extension.

Exercise 2 (see Figure 8.2).

1 Extension: Client crosses arms in lap, with hands in fist.

   a shoulder extension
   b shoulder adduction
   c shoulder internal rotation
   d forearm pronation
   e wrist flexion with ulnar deviation
   f finger flexion and adduction
   g thumb opposition

2 Flexion: Client opens hands, reaching upwards, with the thumbs pointing behind the client.

   a shoulder flexion
   b shoulder abduction
   c shoulder external rotation
   d forearm supination
   e wrist extension with radial deviation
   f finger extension and abduction
   g thumb radial abduction

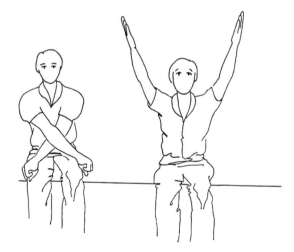

Figure 8.2 Exercise 2: Proprioceptive neuro-muscular facilitation (PNF): Bilateral flexion and extension.

Exercise 3. Client flexes elbows to elbows at 90 degrees, then bends wrists up or back as far as possible and then down as far as possible.

Exercise 4. Client opens and closes fists.

Appendix G: Job rotation protocol

Every person in the group that rotates will change stations according to the following procedure:

Work/job station	Number of hours
Chicken:	
Wings	2
Breasts	2
Legs	2
Carcass	2

Appendix H: Education protocol (supervisors and employees)

Rationale: Increased awareness/knowledge of anatomy, physiology and joint protection decreases the frequency and severity of musculoskeletal problems.

When: During first several days of the study.

Appendix I: Guidelines for intervention at the worksite

1 Basic upper extremity anatomy and physiology.
2 Use the largest joint(s) available whenever possible (i.e. the elbow or shoulder instead of the wrist and fingers).
3 Minimize/avoid repetitive motions of the joints (i.e. the wrists).
4 Minimize/avoid static or holding positions, particularly simultaneous wrist flexion and finger pinching and wrist ulnar deviation with grasp.
5 Instead of pinching, try using a grasp or closed fist with a neutral or wrist extended position.
6 Take informal 'rests' whenever possible (i.e. relax/rest the upper extremities when able).
7 Supervisors should reinforce as indicated.

Appendix J: Stress management protocol

Seven minutes before work, take initial heart rate reading (baseline). Worker then practises Benson Relaxation Response (four steps):

1 Sit down in comfortable position, legs uncrossed.
2 Close eyes.
3 Pay attention to inner breathing.
4 Tell self 'alert mind, calm body'.

Repeat Benson Relaxation Response (5 minutes) during breaks in work schedule. Take heart rate before and after Relaxation Response.

References

Armstrong, T., Foulke, J., Joseph, B. and Goldstein, S. (1982). Investigation of cumulative trauma disorders in a poultry processing plant. American Industrial Hygiene Association Journal, 43, 103–116.

Armstrong, T., Radwin, R., Hansen, D. and Kennedy, K. (1986). Repetitive trauma disorders: Job evaluation and design. Human Factors, 28, 325–336.

Bass-Haugen, J., Henderson, M.L., Larson, B.A. and Matuska, K. (2004). Occupational issues of concern in populations. In C.H. Christiansen, C.M. Baum and J. Bass-Haugen (Eds), Occupational Therapy: Performance, Participation, and Well-being (3rd edn). Thorofare, NJ: SLACK.

Benson, H. (1975). The Relaxation Response. New York: William Morrow.

Blair, S.J. and Bear-Lehman, J. (1987). Prevention of upper extremity occupational disorders. Journal of Hand Surgery, 12, 821–822.

Bloswick, D.S., Villnave, T. and Joseph, B. (1998) Ergonomics. In P.M. King (Ed.), Sourcebook of Occupational Rehabilitation (pp. 145–165). New York: Plenum.

Czaja, S.J. (1999). Promoting employment opportunities for older adults. Paper presented at the International Conference on Aging, Washington, DC, December.

Finkel, M. (1985). The effects of repeated mechanical trauma in the meat industry. Americn Journal of Industrial Medicine, 8, 375–379.

Flood-Joy, M. and Mathiowetz, V. (1987). Grip strength measurement: A comparison of three Jamar dynamometers. Occupational Therapy Journal of Research, 7, 235–243.

Hymovich, L. and Lindholm, M. (1966). Hand, wrist and forearm injuries: The result of repetitive motions. Journal of Occupational Medicine, 8, 573–577.

Kao, S.Y. (2003). Carpal tunnel syndrome as an occupational disease. Journal of American Board of Family Practice, 16, 533–542.

Kaplan, R.M, Sieber W.J. and Ganiats, T.G. (1997). The Quality of Well-Being Scale: Comparison of the interviewer-administered version with a self-administered questionnaire. Psychology and Health, 12, 783–791.

Lopez, M.S. (1998). Musculoskeletal ergonomics: An introduction. In V.J.B. Rice (Ed.), Ergonomics in Clinical Practice: Prevention and Rehabilitation (pp. 155–179). Boston: Butterworth-Heinemann.

McNally, S.A. and Hales, P.F. (2003). Results of 1245 endoscopic carpal tunnel decompressions. Hand Surgery, 8, 111–116.

Madeleine, P., Lundager, B., Voigt, M. and Arendt-Nielsen, L. (2003). The effects of neck-shoulder pain development on sensory-motor interaction among female workers in the poultry and fish industries: A prospective study. International Archives of Occupational Environmental Health, 76, 39–49.

Masear, V.R., Hayes, J.M. and Hyde, A.G. (1986). An industrial cause of carpal tunnel syndrome. Journal of Hand Surgery, 11, 222–227.

Mathiowetz, V., Weber, K., Volland, G. and Kashman, N. (1984). Reliability and validity of grip and pinch strength evaluations. Journal of Hand Surgery, 9, 222–226.

Morse, L. (1986). Repetitive motion musculoskeletal problem in the microelectronics industry. Occupational Medicine, 1, 167–174.

Parker, S. (1972). The Future of Work and Leisure. London: Paladin.

Perry, C.L., Barnowski, T. and Parcel, S. (1997). How individuals, environments, and health behavior interact: Social cognitive theory, In K. Glanz, F.M. Lewis and B.K. Rimer (Eds), Health Behavior and Health Education: Theory, Research and Practice (pp. 39–62). San Francisco, CA: Jossey-Bass.

Pfalzer, L.A. and McPhee, B. (1995). Carpal tunnel syndrome research. In S.J. Isernhagen (Ed.), The Comprehensive Guide to Work Injury Management (pp. 127–191). Gaithersburg, MD: Aspen.

Pheasant, S. (1991). Ergonomics, Work and Health. Gaithersburg, MD: Aspen.

Punnett, L., Gold, J., Katz, J.N., Gore, R. and Wegman, D.H. (2004). Ergonomic stressors and upper extremity disorders in automobile manufacturing: A one year follow up study. Occupational Environmental Medicine, 61, 668–674.

Silverstein, B., Fine, A. and Armstrong, J. (1987). Occupational factors and carpal tunnel syndrome. American Journal of Industrial Medicine, 11, 343–358.

Stein, F. and Associates (2003). Stress Management Questionnaire: An Instrument for Self-regulating Stress. [Individual Version. CD-Rom]. New York: Thomson/ Delmar Learning.

Stein, F. and Cutler, S.K. (2000). Clinical Research in Occupational Therapy (4th edn). San Diego: Singular Publishing Group/Thomson Learning.

Tiffin, R. (1948). Examiner Manual for the Purdue Pegboard. Chicago, IL: Science.

Wellman, H., Davis L., Punnett, L. and Dewey, R. (2004). Work-related carpal tunnel syndrome (WR-CTS) in Massachusetts, 1992-1997, source of WR-CTS, outcomes and employer intervention practices. American Journal of Independent Medicine, 45, 139–152.

CHAPTER 9

A brief history of occupational medicine and ergonomics

In modern industrial medicine the emphasis is upon people, the conditions in which they live and work, their hopes and fears, their abilities, their attitudes towards their job, their fellow workers, and their employers.

D. Hunter, 1978, p. 236

Learning objectives

By the end of this chapter the learner will:

1   Understand the sequential history of ergonomics.
2   Understand the controlling factors in the workplace: employer, government, medical intervention, ergonomist.
3   Understand the laws relating to the workplace.
4   Understand the evolution of the protection of workers.
5   Identify from an historical perspective the factors that cause occupational injury and occupational disease.
6   Understand how vital statistics are used in identifying work injuries.
7   Understand the development of worker's compensation and legislation to protect workers.
8   Identify the purpose of the Occupational Safety and Health Agency (OSHA) and National Institute of Occupational Safety and Health (NIOSH) in the United States of America.
9   Understand the development of the discipline of ergonomics and its relationship to the human factors movement.
10 Recognize ways in which health can be promoted in the workplace.
11 Describe the recent developments in ergonomics and human factors, including certification.
12 Identify future trends in occupational medicine and ergonomics.

History of occupational medicine: Precursors to ergonomics

Ergonomics is a problem-based field that emerged during the Second World War in the design of military equipment and vehicles that enabled the operators to be efficient and safe in carrying out their duties. After the war the principles of ergonomics were incorporated into work environments as a method and philosophy of good environmental design. The basic principles of ergonomics are inherent in the philosophy of occupational therapy and in the application of occupational medicine.

The history of ergonomics is explored in this chapter from the beginnings in occupational medicine and its recent application to human factors psychology. The history of ergonomics is seen as an extension of occupational medicine (see Figure 9.1). In this chapter we explore how concern for the worker in the work environment evolved from abuse, neglect and exploitation to the current state in industrial nations where the worker is protected legally from harmful and disease-generating environments. This evolution towards worker safety is a dynamic process where the work environment is in a continual state of change as workers have to handle toxic substances and keep up with production demands. The ergonomist in alliance with physicians, research scientists, employers

ANTIQUITY	MEDIEVAL GUILDS	APPRENTICESHIP SYSTEM
• Development of work in hunter-gatherer societies • Stigma of manual labour • Occupational diseases ignored	• Voluntary associations formed for mutual aid protection of tradesman • Assist worker with disabilities and funeral expenses • Honest workmanship	• Establishment of apprenticeship system • Provided training and standards for craftsmen
PROTECTION OF MINERS (Sixteenth Century) • Ventilating machines for mines	OCCUPATIONAL MEDICINE (Established Seventeenth Century) • Relationship between occupation and disease investigated medically • Prevention measures introduced rest - intervals, positioning, cleanliness, protective clothing	COMPILING OF VITAL STATISTICS ON OCCUPATIONAL DISEASE (Eighteenth Century) • Use of medical inspectors
PROTECTION OF VULNERABLE WORKERS IN DANGEROUS TRADES (Nineteenth Century) • Public health legislation to regulate child labour • Work day reduced to 10 hours	WORKERS' COMPENSATION (Twentieth Century) • Compensate workers for occupational accidents and diseases	WOMEN'S TRADE UNION MOVEMENT (1875–1903) • Protection of women from exploitation and exposure to dangerous industries
SOCIAL SECURITY LEGISLATION (1930s) • Place safety and health activities within Labor Department	OCCUPATIONAL SAFETY AND HEALTH AGENCIES (Established 1970) • On site inspections, regulations and enforcement of laws relating to dangerous and unhealthy conditions in all industries	AMERICANS WITH DISABILITIES ACT (1990) • Extended Section 504 of the Rehabilitation Act of 1973 to the private sectors • Established comprehensive prohibition of discrimination based on disability
FUTURE TRENDS IN OCCUPATIONAL MEDICINE IN TWENTY-FIRST CENTURY • Occupational health teams • Investigation of physical, chemical, biological and psychological factors in work environment • Investigation of long-term effects of exposure to toxic chemicals, repetitive motion, vibration, excessive noise, extreme temperature, radiation, dust, bacteria		

Figure 9.1 History of occupational medicine: Progress towards social reform in occupational health and safety. Adapted from Clinical Research in Occupational Therapy (4th edn), F. Stein and S.K. Cutler (2000), San Diego: Singular Publishing/Thompson Learning.

and governmental agencies need to be vigilant in protecting the worker as new conditions and equipment are introduced into the work setting. Ergonomics is an emerging field that adapts new solutions to the changes and modernization of the workplace.

How did work unfold in the history of mankind? When did manual labour that was considered slavery become paid work? When did workers organize into guilds and unions? How did these organizations protect the worker? How did workers receive protection from working in dangerous occupations such as mining? When did workers first receive compensation for injuries sustained while working? How does social security legislation impact on retired workers? What are the roles of OSHA and NIOSH in preventing and reducing work injuries in the USA?

Antiquity

Archaeological evidence has shown that work first evolved from hunter-gatherer societies where the division of labour was assigned to certain individuals (Coon, 1955). For example, those who had skill in manual activities (e.g. toolmaking) imparted the skills to the next generation (Felton et al., 1963). Hunting, which was considered a male activity, was related to speed and dexterity. The skills used in hunting were also used in war and fighting (Hunter, 1978). Food gathering was traditionally assigned to women who incorporated this as a domestic activity. Later on, in the development of more advanced societies (e.g. Egyptians, Greeks and Romans), manual labour was assigned only to slaves or prisoners who were supervised by citizens or aristocrats. Most of the workers in these socities consisted of slave labourers and household servants (Rosen, 1943). For example, in Egypt, slaves were dispensable and offered no compensation or consideration of heath needs. The following quote, written by Diodorus Siculus (circa 90–21 BC), a Greek historian who visited a gold mining operation in Egypt in 50 BC, described the conditions under which the slaves worked. This description of manual work by slaves is probably typical of the conditions that occurred during antiquity. It is ironic that almost 2000 years later, the Nazis used slave labourers in forced labour camps similar to conditions described by Siculus.

> [T]hose who have charge of the mining operations obtain the gold by means of a large number of workers, for the kings of Egypt collect condemned prisoners, prisoners of war and others who, beset by false accusations, have been in a fit of anger thrown into prison; these, sometimes alone, sometimes with their entire families, they send to the gold mines; partly to exact a just vengeance for crimes committed by the condemned, partly to secure for themselves a big revenue through their toil.
>
> Those who have been thus consigned are many, and all are fettered; they are held constantly at work by day and the whole night long without any rest, and are sedulously kept from any chance of escape. For their guards are foreign soldiers, all speaking different languages, so the workers are unable either by speech or by friendly entreaty to corrupt those who watch

them. The hardest of the earth that contains the gold is exposed to a fierce fire, so that it cracks, and then they apply hand labour to it; the rock that is soft and can be reduced by a moderate effort is worked by thousands of the luckless creatures with iron tools that are ordinarily used for cutting stone. The foreman, who distinguishes one sort of rock from another, instructs the workers in the whole business and assigns their tasks. Of those who are condemned to this disastrous life such as excel in strength of body pound the shining rock with iron hammers, applying not skill but sheer force to the work, and they drive galleries, though not in a straight line, but in the direction taken naturally by the glistening stone; these then, on account of the windings of these passages, live in darkness, and carry around lamps attached to their foreheads. In accordance with the peculiarities of the rock they have to get into all sorts of positions and throw on the floor the pieces they detach. And this they do without ceasing, to comply with the cruelty and blows of an overseer. The young children make their way through the galleries into the hollowed portions and throw up with great toil the fragments of broken stone, and bring it outdoors to the ground outside the entrance. . . . As these workers can take no care of their bodies and have not even a garment to hide their nakedness, there is no one, who seeing these luckless people would not pity them because of the excess of their misery, for there is no forgiveness or relaxation at all for the sick, or the maimed, or the old, or for women's weakness, but all with blows are compelled to stick to their labour until, worn out, they die in servitude. Thus the poor wretches ever account the future more dreadful than the present because of the excess of their punishment and look to death as more desirable than life.

Rosen, 1943 as cited by Hunter, 1978, pp. 8–9

In the Greek, Roman and Egyptian societies, occupational diseases were ignored. 'Roughly speaking, the working man was neglected in ancient medical practice and the occupational disease ignored in medical science' (Hunter, 1978, p. 13).

Medieval guilds

From the end of antiquity to the Middle Ages, manual workers were not protected from work injuries or abuse by their landowners. Not until the beginning of the eigth century did medieval guilds began to protect craft workers. Miners were not protected, however, until the twelfth century. The contributions to the religious arts, such as in building castles, palaces and cathedrals, began to be recognized by the aristocracy and the Church. These artisans included 'sculptors in stone, wood carvers, silversmiths, goldsmith and decorative ironsmiths' (Hunter, 1978, p. 23). Tanners and weavers were also included in a form of industrial organization called the guild. Guilds 'were voluntary associations formed for the mutual aid and protection of their members' (Hunter, 1978, p. 23). These guilds were associated with local town government.

In 1188, Frederick I Barbarossa of Germany (1122–1190) granted a charter of protection to the miners of Goslar in the Harz Mountains. This charter guaranteed workers compensation for injuries and death benefits for families (Hunter, 1978). In spite of this, the work was long and arduous.

> Hours of work were very long, from 5 o'clock in the morning in winter and 6 in summer to 7 at night, with perhaps three hours off for meal-times. Work by artificial light was often prohibited. The desire to shorten the working day showed itself early, and in some ordinances we find work forbidden on one half-day a week. Holidays were fixed by the Church festivals, of which there were plenty. In all there were 275 working days in the year. Work was forbidden on Sundays, on holy days and on the evenings before them. The apprentice had usually to be indoors by 9 o'clock at night.
>
> Hunter, 1978, p. 25

Reform was considered by the Royal Families in order to protect the health of the artisans whose work was greatly appreciated. Because of the scarcity of workers following the Black Death of the fourteenth century, payment for arts and crafts increased greatly and there were occasional worker protests for higher wages (Hunter, 1978; Orth, nd). In order to control the increasing cost of labour, Edward III (1327–1377) of England, enacted the Statute of Labourers, which resulted in recommending a wage rate for labourers for the whole country. In the fifteenth century, during the reign of Elizabeth I (1533–1603) 'the emphasis on national control was even greater and the town economy ultimately gave place to a national economy' (Hunter, 1978, p. 24).

Apprenticeship system

The apprentice system started as a result of the Statue of Artificers in 1563. A craftsman was given seven years to learn his trade under a master craftsman. 'It was based on the supposition that the average man was without sufficient judgment or experience to govern himself until after the age of twenty-four' (Hunter, 1978, p. 24). After completing the apprenticeship, the craftsman was given permission to marry and either to set up a business of his own or become a journeyman for hire. The modern concept of an apprenticeship system has lasted through the Industrial Revolution and up to the present. Artisans in training who completed internships before working, learned their trades while being supervised by skilled workers. The positive outcomes of the apprenticeship system in the Middle Ages were that it (a) created a pool of master craftsmen that filled the needs of the country; (b) ensured quality craftsmanship; (c) provided a system for selecting and training people with potential for becoming quality craftsmen; and (d) the system protected craftsmen from being exploited by employers.

Protection of miners

Mining in the twenty-first century is still considered to be one of the most dangerous occupations. In the sixth century, Georgius Agricola

(1494–1555), in 12 volumes, wrote about the various diseases and accidents related to mining and the means available to prevent them. Agricola was a pioneer in occupational medicine and his contributions were significant. The following quotes are from the fifth and sixth volumes of his book *De Re Metallica*, published posthumously in 1556:

> Air indeed becomes stagnant both in tunnels and in shafts. I will not speak of ventilating machines. If a shaft is very deep and no tunnel reaches to it, or no drift from another shaft connects with it, or when a tunnel is of great length and no shaft reaches to it, then the air does not replenish itself. In such a case it weights heavily on the miners, causing them to breathe with difficulty, and sometimes they are even suffocated and burning lamps are also extinguished. There is therefore a necessity for machines which enable the miners to breathe easily and carry on their work.
>
> Agricola, 1556/1912, as cited in Hunter, 1978, pp. 28–29

> On the other hand some mines are so dry that they are entirely devoid of water and this dryness causes the workmen even greater harm, for the dust, which is stirred and beaten up by digging, penetrates into the windpipe and lungs, and produces difficulty in breathing and the disease which the Greeks called asthma. If the dust has corrosive qualities, it eats away the lungs, and implants consumption in the body. In the mines of the Carpathian Mountains women are found who have married seven husbands, all of whom this terrible consumption has carried off to a premature death.
>
> Agricola, 1556/1912, as cited in Hunter, 1978, pp. 29–30

Paracelsus (1493–1541), a medical reformer who lived in Switzerland, also examined the occupational diseases of miners and smelter workers. His contribution to occupational medicine was to apply the knowledge of chemistry in understanding the link between mining and lung disease.

Occupational medicine (established seventeenth century)

Bernardino Ramazzini (1633–1714) is considered to be the father of occupational medicine. He advised doctors to ask patients about their occupations in the diagnosis and treatment of diseases. This information helped doctors to understand the causes of diseases that are related to occupational hazards.

Ramazzini's (1700) most noted work, *De Morbis Artificum Diatriba* (Diseases of Workers, in Latin), is an extensive and comprehensive description of occupational diseases that existed during the seventeenth and eighteenth centuries. In this book, he examined the chemicals, metals, abrasive agents and work conditions that could cause disease and injury. His work was also revolutionary and visionary in that his views and recommendations for ergonomic interventions were centuries ahead of his time. For example he:

- recommended rest intervals for workers between long shifts
- recognized the need for exercise and change of posture

- identified the relationship between faulty work posture and poor health
- described the need for ventilation machines in mines because of the effect of dust on lungs
- observed that extreme temperatures can cause diseases and illnesses
- suggested that people in dusty environments should wash their faces and rinse out their mouths with water
- advised personal cleanliness and use of protective clothing and boots especially in occupations that expose workers to harmful chemicals (Hunter, 1978).

Compiling of vital statistics on occupational disease (eighteenth and nineteenth centuries)

> In 1851 the work of Farr led to the publication for the first time of the Registrar General's Occupational Mortality Supplement. Such tabulations of occupational mortality have been issued subsequently at ten-year intervals. For the last hundred years in England and Wales it has therefore been possible to tabulate the deaths of men according to the occupations which are recorded on the death certificates. Bringing these numbers of deaths, by age and certified cause, into relation with the numbers of men following different occupations, as recorded in the decennial census, gives, in terms of mortality, some indication and measure of special occupation hazards. In the Supplement to the Thirty-fifth Annual Report Farr pointed out that the mortality of needle manufacturers at 35 to 45 was excessively high and that earthenware manufacture was one of the unhealthiest trades in England.
>
> Hunter, 1978, p. 97

Protection of vulnerable workers in dangerous trades (nineteenth century)

During the nineteenth century, there was a movement in Western Europe and the USA towards the protection of children and women in factory settings. The Factory Act of 1819 passed in England reduced the number of working hours for men, women and children to 10 hours a day, and the restricted the exploitation of child labour. The quote below describes some of the controversy surrounding the Act.

> It is therefore not surprising that in the subsequent *Factory Act, 1819*, few concessions were made. It stipulated nine years as the minimum age for the employment of children and it limited their working hours, but it did not apply to all textile factories. But one important principle it did establish. Parliament, in the teeth of violent opposition, had won the right to extend the law to workers other than bound apprentices, and as the opponents of the Bill so rightly judged, this was indeed the thin end of the wedge. Though the Bill was badly mutilated, the weak and feeble Act which emerged was to become the Magna Carta of childhood; thereafter the protection of the children of the poor, first from toil and then from bodily starvation and ignorance, began.
>
> Hunter, 1978, p. 115

Charles Turner Thackrah (1795–1833), a physician in England, had a strong interest in industrial diseases and advocated social reform in the manufacturing industries where many diseases and injuries occurred. His writings were influential in developing industrial medicine and recognizing the relationship between diseases and occupation.

> Most persons, who reflect on the subject, will be included to admit that our employments are in a considerable degree injurious to health: but they believe, or profess to believe, that the evils cannot be counteracted, and urge that an investigation of such evils can produce only pain and discontent. From a reference to fact and observations I reply, that in many of our occupations, the injurious agents might be immediately removed or diminished.
>
> Thackrah, 1831, as cited in Hunter, 1978, p. 123

Inadequate ventilation and exposure to toxic chemicals in the workplace were recognized as primary causes of pulmonary diseases during the nineteenth century. Examples of such diseases included the rise of pulmonary tuberculosis in tailors and textile workers, black lung disease among miners, and lead poisoning among metal workers. Chimney sweeps were found to have a high incidence of testicular cancer, while workers who worked in pottery factories developed asthma and tuberculosis as well as muscular ataxia caused by the high rate of lead in the ceramics. This relationship between occupation and disease lead to a number of Parlimentary reforms, including the Factories and Workshops Act 1867 and the Factories (Prevention of Lead Poisoning) Act 1883: 'this Act [Factories and Workshops Act of 1867] marks the opening of the modern era in legislation aimed to protect the workers in all dangerous trades' (Hunter, 1978, p. 130).

The rise of textile factories led to the exploitation of child labour. The Factory Act of 1833, also named An Act to Regulate the Labour of Children in the Mills and Factories of the United Kingdom was written to prevent this exploitation:

> It applied to all textile factories where steam or water power was used, including flax, hemp and silk. It forbade night work for those under eighteen and restricted their hours to twelve a day and sixty-nine a week; factory schools were established and all children under the age of thirteen were required to attend for at least two hours a day. The minimum age was set at nine. Prior to the passing of this Act the age of a child was established by a certificate, often very dubious, from the parent; but by the Act of 1833 a certificate of age was required from a medical man to the effect that a child was of the ordinary strength and appearance of a child exceeding nine years or other specified age.
>
> Hunter, 1978, p. 126

Recent example of toxic chemicals in the workplace in Sweden

When a chemical's toxicity is unknown and handled by workers, there can be a risk for disease and illness. In 1997, during the construction of a railway tunnel in the southern part of Sweden, the toxic substance Rocha Gil was used to stop water from flowing into the tunnel. Little was known about the effects of the substance on workers; however, 28 workers showed neurological symptoms of ataxia, loss of sensory function and severe fatigue after handling Rocha Gil. In 2002, four of these workers continued to have neurological symptoms. Moreover, farmers in the region were forbidden to use the ground water after their cows died having consumed the contaminated water and salmon in nearby streams were found dead (Berg, 2002).

Workers' compensation

Added protection for workers occurred when workers' compensation legislation was introduced in Switzerland in 1877, with additional laws enacted in Europe, the USA and Australia in the early twentieth century (Texas Workers' Compensation Commission, nd). Workers' compensation is now recognized throughout the world as an entitlement. (See Table 9.1 for the sequence of historical events that led to Medicaid, Medicare, and Workers' Compensation.)

Table 9.1 History of workers' compensation, health insurance and disability protection

1877	Switzerland enacted the first coverage for occupational diseases
1883	German national compulsory health insurance programme enacted
1890	The Swedish Labour Inspectorate formed. Renamed the Swedish Work Environment Authority in 1949
1906	Workers' compensation provided for certain diseases in Great Britain
1906	First US workmen's compensation law enacted (later declared unconstitutional) because they violated employer property rights without due process of law
1908	Workers' compensation system established in USA for federal employees
1911	British National Health Insurance programme enacted
1911	First state workers' compensation law that held up in court established in Wisconsin, USA
1912	South Africa passed the Miners' Phthisis Compensation Act
1917	US Supreme Court ruled that States could legally require employers to provide compensation to workers injured on the job
1921	Sheppard–Towner Act enacted providing United States Federal subsidies for state-run child and maternal health programmes
1933	Private hospital insurance approved by American Hospital Association (AHA), leading to establishment of Blue Cross
1935	In the USA, Social Security Act signed into law; health insurance excluded
1942	Beveridge Report advocated a comprehensive social welfare system for UK
1946	Hill–Burton Hospital Survey and Construction Act passed in the USA
1949	Swedish National Board of Safety and Health established standards for protection of workers

Table 9.1 History of workers' compensation, health insurance and disability protection (continued)

1950	United States Social Security Act amendments of 1950 include grants to states for 'vendor payments' in behalf of welfare recipients
1956	United States military 'medicare' programme enacted, providing Government health insurance protection for Armed Forces' dependants
1965	Medicare (as part of the Social Security Amendments of 1965) signed into law by President Johnson. Title XIX of the same Act authorized Medicaid
1970	United States Congress passed the Act of 1970, which established the Occupational Safety and Health Administration (OSHA) and the National Institute for Occupational Safety and Health (NIOSH)
1978	The Swedish Working Environment Act enacted, which covered physical as well as psychological disabilities. This Act also required that the working environment adapt to the individual's condition
1990	Passage of the Americans with Disabilities Act
2001	The Swedish National Board of Safety and Health and The Swedish Labour Inspectorate were merged into the Swedish Work Environment Authority.

Adapted from Adapting Work Sites for People with Disabilities: Ideas from Sweden, G. Elmfeldt, C. Wise, H. Bergsen and X. Olsson, 1982, World Rehabilitation Fund: The Swedish Institute for the Handicapped; Occupational Safety and Health Administration (1970). OSH Act of 1970: Introduction. Public Law 91-596, 91st Congress, S.2193, December 29, 1970; 84 STAT.1590 retrieved 22 March 2005, http://www.osha-slc.gov/pls/oshaweb; Peter Coming History of Medicare – Appendix A Chronology of Significant Events Leading to Enactment of Medicare, ndb, the Social Security Administration, retrieved 21 March 2005, www.ssa.gov/history/cornignappa.html; personal communication from Ingela Rönn, Information Secretary for the Swedish Work Environment Authority; Texas Workers' Compensation Commission, retrieved 21 March 2005, www.twcc.state.tx.us/information/historyofwc.html; Texas Health and Human Services Commission, Medicaid History, retrieved 21 March 2005, http://www.hhsc.state.tx.us/Medicaid

Workers' compensation is a government-regulated system that provides workers with monetary compensation, including death and medical benefits for injuries, fatalities, or diseases directly related to the occupation or job. In the USA, employers purchase workers' compensation insurance through (a) a private company; (b) by self-insuring; or (c) by buying insurance from a state insurance fund (New York State Insurance Fund, 2005). In the United States and US Territories, state or territorial boards regulate workers' compensation. All government and public employers in all states require it. Texas is the only state which still allows private employers to choose whether or not to maintain workers' compensation insurance (Texas Worker's Compensation Committee, nd). The terms workers' compensation, worker's compensation, workman's compensation and workmen's compensation are used interchangeably.

There are still questions raised by employers and workers as to what constitutes a work-related injury or disease. For example, stress-related injuries, cardiovascular disorders and psychological illnesses are litigated in courts (e.g. the Swedish labour court) to determine if they are related to a job and therefore can be covered by worker's compensation. Some workers who have been injured on the job and received worker's compensation are covered, in the USA, by the Americans with Disabilities Act (ADA) (US Equal Employment Opportunity Commission, 1997).

Women's trade unions (1875–1903)

In general, women, like children, were exploited in the various industries until the twentieth century. They often worked long hours, under dangerous conditions, and rarely were paid as well as men working in similar jobs. They were also responsible for childcare and household tasks, which increased their risk for illness and disease. In 1875 in England, Emma Paterson formed the first women's trade union, the Women's Protective and Provident League. The name was later changed to the Women's Trade Union League (Simkin, 2005).

> Not only are women frequently paid half or less than half for doing work as well and as quickly as men, but skilled women whose labour requires delicacy of touch, the result of long training as well as thoughtfulness, receive from 11 shillings to 16 or 17 shillings a week, while the roughest unskilled labour of a man is worth at least 18 shillings.
>   Emma Paterson, 1974 as cited in National Grid for Learning, nd

The purpose of this union, as well as other women's trade unions, was to support women's demands for better working conditions, increase pay and to raise awareness about the exploitation of women workers. Improvement in the working conditions for women in the USA was the direct result of unionization and the formation of the National Women's Trade Union League in 1903 during the American Federation of Labor's Boston convention:

> Since colonial times women have participated in the American labor movement, first forming sisterly self-improvement societies, then organizing their own trade unions, and finally demanding full admission, rights, and responsibilities in the national assemblies of brother workers.
>   O'Sullivan and Gallick, 1975, p. 8

Social security legislation in the United States (1930s to present)

'[I]n terms of the eternal problem of economic security, social insurance endeavors to solve it by pooling risk assets from a large social group and providing income to those members of the group whose economic security is being threatened' (Social Security OnLine, 2003, Social Insurance Movement, para 2).

Social security legislation was passed in the United States in 1935 during the Great Depression, in the administration of President Franklin

Roosevelt. The Preamble for the Social Security Act of 14 August 1935 (HR 7260) reads as follows:

> An act to provide for the general welfare by establishing a system of Federal old-age benefits, and by enabling the several States to make more adequate provision for aged persons, blind persons, dependent and crippled children, maternal and child welfare, public health, and the administration of their unemployment compensation laws; to establish a Social Security Board; to raise revenue; and for other purposes.
>
> Social Security OnLine, nda, History: Social Security, para. 1

Originally, the Act benefited the worker by providing a minimum retirement income. Numerous amendments have extended the original Act. The 1939 amendments included benefits paid to the spouse and minor children of a retired worker, and survivor's benefits paid to the family. This extended the Social Security system to a family-based economic security programme. The Cost of Living Adjustments (COLAs) were introduced in the amendments of 1950 to help retirees to keep up with the rising cost of inflation. Amendments of the Social Security Act in 1954 introduced a disability insurance programme to provide benefits to workers aged 50–64 who were permanently disabled and to adult children with disabilities. This was changed in 1960 to provide benefits to workers of any age who had become permanently disabled and to their dependants. In the Social Security Amendments of 1972, Congress created the Supplemental Security Income (SSI), which federalized the financial benefit programmes for individuals with disabilities (Social Security OnLine, 2003).

President Lyndon Johnson signed legislation covering Medicare and Medicaid into law in 1965. This legislation resulted in a major change to the Social Security Act. Medicare provides basic health coverage for almost all Americans ages 65 or older, while Medicaid provides health coverage for individuals below the poverty line, as defined by the Federal Government (Centers for Medicare and Medicaid Services, 2004).

In 1999, the Ticket to Work and Work Incentives Improvement Act (Social Security OnLine ndc; Social Security OnLine, 2003) was enacted to provide resources to adult individuals with disabilities, enabling them to purchase vocational rehabilitation, employment and other support services, in order to return to work. Vocational rehabilitation agencies are given incentive payments when the individual is successfully rehabilitated and can return to work. This law:

- 'increases beneficiary choice in obtaining rehabilitation and vocational services to help them go to work and attain their employment goals;
- removes barriers that require people with disabilities to choose between health care coverage and work; and
- assures that more Americans with disabilities have the opportunity to participate in the workforce and lessen their dependence on public benefits' (Social Security Online, ndc, para. 1).

In 2000, Congress enacted the Senior Citizens Freedom to Work Act, which allowed retirees over age 65 to collect full Social Security benefits without being limited by other income. Previously, retirees between 65 and 70 would have their social security benefits reduced if they earned more than the maximum amount allowed (Social Security OnLine, 2000). In 2005 there has been much controversy regarding Social Security in the USA and other industrial nations where conservative legislators have advocated changes in the system to allow workers to use a portion of their social security taxes to invest in private accounts. However, the original notion of social security as a retirement benefit for a worker has universal support throughout the world.

United States Occupational Safety and Health Agencies (OSHA)

The Occupational Safety and Health Act was passed by Congress in 1970. The mission of OSHA is:

> To assure safe and healthful working conditions for working men and women; by authorizing enforcement of the standards developed under the Act; by assisting and encouraging the States in their efforts to assure safe and healthful working conditions; by providing for research, information, education, and training in the field of occupational safety and health; and for other purposes.
>
> Occupational Health and Safety Administration, 1970, Introduction

On-site inspections, regulations and enforcement of laws relating to dangerous and unhealthy conditions in all industries are the principal activities of OSHA.

The United States Department of Labor has identified characteristics of dangerous and hazardous occupations, and complied statistical data for those occupations with the largest number of fatalities and injuries (see Table 9.2). In 1994, the occupations with the highest risk for injuries were farm occupations, truck-drivers, roofers, construction labourers, taxicab drivers, pilots, lumberjacks and fishermen (Bureau of Labor Statistics, 1996; Toscano, 1997).

> Today, the jobs that have the highest fatality rates and frequency counts are found in outdoor occupations or occupations where workers are not in an office or factory. These include truck drivers, farmers, construction labourers, and airplane pilots. Most of these workers have one thing in common: they are affected by severe weather conditions, while driving on highways, flying airplanes, performing farm chores, or working on construction sites. Highway crashes are the primary cause of trucker fatalities, falls are the leading cause of death for construction labourers, and tractor rollovers account for 1 of every 3 farm worker fatalities.
>
> Homicide is another serious concern in some job settings. In 1995, homicide accounted for 16 percent of job-related fatalities. Workers most at risk are those who work late at night, work alone, and handle money.

Taxicab drivers are the most susceptible and have a relative risk about 10 times higher than the typical worker. Other occupations that have a high relative risk of homicide include police and guards.

For jobs with high numbers of nonfatal injuries and illnesses, overexertion is the leading event. These injuries result from lifting objects or, in the case of nursing aides and orderlies, patients. Injuries from overexertion accounted for about one third of all the nonfatal injuries in 1994; it took a median of 5 days for those injured to recuperate.

Two occupations appear on both the fatal and nonfatal lists: truckdrivers and construction labourers. But the leading event for fatal and nonfatal incidents for each occupation is different. For truckdrivers, 68 percent of the job-related fatalities are from highway crashes, whereas overexertion is the leading nonfatal event, accounting for 29 percent of the incidents. For construction labourers, the leading fatal events are falls and vehicular-related incidents such as being struck by a backhoe. For nonfatal incidents, the leading event is contact with objects, primarily equipment and tools used on construction sites.

This difference between the leading cause of a fatal and nonfatal injury for truck drivers is important because it suggests different kinds of prevention efforts. For example, to reduce highway crashes, driver training and proper maintenance of trucks is essential, whereas, to reduce the incidence of overexertion, proper lifting techniques must be taught along with proper use of lifting equipment. For construction labourers, prevention programmes for fatal events require awareness of the hazards of falling off buildings, ladders, scaffoldings, and other structures while for serious nonfatal injuries, prevention would focus on the proper use of tools.

Toscano, 1997, p 57

Table 9.2 Occupations with largest number of injuries and illnesses, 1994

Occupation	Total non-fatal cases (thousands)	Employment (thousands)	Chance of injury	Leading non-fatal event (percentage)
All occupations	2252.6	92,973	1:41	
Truck drivers	726.5	14,636	1:20	Overexertion (29)
Non-construction labourers	147.3	1137	1:08	Contact with object (35)
Nursing aides and orderlies	101.8	1359	1:13	Overexertion (59)
Janitors and cleaners	60.6	1407	1:23	Overexertion (27)
Construction labourers	55.7	674	1:12	Contact with object (39)
Assemblers	53.0	1167	1:22	Contact with object (31)
Carpenters	37.4	869	1:23	Contact with object (38)
Stock handlers and baggers	37.2	1121	1:30	Overexertion (37)
Cooks	36.3	1838	1:51	Contact with object (33)
Cashiers	35.6	2626	1:74	Overexertion (27)

Adapted from the Survey of occupational injuries and illnesses, 1994, US Department of Labor, Bureau of Labor Statistics, 1996, retrieved 23 March 2005, http://www.bls.gov/iif/oshwc/osh/os/ossm0008.txt.

National Institute for Occupational Safety and Health (NIOSH)

Another Federal agency founded at the same time as OSHA (OSH Act of 1970) is the National Institute for Occupational Safety and Health (NIOSH). The goals of this agency include (a) conducting research on the full scope of occupational disease and injury; (b) disseminating information to prevent workplace disease, injury and disability; (c) developing a system to monitor major occupational illnesses, injuries, exposures and health hazards; and (d) providing training to occupational safety and health professionals. NIOSH consists of employees from diverse disciplines, including industrial hygiene, nursing, epidemiology, engineering, medicine and statistics (NIOSH, nd).

Americans with Disabilities Act of 1990 (ADA)

The Americans with Disabilities Act of 1990 (1991) extended Section 504 of the Rehabilitation Act of 1973, which prohibited discrimination on the basis of disability to any agency receiving federal funds to the private sector. There are five titles in the law: (a) Employment (Title I); (b) Public Services (Title II); (c) Public Accommodations (Title III); (d) Telecommunications (Title IV); (e) Miscellaneous (Title V) (US Department of Justice, Civil Rights Division, Disability Rights Section, 2001).

- *Title 1: Employment.* When there are 15 or more employees in a private business, the employer must provide reasonable accommodations so that the individual with a disability can perform a job. For example, an individual with a spinal cord injury who is in a wheelchair must be given an accommodation that allows him or her access to the building, workstations or bathrooms. Accommodations may include redesigning the job, adding a ramp, rearranging tables and chairs in the workstation or modifying tools and equipment. Discrimination is prohibited in the application process, interview, hiring procedures, wages or benefits, pre-employment medical examination, health insurance, working conditions, promotions and social activities.
- *Title 2: Public Services.* Individuals with disabilities cannot be denied access to public or governmental buildings, programmes or activities (e.g. voting, public meetings, court hearings or health care), recreational facilities or public transportation (e.g. buses, trains, airplanes or commuter facilities) that are accessible to the general public. For example, public auditoriums, such as cinemas, should have special places available for people in wheelchairs.
- *Title 3: Public Accommodations.* Any new construction or modifications to existing buildings open to the public must be made accessible for individuals with disabilities. Examples of these buildings include restaurants, hotels, supermarkets, shopping centres, department stores, zoos, homeless shelters, funeral homes, day care centres or

recreational facilities (e.g. swimming pools, sports stadiums). Parking spaces should be van-accessible, and individuals with disabilities should have access to privately owned transportation systems. Accessibility frequently includes adding lifts, building ramps or ensuring the bathroom is wheelchair accessible. For example, a supermarket should have sufficiently wide aisles so that individuals in wheelchairs can shop easily.

- *Title 4: Telecommunications.* Telephone and television access for individuals with hearing and speech disabilities are covered in this title. Since federally-funded public service announcements must have closed captions, televisions must have this capability. Telephone companies are required to establish interstate and intrastate telecommunications relay services (TRS) 24 hours a day, seven days a week so that telecommunications devices for the deaf (TDDs), such as teletypewriters (TTYs) or voice telephones, can communicate with each other through a third-party communications assistant. All newer television sets have closed caption capability, and many television studios transmit closed captions programmes on a routine basis.

- *Title 5: Miscellaneous.* Included in this title are such provisions as preventing employees or governmental agencies from requiring an individual with disabilities to accept accommodations through coercion, threat or retaliation against either those with disabilities or those trying to help the individual with disability.

While statistics regarding compliance with ADA regulations are not readily available, the National Council on Disability (1996) has accumulated information regarding compliance from the public sector:

Polls repeatedly indicate that employers support the employment of people with disabilities and experience people with disabilities as good employees. A 1995 poll of 300 chief executive officers and human resource managers in Fortune 5000 companies found that 73 percent of the top industries across the country are currently hiring people with disabilities. Most reported that ADA has had a positive impact on corporations; only 16 percent believed it has had a negative effect (President's Committee on Employment of People with Disabilities [PCEPD] 1995). Lou Harris and Associates surveyed employers in 1986 and again in 1995 and found strong support for ADA and the employment of people with disabilities. The employment antidiscrimination provisions of ADA apply to 666,000 businesses employing about 86 million people.

The percentage of companies reporting that they have made accommodations in the workplace increased from 51 percent to 81 percent between 1986 and 1995 (Lou Harris and Associates 1995). Furthermore, the costs of accommodations did not appear significant, with about half of employers saying costs increased a little between 1986 and 1995 and 32 percent reporting no increase. The Job Accommodation Network operated by PCEPD to assist employers in developing specific work accommodations has consistently reported that the majority of accommodations cost less than $500. One case study of Sears, Roebuck and Co. (Blanck 1994a) found that 97 percent of accommodations involved little or no cost.

Analysis of one national data set indicates that between one-fourth and one-third of workers who become impaired on the job are accommodated following onset of disability. Those who are accommodated at work are more likely to stay employed than those who are not. Most who continue to work after the onset of disability remain with their current employers (Burkhauser, Butler and Kim 1994; Daly and Bound 1994).

Despite the positive attitudes of many employers and the effectiveness of job accommodations, many companies are still not hiring people with disabilities. Lou Harris and Associates (1986, 1995) found that the percentage of companies that had hired people with disabilities within the last three years changed only slightly between 1986 and 1995 – from 62 percent to 64 percent. The most commonly cited reason for not hiring people with disabilities, both in 1986 and 1995, was a lack of qualified applicants.

National Council on Disability, 1996, pp. 74–75

Swedish experience in the protection of the worker

The Swedish Labour Inspectorate started in 1890 and National Board of Safety and Health started in 1949. A merger of these two authorities resulted in the formation of the Swedish Work Environment Authority on 1 January 2001. This authority is financially sponsored by governmental agency, the Labour Market Federations of Trade Unions (e.g. The Swedish Trade Union Confederation (LO)), The Swedish Central Organization of Salaried Employees (TCO), The Swedish Employers' Confederation, Agencies for Business Health Services (aimed at protecting workers' health and preventing work hazards) and other Swedish companies (I. Rönn, Information Secretary for The Swedish Work Environment Authority, personal communication, 16 August 2001).

The Swedish Work Environment Authority

Sweden has a reliable tradition for supervising the health and safety of workers in the work environment and of researching factors that relate to health and safety issues, the job market and the work environment. The concepts of work environment and occupational injury are defined more broadly than in most other countries and are closely linked to productivity and efficiency. The term 'work environment' refers not only to traditional physical, technical and chemical health hazards, but also to psychosocial problems, occupational stress, job organization (work systems), job requirements and other labour market-related issues (e.g. job opportunities). The concept of occupational injury also has a wider meaning than in other countries. The focus of the Swedish Work Environment

Authority is not only on job-related accidents or diseases, but also on work-related environment factors that contribute to cumulative effects of illness and environmental toxins.

Swedish Workers' Rights – Labour Law

The following information is taken from Section 3.10 of the Work Environment Act.

The Work Environment Act applies to the entire labour market with the exception of work performed in the employer's own home and aboard privately owned vessels. Special legislation applies to these workplaces.

The Work Environment Act is a framework law, which means that it does not contain any detailed regulations but only specifies the framework for how work concerning the working environment is to be carried out. The detailed regulations are issued by the Swedish National Board of Occupational Safety and Health in the form of directives.

The state of the work environment. The work environment shall be kept in a satisfactory state having regard to the nature of the work involved and social and technological evolution. The work must be adapted to human physical and mental capabilities. It is important that the work be organised so that the employees themselves have the opportunity to influence their work situation.

The Work Environment Act also contains a number of general requirements concerning special work environment factors. As regards the design of the workplace, for example, it is stipulated that ventilation, acoustics, lighting and other conditions must be satisfactory from the point of view of work environment and worker protection.

The employer has the main responsibility. The local health and safety work at the workplace should be carried out by the employer and the employees together. The main responsibility for the working environment, however, rests with the employer. He is obliged to take all necessary action to prevent the employees from being exposed to health and accident risks at the workplace.

The employer is responsible for planning, directing and controlling the work environment regularly and systematically. Measures for protecting the workers must be planned for the future if they are not possible to implement immediately.

The employer is also responsible for ensuring that there are organised work adaptation and rehabilitation activities suitable to the operations.

The responsibility of the employees. The employees also have a responsibility for the work environment. They are obliged to follow given instructions and to use existing protective devices and other safety equipment. In other respects the employees must also show such care at work that ill-health and accidents are avoided.

The manufacturer's responsibility. Anyone manufacturing, importing, selling or hiring out a machine or other technical equipment is obliged to ensure that it is provided with such protective devices that accidents and ill-health are prevented.

Chemical health hazards. Anyone manufacturing, importing or supplying a substance hazardous to health is obliged to take necessary measures to prevent and counteract risks in the intended use of the substance.

Young people. Anyone under the age of 18 is counted as a young person. No-one under the age of 16 years or who has not completed his or her schooling may be employed. The exception is for simple and non-hazardous duties such as light office work.

Children and young people under the age of 13 years may only perform such work as does not entail physical or mental strain, such as selling Mayday pins or Christmas magazines.

Safety delegates. There is to be a safety delegate at all workplaces with at least five employees. The safety delegate is appointed by the local trade union organization. If there are more safety delegates at a workplace, one of them is to be appointed head safety delegate, with the task of co-ordinating the work of the safety delegates and representing the group in certain questions.

A safety delegate represents the employees in matters of safety and is to work for satisfactory safety conditions. For this purpose, in his or her safety area the delegate is to supervise the protection against ill health and accidents.

The delegate shall participate in the planning of new or changed premises, devices, work processes and working methods as well as in the planning of the use of substances that may cause ill-health or accidents.

The safety delegate should also supervise whether the employer fulfils his responsibility of ensuring that the work environment fulfils the requirements of the Work Environment Act by means of internal control and has organized work adaptation and rehabilitation activities suitable to the operations.

The safety delegate may in certain cases be appointed from outside the circle of employees at the place of work, so called regional safety delegates.

Safety committee. At workplaces with at least 50 employees there is to be a safety committee. If the employees so require, such a committee shall, however, be set up even if the number of employees is less than 50.

The safety committee is made up of representatives of both employer and employees. Its task is to supervise the health and safety work and to follow developments in matters concerning prevention of accidents and ill-health.

Supervisory authority. The National Board of Occupational Safety and Health and the regional Labour Inspectorates function as the supervisory authority and their task is to ensure that the Work Environment Act is complied with.

The Labour Inspectorate has the right to issue injunctions on employers if this is necessary to ensure compliance with the Work Environment Act or the National Board of Occupational Safety and Health's regulations. The Labour Inspectorate is also entitled to issue prohibitions, such as against the use of machines that do not meet safety requirements.

The Swedish Labour Market, 1999, pp. 27–35

Health promotion in the workplace

Psychological counselling programmes for workers were started in the 1950s as large numbers of returning veterans from the Second World War became re-employed in factories and corporations. Many of these veterans had developed drug and alcohol dependencies under the duress of war and continued these habits as civilians. Corporations, recognizing that these problems interfered with work production, established on-the-job counselling to help these workers to deal more effectively with drug and alcohol abuse. These programmes later became formalized and supported by US federal funds and were designated Employee Assistance Programs (EAP). Later, during the 1970s and 1980s, there was a growing trend for large companies to initiate health promotion programmes in addition to EAPs, titled Employee Wellness, Health Enhancement or Disease Prevention. These included smoking cessation, physical conditioning, stress management, nutrition and weight management, in addition to alcohol, drug abuse and psychological counseling (Klarreich, 1987). The rationale for developing these programmes was the recognition by large corporations that (a) healthy employees can increase productivity, (b) prevention is cost-effective and (c) personal health can be improved by changing one's lifestyle (Saxl, 1984). Other incentives to develop health promotion programmes in the workplace included reducing absenteeism, enhancing the corporate image and increasing employee morale (Vojtecky, 1987). Over the years, Employee Assistance Programs have evolved into a formal structure and international organization, EAPA International, Inc. Currently EAP services are defined 'as a worksite-based programme designed to assist work organizations in addressing productivity issues, and employee clients in identifying and resolving personal concerns which may affect job performance' (Employee Assistance Professional Association, 2005, para 1.)

The Employee Assistance Professionals Association (2005) has identified the core components that underlie all EAPs:

1 Consult with employers and management, distressed employees and their families regarding the improvement of work environment and job performance.
2 Provide confidential and timely services for identifying and assessing employee concerns.
3 Use psychological counselling techniques that include motivating the client to change self-abusing behaviour that has negatively affected job performance.
4 Refer employee for evaluation and treatment including case management and follow-up.
5 Consult with employer and managers to maintain effective communication between the work organization, employee and referral agency.
6 Inform employers of the availability and access to health benefits that cover services for drug and alcohol abuse and mental health disorders.
7 Evaluate the effectiveness of the EAP on the job performance and employee health, and recommend changes in the workplace if necessary.

A number of research studies have demonstrated the effectiveness of worksite health promotion programmes on the reduction of disabilities and cost-effectiveness.

- Serxner et al. (2001), in a three-year study with over 1600 participants, examined the effectiveness of a worksite health promotion on short-term disability. The programme included health risk assessment, opportunities to take part in wellness and fitness activities, targeted interventions for employees at risk, health brochures and health information counselling. The researchers compared participants in the study with a non-participant control group. They found that the interventions had a significant effect on absenteeism due to illness. The projected savings for a two-year period was US$1,371,600.
- Rahe et al. (2002) studied the effects of a stress-management programme which included both a focus on reducing stress and anxiety, and increasing coping skills in a small group format. Using random allocation to form three groups, they found that those individuals who participated had fewer days of illness and a significant reduction in medical utilization as compared with a wait-list control (a control group that does not receive intervention). In general the results of research on the effects of health promotion programmes in the workplace have demonstrated that these programmes can reduce corporate costs, increase employee health, decrease health insurance costs and enhance performance, productivity and morale.
- An innovative intervention programme for rural female blue-collar workers in North Carolina evaluated the effects of a health promotion programme in smoking cessation, healthy nutrition and physical conditioning. It was concluded that the project was a successful model for achieving positive changes in health behaviour (Campbell et al., 2002).

Controlling factors in the environment

What are the controlling factors in the workplace that influence the onset of injuries and diseases? The employer, government, health professionals and ergonomists have an important role in creating a safe environment for the worker. The employer who provides the opportunities for the worker to gain employment is most concerned with the profitability and productiveness of the worker. It is in the best interests of the employer and the worker for the company or enterprise to be profitable and for the workers to stay healthy. If the working conditions put the worker in a vulnerable position for injuries and diseases, then both productiveness and the worker's health are compromised. The government, through occupational protection agencies such as OSHA, establishes standards in the work environment to prevent work-related illness. These standards are translated into federal or state laws that are enforced through on-site inspections of the workplace. In the medical model, the company doctor or industrial nurse is employed by large corporations to treat the worker in the workplace and to provide consultation. In the ergonomic model the industrial engineer and occupational therapist apply ergonomic principles in the workplace to prevent injuries in the workplace through job analysis, environmental adaptations, tool modifications and changes in the pace of production.

Various models to control factors in the environment, and which impact on work conditions, have evolved. These four models, identified as *laissez-faire, bureaucratic, medical* and *self-regulation*, describe the authority of the employer, government, health professionals, ergonomists and the worker in creating a healthy work environment (see Table 9.3). Each of these models serves to control the worker's productivity and health and safety. Predominantly the employer is most concerned with economic growth and fostering a cost-effective environment for profit. Both the employer and the worker benefit from the economic viability of the company. Governmental legislation through OSHA and NIOSH in the

Table 9.3 Models of controlling factors in the environment

	Employer (*Laissez-faire*)	Public health (Bureaucratic)	Treatment (Medical model)	Human factors (Self-regulation)
Locus of control	Employer	Government	Physician or nurse	Ergonomist and worker
Purpose	Increase profits	Prevent disease or injury	Treat disease	Design healthy environment
Content for innovation	Production methods	Legislation	Medication and surgery	Ergonomics
Methods for change	Cost-effective technology	Worksite supervision	Scientific medicine	Psychophysiological approaches
Potential problems	Worker burn-out	Increase in litigation	Patient dependence on health personnel	Lack of worker compliance and follow-up
Positive effects	Economic growth, production and growth	Protection from abuse and work injury	Prevent recurrence of illness	Increase responsibility of worker for their health

Adapted from Occupational stress, biofeedback and stress management, F. Stein, 2001, *Work: A Journal of Prevention, Assessment and Rehabilitation*, 17, 235–245.

USA and comparable governmental agencies in other countries seek to prevent work-related disease and injury by establishing standards for healthy conditions in the workplace.

In the first model, *laissez-faire*, the employer is given the option to create a safe working environment with the incentive that a safe environment is both beneficial to the employer and the worker.

The second model, *bureaucratic*, is concerned with governmental monitoring of the work environment. Worksite supervision and monitoring of unhealthy or unsafe conditions are used to reduce injuries and disease in the workplace. An increase in litigation has resulted from enforcing work standards and requiring employers to meet minimum standards for safe and healthy work environments. These standards sometimes create an adversarial relationship between the employer and the worker, creating tension and adding to occupational stress.

The third model, *medical*, is the role of the company doctor or industrial nurse in the workplace. In large corporations or industrial plants, on-site medical personnel are used to treat workers for injuries occurring on the job.

The fourth model in preventing occupational injuries in the workplace is the *self-regulatory ergonomics* or human factors approach. In this model the ergonomist seeks to design work environments that prevent injury and occupational disease. Environmental modifications include (a) the redesign of workplaces using the worker's optimal biomechanical posture for avoiding musculoskeletal neck and back pain (Schult et al., 1995); (b) adaptation of tools to prevent hand injuries; (c) job organization and job rotation to decrease boredom and burn-out; (d) optimal work environments (e.g. lighting, temperature, ventilation and avoidance of exposure to toxic or caustic chemicals); (e) floor mats to decrease falls; (f) protective clothing to prevent toxic chemicals from entering the body; and (g) ear protection to prevent loss of hearing. Psychophysiological factors are also considered in preventing occupational stress. For example, relaxation therapy could be recommended to help the worker cope more effectively with stress and to prevent hypertension from arising from added pressure on the worker. In this model, responsibility is put on the worker to comply with recommendations made by the ergonomist. Lack of compliance and follow-up by the worker can compromise the positive benefits from a human factors or psychophysiological approach (Stein, 2001).

Another important factor in reducing ill-health and absenteeism is an optimal work organization with competent and responsible supervisors and managers. Numerous studies of workplaces are viewed according to the workers' self-evaluation where two models are compared. The Job Diagnostic Survey model (Hackman and Oldham, 1976) shows the need for redesigning jobs (Schult and Söderback, 2000). When the job is redesigned, positive work and personal outcomes (e.g. high internal motivation, work satisfaction and quality performance, low absenteeism and low staff turnover) are expected. Another approach is the Demand-Control-Support Model (Karasek, 1979) designed to describe work organizations. Different kinds of psychological work experiences are generated by the interaction of high and low levels of psychological demands, decision latitude and social support (Johnson et al., 1989). A high degree of strain occurs when the level of decision latitude is low or the social support from fellow workers or superiors is poor, leading to an elevated risk of developing a physical illness such as heart diseases (Malinauskiene et al., 2005).

Development of ergonomics and human factors

The concept of ergonomics, of fitting the work environment, machines and tools to the human anatomy and physiology (anthropometry) developed during the Second World War when scientists and psychologists adapted tanks, submarines and planes to the physical capacities of the individual (Meister, 1999). Prior to the Second World War, Fredrick W. Taylor analysed factory jobs and established times for completing specific tasks by developing the Movement Time Measure (MTM). This 'analyzes any manual operation or method into the basic motions required to perform it and assigns to each motion predetermined time standard which is determined by the nature of the motion and the conditions under which it is made' (Jacobs, 1991, p. 24). During the period between 1930 and 1970 the MTM was the basis for determining the piecework rate for different jobs in the labour market. Simulated work tasks used to assess the worker's vocational capacity (e.g. the VALPAR work samples) uses MTMs to determine when the worker meets the criteria for performing the work task compared with a normal worker standard. Taylor also looked at psychological variables, such as encouragement and attention, to increase production. Taylor was also interested in designing tools, such as a shovel, to increase the worker's output. He employed formal methods of data collection and statistical analysis that foreshadowed the current methods used by ergonomists in job analysis (US Department of Labor, Employment and Training Administration, 1991). Taylor's principles of work design and time-and-motion studies are models for practice (Meister, 1999; Taylor, 1919).

Taylor (1919) believed that the main elements of the scientific management were:

- time studies
- functional or specialized supervision
- standardization of tools and implements
- standardization of work methods
- separate planning function
- management by exception principle

- the use of 'slide-rules and similar time-saving devices'
- instruction cards for workmen
- task allocation and large bonuses for successful performance
- the use of the 'differential rate'
- mnemonic systems for classifying products and implements
- a routing system
- a modern costing system. (Taylor, 1919, pp. 129–130)

Two other pioneers in the history of ergonomics were Frank and Lillian Gilbreth. Frank Gilbreth was one of Taylor's students. They initiated time-and-motion studies and used motion pictures for analysing job tasks. Lillian Gilbreth became interested in applying ergonomics to the performance of household tasks, and was one of the first scientists to work in the area of kitchen layouts for individuals with disabilities (International Work Simplification Institute, Inc., 1968).

During the First World War, psychologists were employed to evaluate the capacities of individuals to operate aeroplanes. Aeromedical research, using flight simulators, placed emphasis on fitting the individual to the machine, rather than adjusting or adapting the machine to the physical and psychological characteristics of the individual. During the 1920s, research in behavioural factors in operating an automobile was initiated at Ohio State University. Using driving simulators and analysing psychological and physical factors, the researchers examined factors leading to automobile accidents, accident-prone drivers, perceptual aspects when driving and the social characteristics of traffic violators (Meister, 1999).

During the 1920s and 1930s, at the Hawthorne Plant of the Western Electric Company in New York State, psychologists examined the relationship between lighting and worker productivity. By accident, they discovered that attention to the worker is an important positive motivational factor in human performance (Meister, 1999). This was later coined the 'Hawthorne effect', which states that any positive attention to an individual can increase productivity or job motivation.

During the Second World War the concepts of ergonomics was applied to the selection of personnel and the fitting of men to jobs. The US Department of Defense used psychologists to develop personnel tests to screen out individuals from the armed services with low intellectual capacity and to use the tests to place individuals into various units where specialized training was provided, such as the signal corps, photography, radar detection and mechanical maintenance. The US Army General Classification Test (AGCT) and the mechanical aptitude and radio code tests were standard tests used in the selection process. Ergonomic principles were used in the design and manufacture of aircraft cockpits where experimental psychologists investigated the placement of control knobs (Meister, 1999). Other work during the war examined the 'human tolerance limits for high-altitude bailout, automatic parachute operating devices, cabin pressurization schedules, breathing equipment,

G-suits, and airborne evacuation facilities' (Dempsey, 1985 as cited in Meister, 1999, p. 152). After the Second World War, the fields of psychophysics, human engineering and human factors research expanded and became priorities for funding by governmental agencies.

The major landmarks in the history of ergonomics internationally are given below:

- 1949: The Ergonomics Research Society (ERS) was founded in Great Britain. The name was later changed in 1977 to the Ergonomics Society. Murrell, as one of the founders of this group, defined ergonomics as 'the study of the relationship between man and his working environment' (Ergonomics Society, 2002, para 1).
- 1953: The German Society for Work Science was first formed.
- 1957: The Ergonomics journal under ERS was founded.
- 1957: The Human Factors Society of America was founded. The name was changed to the Human Factors and Ergonomics Society in 1992. 'The Society furthers serious consideration of knowledge about the assignment of appropriate functions for humans and machines, whether people serve as operators, maintainers, or users in the system. And, it advocates systematic use of such knowledge to achieve compatibility in the design of interactive systems of people, machines, and environments to ensure their effectiveness, safety, and ease of performance' (Human Factors and Ergonomic Society, 1995–2004, para 2).
- 1960: The first textbook on ergonomics was published in Great Britain: *Ergonomics: Fitting the Job to the Worker*, by K.F.H. Murrell.
- 1962: International Ergonomics Association (IEA) formed.
- 1969: The journal *Applied Ergonomics* was founded.
- 1969: University College in London offers MSc in ergonomics.
- 1970: Joint meetings were held between the British Occupational Health Society, Society of Occupational Medicine and Ergonomics Research Society, acknowledging the relationship between occupational medicine and ergonomics.
- 1990: Association of Professional Ergonomic Consultancies founded in Great Britain.
- 1990: The Board of Certification in Professional Ergonomics (BCPE), a non-profit organization in the United States, was established to develop certification standards in ergonomics or human factors.
- 2000: The IEA Council defined ergonomics or human factors as 'the scientific discipline concerned with the understanding of interactions among humans and other elements of a system, and the profession that applies theory, principles and methods to design in order to optimize human well-being and overall system performance. Ergonomists contribute to the design and evaluation of tasks, jobs, products, environments and systems in order to make them compatible with the needs, abilities and limitations of people' (International Ergonomics Association, 2003b, para 1–2).

- 2002: There were 38 member countries in the International Ergonomics Association (International Ergonomics Association, 2003a).
- 2006: The International Ergonomics Association's Congress in Maastricht, The Netherlands

Certification of Professional Ergonomists

In the USA, the Board of Certification in Professional Ergonomics (BCPE) certifies human factors/ergonomics practitioners who (a) have a mastery of human factors/ergonomics knowledge; (b) have the ability to design a product, process or environment for ergonomic design; and (c) can apply this knowledge to analyse, design, test and evaluate ergonomic product, processes and environments.

The development of ergonomics certification however dates back to the mid 1980s when committees of the Human Factors and Ergonomics Society, the International Ergonomics Association, the Department of Defense, NATO, and the National Academic of Science/National Research Council performed several reviews of job/task analyses to identify the knowledge, skills, and abilities required of human factors/ergonomics practitioners.

Board of Certification in Professional Ergonomics, 2002–2005b, para 1

There are two levels of certification: Professional and Associate. The Professional certification applies to those individuals who solve complex problems and improves ergonomic technologies and methods. The Associate is an interventionist who applies knowledge in ergonomics to the performance, safety, health and/or quality issues in the workplace (Board of Certification in Professional Ergonomics, 2002–2005a).

The requirements for the Certified Professional Ergonomist (CPE) or Certified Human Factors Professional (CHFP) are:

1 A masters degree in ergonomics or human factors, or an equivalent educational background in the life sciences, engineering sciences and behavioral sciences to comprise a professional level of ergonomic education.
2 Three (3) years of full-time professional practice as an ergonomics practitioner with emphasis on design involvement (derived from ergonomic analysis and/or ergonomic testing/evaluation).
3 A passing score on the BCPE CPE/CHFP written examination.

Board of Certification in Professional Ergonomics, 2002–2005a,
Certification Requirements, para 1

The Certified Ergonomics Associate (CEA), available for the associate practitioner, has the following as criteria for CEA certification:

1 A bachelor's degree from an accredited university.
2 At least 200 contact hours of ergonomics training.

3 Two (2) years of full-time practice in ergonomics
4 A pass score on the CEA written examination.
            Board of Certification in Professional Ergonomics, 2002–2005a, p. 1
                                  Certification Requirements, para 2)

The Oxford Research Institute, located in New Market, Maryland, USA, offers certification as a Certified Industrial Ergonomist (CIE), or Certified Human Factors Engineering Professional (CHFEP). The criteria are as follows:

1 Résumé of experience as a provider of Human Factors Engineering, Engineering Psychology or Ergonomics technical services, documenting

   a Five or more years of experience plus BS, or
   b Four or more years of experience plus Masters, or
   c Three or more years of experience plus a PhD.
2 Evidence of specialized training or formal education in fields directly or closely related with human factors/ergonomics.
3 At least two work samples or technical products that reflect major contributions to the field of human factors/ergonomics.
4 Letters of professional recommendations.
5 Application fee.
6 Passing score on written examination (Oxford Research Institute, 2002).

Future trends in occupational medicine

In the last reported statistics in the USA in 1997, over 32 million injury episodes occurred in the home, work, school and leisure environments. Of these 32 million injury episodes, many could have been prevented by good ergonomic practices. According to the CDC (Warner et al., 2000), the following approximate injury episodes occurred:

• home (inside and outside) 43%
• street/highway 14%
• sports facility 8%
• industrial/construction 7%
• trade/service 7%
• park/recreation 4%
• other public buildings 3%
• others specified and not noted 13%
• Not known 1%

Of these injuries, 7 per cent required help in activities of daily living, such as household chores, shopping or personal care. On the basis of these reported statistics, the need for health professionals to provide ergonomic strategies to redesign environments that prevent accidents and injuries in the home, school, work and leisure environments are essential.

Currently, environmental factors such as inadequate ventilation resulting in poor building air quality, extreme temperature and humidity, inadequate illumination or excessive glare, and excessive noise can lead to disease and injury. In industrial environments, toxic chemicals, repetitive motion, vibration, radiation, dust and bacteria adversely affect workers. Sports injuries, such as muscular sprains and bone fractures, could be the result of poor or ill-fitting equipment, dangerous sports surfaces (e.g. wet or slippery fields) exceeding individual physical limits, lack of physical conditioning, poor instruction, or inattention to safety practices. In the home, injuries can occur because of slippery surfaces or stairs, obstacles, inattention when using sharp objects, inadequate lighting, improper safety practices when cooking (e.g. grease fires), lack of grab bars or bath mats in the bathroom or use of extremely hot liquids. Frequently, injuries occur because of unsafe practices when repairing electrical wiring, plumbing fixtures or roof tiles. The majority of school injuries occur in the playground, often because of inadequate supervision. For example, pupils fall off climbing frames, fall while chasing each other or running, or get hit by swings.

Physical, chemical, biological and psychological factors in work, home, school and leisure environments may cause or aggravate disease or injury in individuals who are vulnerable. For example, an individual with a predisposing condition of stenosis of the spinal column is at risk of developing a back injury if he or she works at task that entails twisting the back. Likewise, an individual with schizophrenia is at risk for exacerbation of psychological symptoms if the job includes high-performance demands or high stress (see Table 9.4).

Physical violence has increased in work settings because of occupational stress and job dissatisfaction. In the home, stress and financial issues,

Table 9.4 Relationship between predisposing and precipitating factors and occupational disabilities

Vulnerabilities (predisposing)	Stresses in workplace (precipitating)	Occupational Disabilities (potential risk)
Respiratory	Toxic fumes	Emphysema
Anatomical/musculoskeletal	Repetitive motion	Carpal tunnel syndrome
	Awkward positioning	Joint disorders
	Manual materials handling	Low back pain
Suppressed immune system	Exposure to pesticides	Neurological disorders
Pregnancy	Temperature extremes	Damage to foetus
Cardiovascular	Job overload	Hypertension
Gastrointestinal	Shift work	Gastric ulcers
Auditory	Excessive noise	Auditory impairment
Psychological	Interpersonal conflict	Depression
		Job burn-out

Adapted from The ergonomic model in occupational therapy, F. Stein, 2002, presentation at the World Federation of Occupational Therapy Congress, Stockholm, Sweden, June.

in combination with drug and alcohol use, are related to increases in the number of cases of physical abuse. Emotional disturbance and hopelessness have led to student violence.

In the future, ergonomic specialists using a systems approach will be employed to prevent and reduce the causes of injuries and disease previously listed. Interventions may include (a) modification of tools and equipment; (b) psychoeducational instruction; or (c) the development of healthy and safe environments. A biopsychosocial model will be employed in the evaluation and assessment of environmental factors; worker, homemaker and student characteristics; and organizational structure. For example, in the home, the ergonomic specialist may propose a kitchen layout that considers energy conservation, access to frequently used appliances, and lighting and ventilation. Another example might involve an individual in a wheelchair who requires changes in the heights of tables and more floor space in which to operate.

Within the psychosocial aspect, ergonomic principles will be used to decrease occupational stress, increase job satisfaction and manage anger, while increasing the worker's autonomy and participation in decision-making. Intervention programmes will include relaxation therapies (Benson, 1975), prescriptive exercise (Stein and Cutler, 2001), biofeedback (McGrady et al., 1995) and psychosocial techniques (Courtney and Escobedo, 1990; Stein and Nikolic, 1989; Taylor, 1988).

Summary

Progress towards creating a healthy environment for workers began in the seventeenth century with the work of Ramazzini who originated the field of occupational medicine. Ramazzini identified the relationship between hazards in the workplace and the onset of disease, and as a result, recommended cleanliness and healthy practices in the work environments. The industrial revolution that followed in the eighteenth and nineteenth centuries led to governmental regulations that enforced many of the recommendations of Ramazzini. Reforms in the workplace were the result of social movements and the collective action of women and unions. Government, employers, workers and health professionals all have been instrumental in creating a healthy work environment. Governmental agencies in industrial nations throughout the world, such as OSHA and the Department of Labor in the United States and the Work Environment Authority in Sweden, have recommended standards of practice to prevent injuries and illnesses. Employers are not only concerned with increasing production but with maintaining a healthy workforce. This has resulted in the creation of employee assistance programmes and the promotion of health in the workplace.

Workers have also enhanced their own safety by advocating the reduction of risks in the workplace and the protection of the health of children and women in dangerous occupations. Healthcare workers, including occupational physicians, ergonomists, industrial engineers and occupational and physical therapists, have brought their understanding of universal design, biomechanics, occupational diseases, kinesiology and stress management to develop occupational health programmes. These programmes aim at preventing occupational disease and injury, accommodating workers with disabilities and restoring function in workers injured on the job. The progress towards creating a ergonomically sound work environment where production is efficient and the worker is protected from injury is an ongoing activity that involves a multidisciplinary team. The influence of evidenced-based practice supported by clinical research will definitely affect the work of the occupational therapist incorporating ergonomics into everyday practice (Jacobs, 1999).

Review questions

1   Why is the history of ergonomics important in understanding current concepts in the discipline?
2   Why is occupational medicine included as part of the ergonomics history?
3   What role did occupational medicine play in the development of the field of ergonomics?
4   What is the relationship between ergonomics and human factors?
5   How does ergonomics relate to occupational therapy?
6   What are the diseases and injuries relevant to ergonomics and occupational medicine?
7   How does ergonomics as a problem-solving discipline examine factors in the environment that cause occupational diseases?
8   What are the controlling factors in the environment that pertain to ergonomics?
9   What are the major roles of the employee assistance programmes?
10   What is the effect of health promotion programmes in the workplace?
11   What are the certification requirements in ergonomics and human factors?

References

Agricola, G. (1912). De re metallica, Basil (H.C. Hoover and L.H. Hoover, Trans.). London: The Mining Magazine. (Original work published 1556.)
Americans with Disabilities Act of 1990, Pub. L. No. 101-336, 2, 104 Stat. 328 (1991).
Benson, H. (1975). The Relaxation Response. New York: William Morrow.
Berg, A. (2002). Skanskadirektörer fällda för arbetsmiljöbrott i förgiftningsfallet vid Hallandsåsen. [Skanska managers found guilty of work environment crime].

Retrieved 22 March 2005, http://www.eiro.eurofound.ie/about/2002/02/feature/ SE0202106F.html

Board of Certification in Professional Ergonomics (BCPE) (2002–2005a). Certification information. Retrieved 24 March 2005, http://www.bcpe.org/info/ default.asp

Board of Certification in Professional Ergonomics (BCPE) (2002–2005b). History of BCPE. Retrieved 24 March 2005, http://www.bcpe.org/aboutus/default.asp.

Bureau of Labour Statistics (1996). Survey of occupational injuries and illnesses, 1994. Retrieved 23 March 2005, http://www.bls.gov/iif/oshwc/osh/os/ ossm0008.txt.

Campbell, M.K, Tessaro, I., DeVellis, B., Benedict, S., Kelsey, K., Belton, L. and Sanhueza, A. (2002). Effects of a tailored health promotion programme for female blue-collar workers: Health works for women. Preventative Medicine, 34, 313–323.

Centers for Medicare and Medicaid Services (2004). Medicaid home page. Retrieved 23 March 2005, http://www.cms.gov/medicaid/

Coon, C.S. (1955). The Story of Man. New York: Knopf.

Courtney, C. and Escobedo, B. (1990). A stress management of inpatient to outpatient. American Journal of Occupational Therapy, 44, 306–310.

Elmfeldt, G., Wise, C., Bergsen, H. and Olsson. (1982). Adapting work sites for people with disabilities. Ideas from Sweden. World Rehabilitation Fund: The Swedish Institute for the Handicapped.

Employee Assistance Professionals Association (2005). What's an EAP? Retrieved 23 March 2005, http://www.eapassn.org/public/pages/index.cfm?pageid=507

Ergonomics Society (2002). Chronology of the society. Retrieved 23 March 2005, http://ergonomics.org.uk/society/history/chronology1.htm.

Felton, J.S., Newman, J.P. and Read, D.L. (1963). Man, Medicine, and Work: Historic Events in Occupational Medicine. [Public Health Service Publication Number 1044]. Washington, DC: US Department of Health, Education and Welfare, Public Health Service, Division of Occupational Health.

Hackman, J. and Oldham, G. (1976). Motivation through the design of work: Test of a theory. Organizational Behaviour and Human Performance, 16, 250–279.

Human Factors and Ergonomic Society (1995–2004). About the HFES. Retrieved 25 March 2005, http://hfes.org/About/Menu.html

Hunter, D. (1978). The Diseases of Occupations (6th edn). London: Hodder and Stoughton.

International Ergonomics Association. (2003a). IEA history. Retrieved 23 March 2005, http://www.iea.cc/about/history.cfm

International Ergonomics Association (2003b). The discipline of ergonomics. Retrieved 23 March 2005, http://www.iea.cc/ergonomics

International Work Simplification Institute (1968). Pioneers in improvement and our modern standard of living. IW/SI News, 18, 37–38. Retrieved 23 March 2005, http://gilbrethnetwork.tripod.com/bio.html

Jacobs, K. (1991). Occupational Therapy. Work-related Programs and Assessments. Boston: Little, Brown.

Jacobs, K. (1999). Ergonomics for Therapists (2nd edn). Boston: Butterworth-Heinemann.

Johnson, J., Hall, E. and Theorell, T. (1989). Combined effects of job strain and cardiovascular disease research. Journal of Work Environment Health, 15, 271–279.

Karasek, R. (1979). Job demands, job decision latitude and mental strain: Implication for job redesign. Administration Science Quarterly, 24, 285–307.

Klarreich, P.R. (1987). Health promotion in the workplace: A historical perspective. In S.H. Klarreich (Ed.) Health and Fitness in the Workplace (pp. 5–12). New York: Prager.

Malinauskiene, V., Theorell, T., Grazuleviciene, R., Azaraviciene, A., Obelensis, V. and Azelis, V. (2005). Psychosocial factors at work and myocardial infarction among men in Kaunas, Lithuania. Scandinavian Journal of Work Environment and Health, 31, 218–223.

McGrady, A., Olson, R.P. and Kroon, J.S. (1995). Biobehavioural treatment of essential hypertension. In M.S. Schwartz and Associates (Eds), Biofeedback: A Practitioner's Guide (pp. 445–467). New York: Guilford Press.

Meister, D. (1999). The History of Human Factors and Ergonomics. Mahwah, NJ: Lawrence Erlbaum.

National Council on Disability (1996). Achieving independence: The challenge for the 21st century. Retrieved 23 March 2005, http://www.ncd.gov/newsroom/publications/1996/pdf/achieving.pdf

National Grid for Learning (nd). Article written by Emma Paterson in 1874. Retrieved 22 March 2005, http://www.learningcurve.gov.uk/victorianbritain/divided/source7.htm

National Institute of Occupational Safety and Health (NIOSH) (nd). About NIOSH. Retrieved 23 March 2005, http://www.cdc.gov/niosh/about.html

New York State Insurance Fund (2005). General information: About worker's compensation. What is worker's compensation? Retrieved 23 March 2005, http://www.nysif.com/general/workerscompensation.asp

Occupational Health and Safety Administration (OSHA) (1970). OSH Act of 1970: Introduction. Public Law 91-596, 91st Congress, S.2193, 29 December, 1970; 84 STAT.1590. Retrieved 22 March 2005, http://www.osha-slc.gov/pls/oshaweb

Orth, S.P. (nd). The armies of labour. Retrieved 23 March 2005, http://www.black-mask.com/books14c/labour.htm

O'Sullivan, J. and Gallick, R. (1975). Workers and Allies: Female Participation in the American Trade Union Movement, 1824–1976. Washington, DC: Smithsonian Institution Press.

Oxford Research Institute (2002). Certification applications. Retrieved 24 March 2005, http://www.oxfordresearch.org/oriappnew.html

Rahe, R.H., Taylor, C.B., Tolles, R.L., Newhall, L.M., Veach T.L. and Bryson, S. (2002). A novel stress and coping workplace programme reduces illness and health-care utilization. Psychosomatic Medicine, 64, 278–286.

Rosen, G. (1943). The History of Miners' Diseases. New York: Shumans.

Saxl, L.R. (1984) The picture of health in the workplace. Training and Development Journal, 38, 44–45.

Schult, M.-L. and Söderback, I. (2000). A method for 'diagnosing' jobs before redesign in chronic-pain patients: Preliminary findings. Journal of Occupational Rehabilitation, 10, 295–307.

Schult, M.-L., Schüldt, K. Söderback, I., and Ekholm, J. (1995). Work technique training for patients with chronic pain in neck, shoulder and arm: A questionnaire pilot study after a comprehensive exercise-oriented rehabilitation programme. Work: A Journal of Prevention, Assessment and Rehabilitation, 5, 173–183.

Serxner, S., Gold, D., Anderson, D., and Williams, D. (2001) The impact of a worksite health promotion programme on short-term disability usage. Journal of Occupational Environmental Medicine, 43, 25–29.

Simkin, J. (2005). Women's trade union. Retrieved 23 March 2005, http://www.spartacus.schoolnet.co.uk/USAWtu.htm

Social Security OnLine (nda). History: Legislative History: Social Security Act of 1935 Preamble. Retrieved 23 March 2005, http://www.ssa.gov/history/35act-pre.html

Social Security OnLine (ndb). Peter Coming history of medicare – Appendix A Chronology of significant events leading to enactment of Medicare. Retrieved 29 December 2003, www.ssa.gov/history/cornignappa.html

Social Security OnLine (ndc). The workplace: Ticket to work and work incentives improvement act of 1999. [Fact Sheet]. Retrieved 23 March 2005, http://www.ssa.gov/work/ResourcesToolkit/legisregfact.html

Social Security OnLine (2000). The President Signs the 'Senior Citizens' Freedom to Work Act of 2000'. Social Security Legislative Bulletin, 106–20. Retrieved 23 March 2005, http://www.ssa.gov/legislation/legis_bulletin_040700.html

Social Security OnLine (2003). Brief history. Retrieved March 23, 2005 from http://www.ssa.gov/history/briefhistory3.html

Stein, F. (2001). Occupational stress, biofeedback and stress management. Work: A Journal of Prevention, Assessment and Rehabilitation, 17, 235–245.

Stein, F. (2002). The ergonomic model in occupational therapy. Presentation at the World Federation of Occupational Therapy Congress, Stockholm, Sweden, June.

Stein, F. and Cutler, S. (2001). Psychosocial Occupational Therapy: A Holistic Approach (2nd edn). San Diego: Singular Publishing Group/Delmar.

Stein, F. and Nikolic, S. (1989). Teaching stress management techniques to a schizophrenic patient. American Journal of Occupational Therapy, 43, 162–169.

Swedish Labour Market (1999). Facts and Figures (pp. 27–35). Retrieved 23 March 2005, http://www.lo.se/home/lo/home.nsf/unidView/D24CC7E9 41A888DDC1256E7E0039FABD/$file/LOThe20SwedisLabourmarket.pdf#sear ch='The%20State%20of%20the%20Work%20Environment.%20Sweden"

Taylor, E. (1988). Anger intervention. American Journal of Occupational Therapy, 1, 147–155.

Taylor, F.W. (1919). Principles of Scientific Management. New York: Harper.

Texas Workers' Compensation Commission (nd). About worker's compensation. Retrieved 29 December 2003, http://www.twcc.state.tx.us/information/aboutwc.html

Texas Health and Human Services Commission (1999–2003) Medicaid history. Retrieved 23 March 2005, http://www.hhsc.state.tx.us/medicaid/

Thackrah, C.T. (1831). The Effects of the Principle Arts, Trades and Professions.

Toscano, G. (1997). Dangerous jobs. Compensation and Working Conditions Online, 2(2), 57–60. Retrieved 23 March 2005, http://www.bls.gov/opub/cwc/archive/summer1997brief3.pdf

US Department of Justice, Civil Rights Division, Disability Rights Section (2001). A guide to disability rights laws. Retrieved 23 March 2005, http://www.usdoj.gov/crt/ada/cguide.htm#anchor62335

US Department of Labor, Employment and Training Administration (1991). The Revised Handbook for Analyzing Jobs. Indianapolis: JIST Works.

US Equal Employment Opportunity Commission (1997). EEOC Enforcement Guidance: Worker's Compensation and the ADA. Retrieved 23 March 2005, http://www.eeoc.gov/policy/docs/qidreps.html

Vojtecky, M.A. (1987). Worker education and training in health and safety in the United States. In S.H. Klarreich (Ed.) Health and Fitness in the Workplace (pp. 13–28). New York: Praeger.

Warner, M., Barnes, P.M. and Fingerhut, L.A. (2000). Injury and poisoning episodes and conditions; National Health Interview Survey, 1997. Vital Health Statistics, 10(202). Retrieved 24 March 2005, http://www.cdc.gov/nchs/data/series/sr_10/sr10_202.pdf.

Glossary

Ability is 'the individual's potential (mental and physical capacity, and skill required) to perform a task or an action' (World Health Organization, 2001, p. 159). The individual's abilities can be realized depending on the individual's motivation, interests and determination to succeed.

Accessibility is gaining access to the environment, products and services that are available to all people. It is related to universal design that implies that the environment be usable to all persons without special adaptations, for example elevators make a building accessible to people in wheelchairs as well as being used by those without disabilities.

Accommodation is the process of adapting or adjusting work, home and leisure environments to meet the psychological or physical needs of the individual. Successful accommodations and assistive technology can increase the individual's function and quality of life (Cook and Hussey, 2002).

Accommodations are the specific environmental changes or tools that are used in helping the individual with a disability to be independent in the activities of daily living. These accommodations can include a built-up handle for a pencil, as well redesigning a kitchen or fabricating special hand controls in a car or use mechanical life systems (Edlich et al., 2004).

Activities or occupations are the tasks that an individual performs in the home, work, school and leisure environments. Meaningful and purposeful activities help an individual to develop sensory, cognitive, motor, social and psychological functions. Occupations are important in developing skills for occupational roles and creating competence.

Activity limitations are the difficulties an individual may have in carrying out activities of daily living in the home, work, school and leisure environments (World Health Organization, 2001).

Adaptation is the process of attaining a good fit between the person and the environment so that the person reaches an optimal level of

315

competence (Law et al., 1994). Adaptation can involve the modification of a home environment such as a wheelchair ramp, modification of an ADL device such as a built-up handle for a toothbrush or adapting a portion of the work environment so that the work is performed in a neutral position.

Americans with Disabilities Act (ADA) of 1990 was enacted to protect the civil rights of people with disabilities from discrimination in all aspects of everyday life including employment, transportation, education, housing, medical care and accessibility. The ADA defines an individual with a disability as a person who has a physical or mental impairment that substantially limits one or more major life activities, such as having a spinal cord injury, being visually impaired or having a diagnosis of schizophrenia. In addition, the ADA covers all aspects of employment such as applying for a job, training on the job and compensation.

Anthropometry is the study of human body measurements and physical dimensions. It is used in ergonomics to determine standards of practice such as the amount of weight that an average individual should lift without causing bodily injury. Anthropometry measurements are also used to create safe environments such as heights and widths of doors, size of furniture and the positioning of controls in cars and planes.

Aptitude is the inherent, natural or acquired ability that indicates an individual's capacity to learn or perform in a specific area (Stein and Cutler, 2000). A vocational assessment usually includes the following aptitudes: (G) intelligence or general learning ability, (V) verbal aptitude, (N) numerical aptitude, (S) spatial aptitude, (P) form perception, (Q) clerical perception, (K) motor coordination, (F) finger dexterity, and (M) manual dexterity (Power, 2000).

Architectural barriers are structures and buildings that prevent a person with a disability from using a facility such as a restroom, lift, building or office.

Assessment is the process by which an individual is evaluated. In this process data are gathered, such as vocational interests, hypotheses formulated, such as the individual has major interests in social service activities, and decisions are made, such as recommending further education for a client or return to work. Assessment also refers to the specific procedures or tools that are used in evaluating a client.

Assistive devices are specially designed for a person with a disability, are usually available commercially and consequently of value for people with disabilities (Burt, 2000). Assistive devices, tools for living, adaptive equipment or self-care aids are used interchangeably and can include orthotic and prosthetic devices (Gitlin, 1998). Assistive devices are not affixed to the body and are designed to help persons having musculoskeletal or neuromuscular disabilities to perform activities involving movement (National Library of Medicine, 2002).

Assistive technology is a broad term to designate strategies, practices or equipment that are used to improve functional capabilities in performing motor activities for individuals with musculoskeletal or neuromuscular disabilities (Cook and Hussey, 2002; Foti, 2000). Assistive technologies include the MeSH search terms self-help devices, protective devices, orthotic devices, prosthesis and implants.

Awkward posture is the deviation from the neutral position in performing work tasks, such as reaching above the shoulders, reaching behind for objects, twisting the back and squatting for extended periods of time. Researchers have examined how awkward posture contributes to musculoskeletal injuries (Earle-Richardson et al., 2004).

Back school is an educational programme at a worksite or in an occupational rehabilitation programme, where clients are taught prevention and management of back pain (information about posture, anatomical and physiological characteristics of the spine, exercise, proper body mechanics, job-site ergonomics, pain management and stress management. For example, Guthrie et al. (2004) applied back school education in conjunction with lifting devices to prevent work-related injuries in nurses.

Baltimore Therapeutic Equipment (BTE) Work Simulator (Baltimore Therapeutic Equipment Company, 1992) is a functional capacity evaluation tool, which is computerized and assesses physical tasks that underlie many manual jobs.

Barrier-free accessibility refers to buildings, houses and gardens that are free from physical barriers. An architectural barrier, on the other hand, is a structural impediment to the approach, mobility and functional use of an interior or exterior environment (World Health Organization, 2001). Cardinal and Spaziani (2003) investigated the accessibility of physical activity facilities to determine if they were accessible to students with disabilities.

Basic Activities of Daily Living (ADL) are tasks that pertain to self-care (e.g. grooming, bathing, dressing and undressing), mobility and communication as compared with instrumental ADL, which refers to higher level tasks such as cooking and driving.

Biofeedback is a treatment method that is commonly used in conjunction with relaxation therapy in which the client is taught to enhance control of the autonomic (involuntary) nervous system and become aware of internal processes by monitoring biological signals, e.g. heart rate, blood pressure, muscle tension and finger temperature (Engel et al., 2004).

Biomechanical principles refer to the laws of physics that govern the movement and posture of humans. It is used in designing seating systems such as wheelchairs. Terms such as centre of gravity, force, pressure and laws of motion are applied in assisting an individual in maintaining functional body postures and to reduce the stress placed on the spine or other joints. Proper body mechanics may maximize the performance, decrease pain or vulnerability to injury, conserve energy and prevent skeletal disorders. Biomechanical analysis is used to assess work injuries (Ulin and Keyserling, 2004).

Body mechanics involves the body tissues and structures (e.g. bone, tendons, ligaments and muscles), the physical principles of movement (i.e. the size and directions of the vectors, centre of gravity, torque; that is, the amount of force required to produce a rotation around an axis). These factors influence the individual's load in occupational performance (Jacobs and Bettencourt, 1995).

Classification of jobs includes the International Standard Classification of Occupations of the International Labor Organization (IISCO-ILO) and is a nine-category simple classification (Spenner, 1990). The *Dictionary of Occupational Titles* (*DOT*) US Department of Labor, Employment and Training Administration, 1991a) describes more than 22, 000 jobs, classified into nine categories. Each work is defined in 96 variables, which determines the requirements of the specific work (ONET Consortium, 2005).

Cluster trait work sample refers to worker traits or characteristics that are related to a number of jobs or occupations such as hand dexterity or social service skills. These traits can underlie a number of occupations such as assembly work or nursing. 'Based upon an analysis of occupational grouping and the traits necessary for successful performance, it is intended to assess the individual's potential to perform jobs having a common set of performance requirements' (Dowd, 1993, p. 6).

Cognitive workload is the worker's perception of the strain and effort required for the work being completed (e.g. the demand of the worker and the amount of control the worker has over the work to be completed) (Karasek, 1990). Cognitive workload can also cause stress (Leyman et al., 2004) and work-related injuries (Folts et al., 1995).

Commercial work evaluation systems (CWE) are multi-cluster job samples that systematically and objectively evaluate an individual's ability to work. Brown et al. (1994) evaluated a number of the vocational evaluation systems that are available for purchase.

Context is the temporal and the environmental circumstances in which activities, occupations or tasks are performed or take place.

Criterion is a factor, a variable, an observation or an index that constitutes a standard of performance or outcome (set of scores, rating) by which a client may be judged or evaluated and which is the basis or yardstick for comparisons (Dowd, 1993; Stein and Cutler, 2001) or an empirical measure (Scriven, 1991). For example, the criterion is met if the worker's output corresponds to the requirements of the work demands.

Criterion-referenced test or assessment evaluates specific skills or knowledge 'based on a standard of performance, competence, or mastery' (Stein and Cutler, 2000, p. 501). 'An individual's performances on a given task or series of tasks is observed and assessed at different times to determine whether learning is taking place and whether skills are being either acquired or maintained. These assessments are used to compare the individual's performance to him- or herself across time' (Wheeler et al., 1994).

Cumulative trauma disorders (CTD) are workplace-related injuries that are caused by repetitive motion or overuse of regions of the body such as back, neck, shoulder, arms, wrist and hands. The symptoms of CTD include muscle and joint pain, fatigue, inflammation, swelling and numbness. Other terms such as repetitive-stress injuries and musculoskeletal disorders are synonymous with CTD (Novak, 2004).

Decubitus ulcer is a sore that can develop usually on the buttocks area from the pressure when seated in a wheelchair or in a bed for extended periods of time. Pellerito (2003) investigated whether computer-aided instruction is effective in reducing pressure sores in clients with paraplegia.

Dictionary of Occupational Titles (DOT) (US Department of Labor, Employment and Training Administration, 1991a) defines each of about 20,000 occupations which are classified on the basis of the work functions and what is produced (e.g. data, people, things) using a unique job code.

Disability is an umbrella term which covers impairments, activity limitation and participation restrictions. Disability limits participation in activities in daily life and/or restrictions to participate in life situations. Disability concerns (a) difficulties in learning and applying knowledge, communication or mobility (e.g. moving and handling objects, maintaining body positions, moving around, using transportation); (b) a psychosocial illness, such as depression, which may result in an inability to cope with the everyday activities; (c) learned helplessness; or (d) negative attitudes or stigmas attached to the disability. Disability affects an individual's capacity to function (World Health Organization, 2001).

Employability is an important issue in vocational rehabilitation and refers to the client's readiness for work. Factors related to employability include, vocational interests, job skills, ability to apply for a job, interview skills, work performance skills, social skills and decision-making skills.

Energy conservation refers to intervention techniques to help the client use energy efficiently without fatigue while engaged in occupational performances. Branick (2003) describes how energy conservation techniques can be applied in the home to help a client with a disability to carry out activities of daily living. Ergonomic strategies are applied in conjunction with energy conservation.

Engineering controls are methods of reducing risk factors in the work environment by redesigning equipment, tools and workstations. An example of an engineering control device is the use by nursing personnel of mechanical hoists in lifting and transferring patients (Edlich et al., 2004).

Environment is the external elements and conditions that surround, influence and affect the life and development of an organism or population (World Health Organization, 2001). The environment is composed of concentric layers comprised of (a) physical characteristics (e.g. natural terrain, plants, animals, architectural designs of landscape, buildings, furniture, objects, tools, devices); (b) social characteristics (e.g. availability and expectations of significant individuals and also includes larger social groups that are influential in establishing norms, role expectations and social routines); and (c) culture (e.g. economic considerations, customs, beliefs, activity patterns and expectations accepted by the society of which the individual is a member) (Christiansen, Baum, and Bass-Haugen 2005).

Environmental barrier is an obstacle in the environment that restrict the individual's occupational performances, independent living and interferes with family life and social activities (World Health Organization, 2001).

Environmental conditions are those environmental components and demands of work that could affect ergonomic interventions, including (a) physical demand factors (e.g. position, weight/force: sedentary, light, medium, heavy), (b) climbing, (c) balancing, (d) stopping, (e) kneeling, (f) crouching, (g) crawling, (h) reaching, (i) handling, (j) fingering, (k) feeling, (l) talking, (m) hearing, (n) tasting/smelling, (o) near acuity, (p) far acuity, (q) depth perception, (r) accommodation, (s) colour vision, (t) field vision, (u) weather exposure, (v) extreme cold, (w) extreme heat, (x) dampness and/or humidity, (y) noise intensity level, (z) vibration, (aa) atmospheric conditions, (bb) proximity to moving mechanical parts, (cc) exposure to electrical shock, (dd) working in high, exposed places, (ee) exposure to radiation, (ff) working with explosives, (gg) exposure to toxic or caustic chemicals, (hh) other environmental conditions (US Department of Labor, Employment and Trainig Administration, 1991b).

Environmental facilitators are factors in the home, work or public environment that enable the client to perform occupations and activities of daily life and to participate in family life as independently as possible (World Health Organizations, 2001).

Environmental factors are 'extrinsic to the individual' (World Health Organization, 2001, p. 16), and include the person's immediate surroundings and social interactions with other people.

Ergonomic design is the biomechanical and ergonomic construction of furniture, tools, equipment and machines that fit the individual (Mace, 1998). Ergonomic redesign of workstations has been shown to decrease upper back pain (May et al., 2004).

Ergonomic job analysis is an open-ended process that includes a detailed inspection, description and evaluation of the workplace, equipment, tools, work methods and the human factors that impact on performing the job (Keyserling et al., 1991).

Ergonomic risk factors are variables related to performing a job that can potentially lead to injuries, illness or disease. These factors can include the environment, such as extreme temperature, the tools, such as poorly designed knives, an uncomfortable chair, work methods, such as using poor lifting techniques, undue or continual stress and repetitive motions. In a related study, Chee et al. (2004) examined the relationship between job tasks of workers in a semiconductor factory and ergonomic risk factors. They found that the job tasks that included heavy lifting, repetitive motion and standing for prolonged periods placed the worker at risk of injury.

Ergonomics is the study of fitting the environment to the individual in his or her everyday activities. The word ergonomics is derived from the Greek words 'ergon' meaning work, and 'nomos' meaning law. Health professionals apply ergonomic principles and human factors to design tools, equipment, consumer products, machines, systems and workstations as well as work methods and work organization for performance of work tasks. The term human factors is interchangeable with ergonomics.

Evaluation is an 'analysis of an individual's behavior, characteristics, aptitudes and present functioning gained through specific tests, clinical observation, and procedures that can be used for treatment planning or discharge recommendations' (Stein and Roose, 2000, p. 102).

Evidence-based practice (EBP) is founded on research data that is the rationale for clinical interventions. As applied to ergonomics it is the application of research findings in designing the most functional environments so as to prevent injuries in workers and to enable individuals with disabilities to be independent in their everyday activities.

Feedback is the information that is given to the worker, homemaker or client to effect change. It reinforces the client's awareness, knowledge and behaviour in a desirable direction.

Forceful exertions are work activities that put significant pressure on the hands and arms (e.g. carrying heavy tools, using strong force with wrenches, scissors and pneumatic tools) and increase the risk of upper extremity cumulative trauma disorders (Keyserling, 2000a, 2000b; Marshall and Armstrong, 2004).

Functional assessment is the measurement of purposeful behaviour (ability, competence, performance) in interaction with the environment, which is interpreted according to the assessment's intended uses (Dowd, 1993).

Functional capacity (assessment) evaluation (FCE), e.g. physical capacity evaluation (Dowd, 1993) or work tolerance screening, 'is a comprehensive and systematic approach that measures the client's/worker's overall physical capacity such as muscle strength and endurance' (Stein and Cutler, 2000, p. 503) and the ability to carry out work tasks in a safe way. The results provide information about the individual's physical work tolerance and preparedness for returning to work. Harbin and Olson (2005) used functional capacity evaluation with a large group of healthy workers who had been recently hired by a food production plant to determine whether the functional assessment was effective in predicting work-related injuries. They found that the FCE was a cost-effective method to lower the incidence of work-related injuries.

Goal attainment scaling (GAS) is an outcome measure that is based on multiple individual patient goals. The GAS requires (a) measurable goals (e.g. time, frequencies, functional status, status of well-being or compliance with a disability); (b) the direction of the goal (e.g. maintain, improve); and (c) in advance determining the period or number of occasions needed for attaining the goal (Kiresuck et al., 1994). Gordon et al. (1999) applied goal attainment scaling in measuring the effectiveness of a cognitive rehabilitation programme. They found that the GAS was a sensitive tool in measuring change in the client's health status.

Guide for occupational exploration (GOE) (Farr et al., 2001) contains a classification of the job's sphere of interest (12 interest areas, 66 work groups and 348 subgroups).

Hazard prevention and control is the elimination or minimizing of potential risks in the work environment by job modification, job rotation, redesign of tools and equipment, pacing and through protective clothing.

Health in the perspective of occupation connotes the performance of occupations as valuable for the maintenance of health and for the restoration of health and wellness after illness and disability. A client's engagements in meaningful, purposeful occupations facilitate a change toward health and well-being (Breines, 2001).

Home evaluation is an assessment of the client's functional living at home. The client and the caregiver are provided with recommendations for redesigning the home environment, prescribing assistive devices and adapting tools and equipment with purpose of simplifying performance of tasks and removing environmental obstacles. During a home evaluation, the client performs personal or intermediate activities of daily life demonstrating whether the current environment is appropriate and acceptable or not. Below are components in the home environment to be evaluated (Iwarsson, 1999):

- The client's mobility status and devices used (e.g. wheelchairs, quad cane)
- Type of home and number of levels within home, including basement where applicable
- Access from the driveway and/or the garage to the house
- Number of steps at entrance to home, the steps' dimensions, and if railing is installed
- Ramp location and dimensions if applicable
- Size of the threshold at the entrance
- Size of door at entrance and the direction it opens
- Type of floor covering in rooms used by the client
- Living room arrangement conducive to client's mobility status
- Height and firmness of furniture used by client
- Dimensions of hallways and if sharp turns are necessary when entering various rooms
- Dimensions of bedroom door and direction it opens
- Type and height of bed, including client's ability to transfer to/from bed
- Space in bedroom, including room for wheelchair or special bed
- Accessibility of dressers and closet
- Dimensions of bathroom door and direction it opens, including threshold height
- Dimensions of door and height of threshold of walk-in shower
- Height of sink and type of taps
- Height of toilet, toilet paper location, or location near cabinet-type sink to assist client with standing, including his/her ability to transfer
- Accessibility and location of hinge on refrigerator
- Availability for grab bar installation if not currently installed
- Dimensions of kitchen door and direction it opens, including threshold height
- Height of hob, location of oven, location of controls, and accessibility
- Height of sink, type of taps, and availability for wheelchair to fit beneath if applicable
- Accessibility, type and location of cupboards
- Accessibility and locations of necessary switches and outlets
- Height of kitchen table and countertops
- Height of kitchen table and countertops
- Dimensions of laundry room door and direction it opens, including threshold height
- Dimensions and number of steps to laundry facilities. Accessibility and type of washing machine

- Accessibility and type of dryer
- Location of any scatter rugs
- Location of phone, emergency call system or list of emergency numbers
- Location of letterbox
- Location of thermostat
- Note of any unsafe situations like sharp-edged furniture, uninstalled hot water pipes or uneven floors
- Note of cluttered areas
- Whether client has a fire extinguisher and its location. List of equipment the client currently has
- List of problem situations and areas to be rectified. Recommendations for adaptations to be made
- Recommendations for equipment to be purchased

Stein and Roose, 2000, pp. 121–123

Human factors ergonomics (HFE) is a branch of psychology that studies the interactions between humans and technology. The purposes of HFE are to improve system productivity, increase human comfort and safety and add to the knowledge base of human-technology interactions (Meister, 1999).

Impairment denotes changes in body functions or body structures such as a significant damage or loss (physiological, psychological or anatomical), and may influence functioning and social life (World Health Organization, 2001).

Incidence is the rate or frequency of new injuries and illnesses that occur during a year or specified period.

Individuals with disabilities are restricted in their ability to perform activities of daily living (ADL) (World Health Organization, 2001).

Instrumental activities of daily living (IADL) include high-level executive functioning and decision-making abilities necessary to perform activities such as shopping, budgeting (money management), baking, cooking (meal preparation), laying the table and cleaning the house, clothing care and care of others (Foti, 2000; Söderback, 1988) as well as 'stress management' (Stein, 2002).

International Classification of Functioning, Disability and Health (ICF) is a conceptual model and a system for classification of human functioning and disability (World Health Organization, 2001).

Job accommodation involves adjusting the work environment to meet the needs of the worker. For example, when a worker has a disability, the work environment is modified to enable the worker to perform at his or her maximum level. Wang et al. (2004) in a Canadian study concluded that adequate workplace accommodation is helpful for enabling individuals with disabilities and activity limitations to be fully employed.

Job analysis is 'the gathering, evaluating and recording of accurate, objective and complete job data' (Dowd, 1993, p. 15), including (a) what the worker does in terms of activities or function, (b) how the work is performed (methods, techniques, or processes involved and the work devices used), (c) the results of the work, (d) worker characteristics (skills, knowledge, adaptations needed to accomplish the work task), and (e) environmental and organizational factors (Dowd, 1993; US Department of Labor, Employment and Training Administration, 1991b).

Job burn-out is characterized by a worker's low motivation, inefficiency, absenteeism, job dissatisfaction, depleted energy and vulnerability to injury and disease. Chronic stress, poor management and lack of challenges or opportunities on the job can cause boredom and job burn-out.

Job coach is a counsellor or therapist who provides one-to-one support on-site to the employed client for skill training, travel assistance and job placement.

Job demand–control–strain is a three-dimensional model used to describe how the psychosocial work environment predicts stress-related risk factors that affect an individual's health negatively as well as the degree of desirable stress at work. The ratio between the work demands and the degree to which the worker has control over the work task shows how much psychological strain the work task requires to be performed. The operationalization of the model is the job content questionnaire (JCQ) (Karasek, 1990), which includes the dimensions of (a) *decision latitude* (measure the dimensions skill discretion and skill decision authority, that is, how much control the worker has over the work tasks); (b) *psychological demands* (measure the mental workload that reflect the worker's perception of himself or herself as a worker); and (c) *social support* (a measure of the worker's perception of the amount of support that is given to him or her from fellow workers and supervisors).

Job diagnostic survey (JDS) is the theory of diagnosing *how* an actual work environment influences of the worker's job motivation, job satisfaction and the quantity of the productivity, level of absenteeism and staff turnover. The JDS theory is measurable by the assessment instrument job diagnostic scores (JDS) (Hackman and Oldham, 1975) including the following job dimensions (sub-scales): skill variety, task significance, autonomy, feedback from the job itself, feedback from agents and dealing with other.

Job fatigue is the body's response to excessive physical or psychological activity without enough time to recover. It may be an early symptom of a job design problem. It can affect the whole body or a particular part of the body that is being stressed. The whole-body fatigue affects the whole body as a result of continuous or repeated activities (UAW-Ford National Joint Committee on Health and Safety, 1996).

Job modification is the process of changing a job to meet the needs of the worker through environmental adaptations, adaptive equipment or job strategies.

Job satisfaction is the worker's feeling about his or her job reflecting (a) job security, (b) pay, (c) supervision, (d) relationships with co-workers. Lamberth and Comello (2005), in a study investigating the relationship between job satisfaction and retention among nurses, identified money, work environment, performance feedback, advancement opportunities, group cohesion and relationship with management as important factors in defining job satisfaction in their research sample.

Mechanical contact stress is the physical contact between soft body tissues and a tool, work surface or work object such as when a fist is used as a hammer, or pressure is put on the fingers when using scissors (Keyserling, 2000a, 2000b).

Methods-time Measurement (MTM) is used as a standard to ascertain the time it would take the average, well-trained worker to complete the work sample tasks if they were carried out over the eight-hour work day in a typical industrial context (Farrell, 1993).

Musculoskeletal disorders include damage to the muscles, ligaments, cartilage, connecting nerves and blood vessels, tendons, joints and bones of the individual's anatomy. These disorders can be aggravated by repetitive motion. Musculoskeletal disorders are characterized by symptoms of pain, stiffness, restricted range of joint motion and muscle weakness, and include (a) rheumatoid arthritis; (b) ankylosing spondilitis; (c) muscular dystrophy; (d) osteoarthritis; and (e) herniated disc resulting in low back pain. Individuals with amputations (e.g. removal of pelvises, parts of the legs or parts of the arms).

Neurological disorders are impairments of the nervous system that can lead to a disability. Examples of neurological disorders include (a) stroke or traumatic brain injury resulting in pareses or hemiplegia; (b) spinal cord injuries (paraplegia, quadriplegia or tetraplegia); (c) post-polio syndrome; and (d) progressive degenerative disease (e.g. multiple sclerosis, Parkinson's disease).

Neutral position is the most comfortable and efficient anatomical position for the human in engaging in an occupation, or physical activity. The position reduces the risk for musculoskeletal injuries where there is minimal stress on the muscles and joints.

Norms are the values that describe the performance on an assessment or test outcome for a specified group. In an evaluation, the norms of a test are used to compare a client's competence for a task or level of functioning (Lyman, 1991).

Occupational medicine is the medical specialty concerned with preventing and treating illnesses and diseases that are related to work.

Occupational performance is related to the dynamic interaction between the client, environment, interventions and social/cultural norms. Occupational performance is (a) the domain of concern in occupational therapy; (b) the outcome of the interactive process of the triad of components: person, environment and occupations; and (c) concern the description of the content of the occupational therapy process (Pedretti and Early, 2001).

Occupational stress is the body's reactions to workplace stressors. They can be (a) physical, such as excessive heat, cold, noise, chemical pollutants; (b) job conditions, such as repetitive motion, job overload, job dissatisfaction or shift work; or (c) social and economic conditions, such as unemployment or underemployment, sexual harassment or discrimination because of race, religion or sexual orientation. The body's reactions to these stressors can be (a) psychological, such as depression or anxiety; (b) physiological, such as hypertension; (c) cognitive, such as poor concentration; or (d) behavioural, such as insomnia (Stein and Associates, 2003).

Occupational therapy is the application of purposeful and meaningful occupation to restore functions, develop independence and enable functional performances in individuals who are disabled, and to prevent injury and disability in people who are at risk. Functional activities include the ability 'to work, to be independent in self-care, to engage in leisure activities and to be effective in social interactions. The effectiveness of occupational therapy will depend on the therapist's ability to establish a therapeutic relationship and to select a purposeful activity that is meaningful to the client in producing a desired outcome' (Stein and Roose, 2000, p. 200).

Occupational therapy practice framework is the most up-to-date guide for the practice of occupational therapy. It divides practice into evaluation, intervention and outcome. Evaluation includes the occupational profile (client's demographics, reasons for seeking therapy and client's occupational history); intervention plan (goals, discharge plans, outcome measures) and outcomes (related to engagement in occupation) (American Occupational Therapy Association, 2002).

Occupations are 'the culturally and personally meaningful and purposeful activities that humans engage in during their everyday lives' (Stein and Roose, 2000, p. 201).

On-the-job site evaluation is carried out at the actual place of work with a systematic observation of the worker's capability to perform the required work tasks following, for example, the *Revised Handbook of Analyzing Jobs* (US Department of Labor, Employment and Training Administration, 1991b).

Outcome is the measured results of an intervention. The client's outcome may be evaluated through a number of assessments such as the Goal Attainment Scale (Kiresuck et al., 1994).

Participatory ergonomics is a group dynamics approach to making ergonomic improvements by involving management and employees in identifying and implementing ergonomic changes in the workplace (King, 1994).

Personal activities of daily living (PADL) include basic activities requiring cognitive and motor planning used in (a) *self-care or self-maintenance*: feeding and eating, medication routine, grooming, oral hygiene, toileting and toilet hygiene, dressing and undressing, health maintenance, emergency response; (b) *functional mobility*: bed mobility, wheelchair mobility, transfer, functional ambulating; (c) *functional communication*: writing, typing, telephoning, argumentative communication devices; and (d) *functional handling of environmental facilitators*, such as keys, switchers, door and window openings, telephones and computers (Foti, 2000).

Personal factors 'are the particular background of an individual's life and living, and are composed of features of the individual that are not part of a health condition or health states. These factors may include gender, race, age, fitness, lifestyle, habits, upbringing, coping styles, social background, education, profession, past and current experience, overall behavior pattern and character style, individual psychological assets and other characteristics all that may play a role in disability at any level' (World Health Organization, 2001, p 15).

Physiological adaptation is the adjustment of a person's physiological responses to environmental stimuli, measured by, for example, body temperature, heart rate, blood pressure and biomechanical load.

Prescreening interview is used by an employer to screen in a candidate for a job who will be successful in the job or to screen out applicants who do not have the qualifications for doing the job or are at risk physically in developing an injury on the job. Pre-employment physicals are used to determine the worker's physical potential to perform the work tasks. Employees with disabilities cannot be discriminated against solely on the basis of their disability. The employer is required to make reasonable accommodations to enable the individual with a disability to perform the job as required by the ADA.

Prevocational evaluation assesses a client's ability to work (Jacobs, 1994) such as in sheltered workshop, competitive employment or as a homemaker. Various tasks are used in a prevocational evaluation.

Protective devices are 'designed to provide personal protection against injury to individuals exposed to hazards in industry, sports, aviation, or daily activities such as smoke alarms, helmets, glasses and ear protections' (National Library of Medicine, 2002).

Psycho-educational approach includes teaching and mentoring the client using educational technology (role playing, group therapy, video feedback, films, biofeedback) for instruction of how to use proper lifting techniques (e.g. lifting objects from the floor by bending knees and keeping object close to the body in a squat position); preventative exercises that stretch back muscles while increasing muscle strength and which include a variety of movements, micro-pauses and stretch breaks at work and at home and other biomechanical principles in performing ADL activities (Stein and Roose, 2000).

Psychometric tests are an essential part of vocational evaluations assessing personality, general intelligence, achievement, interest, abilities and aptitude. Psychometric tests can be used in the assessment of an individual's capacity for returning to work.

Psychosocial impairments include individuals with severe mental illness such as schizophrenia, depression, bipolar mental disorders or other diagnoses that interfere with everyday functioning (World Health Organization, 2001).

Psychosocial work environment are the psychological factors in the work environment such as cognitive workload, occupational stress, worker motivation, job satisfaction, morale and burn-out that can contribute to the quality of work and worker productivity (Hackman and Oldham, 1975).

Quality assurance is a method to determine, for example, the quality of a healthcare programme. It is a continuously on-going process for measuring, controlling and evaluation of the quality and effectiveness of a programme based on standards such as JCAHO (Joe, 1991).

Quality of life 'is the concept that implies that individuals have the capacity to determine what brings them most happiness in their lives' (Stein and Roose, 2000, p. 245). Satisfaction with life in general or satisfaction with the job situation is how people evaluate their self-valued important life situations. The term is closely related to the concept of life values (Montgomery and Johansson, 1988).

RUMBA is 'an acronym for Relevant, Understandable, Measurable, Behavioral and Achievable which is used as a guide in writing operational intervention objectives for clients' (Stein and Roose, 2000, p. 267).

Sheltered workshop 'provides transitional and/or long-term employment in a controlled and protected working environment for those individuals who are unable either to compete or to function in competitive employment. It may provide vocational evaluation, work adjustment, and supported employment services' (Dowd, 1993, p. 25)

Situational assessment is 'the systematic observation process or evaluating work-related behaviors in a controlled or semi-controlled work environment whereas any type of real work task or work situation may be used' (Dowd, 1993, p. 25).

SOAP is an acronym for 'subjective, objective, assessment and plan. It is an 'organized method for recording a client's progress'. The acronym 'stands for Subjective findings which are the reported symptoms of the client; Objective findings reported by the therapist; Assessment, which is the documented analysis and summary of the findings; and Plan, which are the recommended therapeutic interventions, and further diagnostic tests, if necessary' (Stein and Roose, p. 294)

Socratic Case Study Method (SCSM) also entitled The Case Study Method (which is the specific search term when using the database ERIC) and The Harvard Case Method (Egidius, 1999, p. 56). SCSM is the practice of using cases as a pedagogical tool in fields such as law, business, medicine or education – cases may include real and imaginary scenarios, critical incident analysis, case studies, vignettes and anecdotal accounts (Educational Resources Information Center (ERIC) 2002).

Standard is the expected level of goal attainment. The term standard belongs to performance of quality assurance (Parenté and Anderson-Parenté, 1986). A standard of work performance such as published by OSHA regulations include acceptable physical limits in performing a job or the equipment necessary in installing equipment.

Stress management 'is a general term that includes systematic interventions aimed to reduce the hyper-arousal of the sympathetic nervous system' (Stein and Roose, 2000, p. 301). Examples of techniques used are biofeedback (Norris and Fahrion, 1993), relaxation response, meditation, yoga, T'ai-Chi, music therapy. The choice of technique is related to the target population, the specific context, modalities and the goals.

Stressful postures are work positions that place individuals at risk from musculoskeletal injuries. Examples include working continuously with hyper-extension or hyper-flexion in the wrist, radial deviation, working with arms over head, working with arms extended for long periods, bending sidewards more than 20 degrees, lifting heavy objects from the floor, twisting the trunk and or working too high at a work surface (UAW-Ford National Joint Committee on Health and Safety, 1996).

Supported employment is paid employment for people with disabilities who need a transitional work experience such as sheltered workshops and who could benefit from support services such as on-the-job counselling, environmental adaptations, job-coaching and work simplification methods to perform job-related tasks.

Symptom magnification syndrome was a term identified by the psychologist Leonard Matheson in the early 1980s. He defined it as 'a conscious or unconscious self-destructive socially reinforced behavioral response pattern consisting of reports or displays of symptoms which function to control the life circumstances of the sufferer' (Matheson, 1998, p. 257). Symptom magnification can be caused by factors in the worker's daily setting or by factors in family that are carried over to the work setting. The effects of symptom magnification result in the worker's inability to perform his or her job at an optimal level. The worker's reporting of exaggerated pain, for example, is often difficult to diagnose and treat.

Task is viewed as an objective set of behaviours necessary to accomplish a goal (Neistadt and Crepeau, 1998). Tasks relate to work, leisure, school and social interactions, such as in forming a job, or engaging in leisure activity.

Task analysis is 'the breakdown of a particular occupation/ activity into its components' (Dowd, 1993, p. 27). It is a critical part of the occupational therapy evaluation and intervention process (Watson, 2003).

Test battery is a group of tests selected to comprehensively measure an individual's capacity such as work capacity, self-care or ability return to work.

Therapeutic intervention is 'the use of strategies (e.g. teaching, healing, adapting) which are directed at meeting the client's need for establishing or restoring or developing or improving occupational performances, in collaboration between the client, the occupational therapist and significant others' (Neistadt and Crepeau, 1998, p. 533).

Universal (ergonomic) design is 'based on sound biomechanical principles applied to the manufacture of utensils and tools used for self-care and housework to make them useful for all people including individuals with disabilities' (Anson, 1994, p. 258) and in housing adaptations (Mace, 1998).

Usability testing (user-acceptance testing) for assistive devices is the process of product development and determination of its efficacy including product description (load, height, weight, material, stability, comfort, adjustment regarding anthropometric principles) (Jacobs and Bettencourt, 1995).

Vibration is a risk factor for cumulative trauma disorders, decreased manual dexterity and grip strength. It can be caused by repetitive use of chainsaws, pneumatic drivers, grinders and jack hammers (Keyserling, 2000a, 2000b).

Vocational assessment is a comprehensive interdisciplinary process, which comprises gathering and analysing information by using real or simulated work. The individual's characteristics, education and work history is obtained and physical, mental and emotional function, capacity for work, work tolerance and work limitations are assessed. The purpose is to guide the individual's preparation to an affiliation, and provide him or her with insight into his or her vocational potential (Dowd, 1993).

Vocational interest test measures 'an individual's preferences toward occupation-related tasks or jobs' (Stein and Cutler, 2000, p. 512).

Vocational rehabilitation 'is the restoration of work function in client's with mental or physical disabilities' (Stein and Roose, 2000, p. 324).

Work is paid or unpaid activity that contributes to subsistence, produces a service or product, and is culturally meaningful to the worker.

Work adjustment is 'any individualized series of techniques, methods, and processes utilized to enable an individual to achieve harmony between self and work environment' and includes '(a) the process of adjusting to work versus the outcome of adjusting to work; (b) individual versus external support; (c) daily versus life-time commitments; and (d) simple versus complex criteria that are needed for job satisfaction' (Dowd, 1993, p. 31).

Work capacity comprises the worker's physical, cognitive and social abilities, behaviour in work, tolerance of the work, competence and professional skill that he or she uses for carrying out a specific work task and which is the equivalent of the worker's duties.

Work conditioning is used to enable a client with a work-related injury to return to work as part of a comprehensive occupational rehabilitation programme. Traditionally work conditioning includes physical therapy activities to increase muscle strengthening, endurance, range of motion, coordination, cardiovascular capacity and body mechanics. Schonstein et al. (2003), in reviewing the efficacy of work conditioning for workers with back pain, they found that researchers used the terms work conditioning, work hardening, physical conditioning and functional restoration/exercise programmes interchangeably to identify return-to-work programmes that aimed to improve work status and function.

Work hardening is an interdisciplinary team approach that applies a highly structured environment with supervised, goal-oriented real or simulated work activities designed to maximize the injured worker's return to work. The activities include exercises to increase muscle strength, range of motion and graded activities to improve function in biomechanical, neuromuscular, cardiovascular and psychosocial areas. The work tasks simulate bending, lifting, carrying, standing and sitting positions often applied by using functional capacity evaluations. Work hardening concerns productivity, safety, physical tolerances, stamina, endurance and worker behaviours (Dowd, 1993; Ogden Niemeyer and Jacobs, 1989).

Work samples are well-defined work activities involving tasks, materials and tools that are identical or similar to those in an actual job or cluster of jobs (Dowd, 1993). Work sample are used to assess an individual's vocational aptitudes, work characteristics and/or vocational interests (Dowd, 1993). Examples include the VALPAR Component Work Samples (Valpar International Corporation, 1993).

Work simplification is 'a technique that divides tasks into smaller steps or uses simple methods to make activities easier' (Stein and Roose, 2000, p. 329).

Work standards:

- Sedentary work is defined by the Department of Labor (US Department of Labor, Employment and Training Administration, 1991a) as exerting up to 10 pounds of force approximately one-third of the worker's time, to lift, carry, push, pull or move objects. Sedentary work is mostly sitting at a desk with walking and standing occasionally.
- Light work according to the US Department of Labor, Employment and Training Administration (1991a) is exerting up to 20 pounds of force occasionally. It requires sitting most of the time. Work demands exceed sedentary work.
- Medium work is exerting 20–50 pounds of force occasionally and 10–25 pounds of force frequently (US Department of Labor, Employment and Training Administration, 1991a).
- Heavy work is exerting 50–100 pounds of force occasionally (US Department of Labor, Employment and Training Administration, 1991a).

Worker Traits Data Book (WTDB) contains definitions and ratings of work requirements of each of about 20,000 occupations. These requirements are defined as general educational development (GED) (three factors; scale 6 = high to 1 = low); training time (four time periods); aptitudes (11 factors; scale 1 = high to low = 5); temperaments (11 factors; scale yes – no); physical demands (20 items; scale yes – no; apart from strength = 5-degree scale); and environmental conditions (14 factors; scale not present – continuously present, apart from noise = 5-degree scale) (Myall, 1994).

References

American Occupational Therapy Association (2002). Occupational therapy practice framework: Domain and process. American Journal of Occupational Therapy, 56, 609–639.

Americans with Disabilities Act of 1990 (1991). 28 CFR Part 36: ADA standards for accessible design (Rev. July 1, 1994). Retrieved 24 January 2004, http://www.usdoj.gov/crt/ada/adastd94.pdf

Anson, D. (1994). Finding your way in the maze of computer access technology. American Journal of Occupational Therapy, 48, 121–129.

Baltimore Therapeutic Equipment Company (1992). Clinical application model: A conically oriented reference model for users of the BTE work simulator. Baltimore: Baltimore Therapeutic Equipment Company.

Branick, L. (2003). Integrating the principles of energy conservation during everyday activities. Caring, 22, 30–31.

Breines, E.B. (2001). Occupational therapy interventions. The biomechanical approach. In L.W. Pedretti and M.B. Early (Eds). Occupational Therapy: Practice Skills for Physical Dysfunction (5th edn; pp. 503–529). St Louis: Mosby.

Brown, C., McDaniel, Couch R. and McClanahan, M. (1994). Vocational Evaluation Systems and Software: A Consumer's Guide. Menomonie. Stout, WI: Materials Development Center, University of Wisconsin.

Burt, C.M. (2000). Work evaluation and work hardening. In L.W. Pedretti and M.B. Early (Eds). Occupational Therapy: Practice Skills for Physical Dysfunction (5th edn; pp. 226–236). St Louis: Mosby.

Cardinal, B.J. and Spaziani, M.D. (2003). ADA compliance and the accessibility of physical activity facilities in western Oregon. American Journal of Health Promotion, 17, 197–201.

Chee, H.L., Rampal, K.G. and Chandrasakaran, A. (2004). Ergonomic risk factors of work processes in the semi-conductor industry in Peninsular Malaysia. Industrial Health, 42, 373–381.

Christiansen, C., Baum, C. and Bass-Haugen J. (2005). Occupational Therapy: performance, participation, and well-being. Thorofare: SLACK.

Cook, A.M. and Hussey, S.M. (2002). Technologies that enable mobility. In A.M. Hussey and S.M. Hussey (Ed.), Assistive Technology: Principles and Practices (pp. 329–373). St Louis: Mosby.

Dowd, L. (1993). Glossary of Terminology for Vocational Assessment, Evaluation, and Work Adjustment. Menomonie, WI: Material Development Center, Stout Vocational Rehabilitation Institute.

Earle-Richardson, G., Fulmer, S., Jenkins, P. Mason, C., Bresee, C. and May, J. (2004). Ergonomic analysis of New York apple harvest work using a Posture-Activities-Tools-Handling (PATH) work sampling approach. Journal Agriculture Safety Health, 10, 163–176.

Educational Resources Information Center (ERIC) (2002). Scope note for case study as a teaching method. [Data-base]. Lanham, MD: Educational Resources Information Center.

Egidius, H. (1999). PBL och casemetodik. Hur man gör och varför. (In Swedish). [PBL and case method. How you act and why]. Lund: Studentlitteratur.

Engel, J.M., Jensen, M.P. and Schwartz, L. (2004). Outcome of biofeedback-assisted relaxation for pain in adults with cerebral palsy: preliminary findings. Applied Psychophysiological Biofeedback, 29, 135–140.

Farr, M., Ludden, L.L and Shatkin, L. (2001). Guide for Occupational Exploration (3rd edn). Indianapolis: JIST.

Farrell, J. (1993). Predetermined Motion–Time standard in rehabilitation. A review. Work. A Journal of Prevention Assessment and Rehabilitation, 3, 56–72.

Folts, D.J., Giannini, A.J. and Otonicar, B. (1995). Cognitive workload. In K. Jacobs and C.M. Bettencourt (Eds), Ergonomics for Therapists (pp. 43–54). Newton, MA: Butterworth-Heineman.

Foti, D. (2000). Activities of daily living. In L.W. Pedretti and M.B. Early (Eds), Occupational Therapy: Practice Skills for Physical Dysfunction (pp. 124–171). St Louis: Mosby.

Gitlin, L.N. (1998). Testing home modification interventions: Issues of theory, measurement, design, and implementation. Annual Review of Gerontology and Geriatrics, 18, 190–246.

Gordon, J.E., Powell, C. and Rockwood, K. (1999). Goal attainment scaling as a measure of clinically important change in nursing-home patients. Age and Aging, 28, 275–281.

Guthrie, P.F., Westphal, L., Dahlman, B., Berg, M., Behnam, K. and Ferrell, D. (2004) A patient lifting intervention for preventing the work-related injuries of nurses. Work. A Journal of Prevention Assessment and Rehabilitation, 22, 79–88.

Hackman, J. and Oldham, G. (1975). Development of the Job Diagnostic Survey. Journal of Applied Psychology, 60, 159–170.

Harbin, G. and Olson, J. (2005). Post-offer, pre-placement testing in industry. American Journal of Industrial Medicine, 47, 296–307.

Iwarsson, S. (1999). The Housing Enabler: An objective tool for assessing accessibility. British Journal of Occupational Therapy, 62, 491–497.

Jacobs, K. (1994). Job analysis: Equipping therapists to deal with the increasing number of work-related injuries. Rehabilitation Management, 7, 113–114.

Jacobs, K. and Bettencourt, C.M. (1995). Ergonomics for Therapists. Boston: Butterworth-Heinemann.

Joe, B.E. (1991). Quality assurance in occupational therapy: A practitioner's guide to setting up a QA system using three models. Rockville, MD: The American Occupational Therapy Association.

Karasek, R.T.T. (1990). Health, Work, Stress, Productivity and the Reconstruction of Working Life. New York: Basic Books.

Keyserling, W.M. (2000a). Workplace risk factors and occupational musculoskeletal disorders, Part 1: A review of biomechanical and psychophysical research on risk factors associated with low-back pain. AIHAI: A Journal for the Science of Occupational and Environmental Health and Safety, 61, 39–50.

Keyserling, W.M. (2000b). Workplace risk factors and occupational musculoskeletal disorders, Part 2: A review of biomechanical and psychophysical research on risk factors associated with upper extremity disorders. AIHAJ : A Journal for the Science of Occupational and Environmental Health and Safety, 61, 231–243.

Keyserling, W.M., Armstrong, T.J. and Punnett, L. (1991). Ergonomic job analysis is a structured approach for identifying risk factors associated with overexertion injuries and disorders. Applied Occupational Environment Hygiene, 6, 353–363.

King, P.M. (1994). Participatory ergonomics: A group dynamics perspective. Work. A Journal of Prevention Assessment and Rehabilitation, 4, 195–198.

Kiresuck, T., Smith, A. and Cardillo, J.E. (1994). Goal Attainment Scaling: Application and Measurement. London: Lawrence Erlbaum.

Lamberth, B. and Comello, R.J. (2005). Identifying elements of job satisfaction to improve retention rates in healthcare. Radiological Management, 27, 34–38.

Law, M., Acheson, C.B., Steward, D., Letts, L., Rigby, P. and Strong, S. (1994). Person–environment relations. Work, 4, 228–238.

Leyman, E., Mirka, G., Kaber D. and Sommerich, C. (2004). Cervicobrachial muscle response to cognitive load in a dual-task scenario. Ergonomics, 47, 625–645.

Lyman, H.B. (1991). Test Scores and What They Mean (5th edn). Boston: Allyn and Bacon.

Mace, R.L. (1998). Universal design in housing. Assistive Technology, 10, 21–28.

Marshall, M.M. and Armstrong, T.J. (2004). Observational assessment of forceful exertion and the perceived force demands of daily activities. Journal of Occupational Rehabilitation, 14, 281–294.

Matheson, L.N. (1998) Symptom magnification syndrome. In S.J. Isenhagen (Ed.), Work Injury: Management in Prevention (pp. 257–270). Rockville, MD: Aspen.

May, D.R., Reed, K., Schwoerer, C.E. and Potter, P. (2004). Ergonomic office design and aging: A quasi-experimental field study of employee reactions to an ergonomic intervention program. Journal Occupational Health Psychology, 9, 123–135.

Meister, D. (1999). The History of Human Factors and Ergonomics. Mahwah, NJ: Lawrence Erlbaum.

Montgomery, H. and Johansson, U.S. (1988). Life Values: Their Structure and Relation to Life Situations. Göteborg: Department of Psychiatry, University of Göteborg.

Myall, D. (1994). The Worker Traits Data Book. Indianapolis: JIST Works.

National Library of Medicine (2002). MeSH subject headers. Available at http://www.ncbi.nlm.nih.gov/entrez/query.fcgi?db=mesh, retrieved 20 september, 2005

Neistadt, M.E. and Crepeau, E.B. (1998). Theories that guide practice. In Willard and Spackman's Occupational Therapy (9th edn; pp. 525–535). Philadelphia, PA: Lippincott.

Norris, P.A. and Fahrion, S.L. (1993). Autogenic biofeedback in psychophysiological therapy and stress management. In P.M. Lehrer and R.L. Woolflolk (Eds), Principles and Practice of Stress Management (2nd edn; pp. 231–262). New York: Guilford.

Novak, C.B. (2004). Upper extremity work-related musculoskeletal disorders: a treatment perspective. Journal of Orthopedic and Sports Physical Therapy, 34, 628–637.

ONET Consortium (2005). Occupational Information Network (ONET online). Available at http://online.onetcenter.org, retrieved 20 September 2005.

Ogden Niemeyer, L. and Jacobs, K. (1989). Work Hardening: State of the Art. Thorofare: SLACK.

Parenté, R. and Anderson-Parenté, B. (1986). Alternative research strategies for occupational therapy, Part 2: Ideographic and quality assurance research. American Journal of Occupational Therapy, 40, 428–431.

Pedretti, L.W. and Early, M.B. (2001). Occupational performance and models of practice for physical dysfunction. In L.W. Pedretti and M.B. Early (Eds),

Occupational Therapy: Practice Skills for Physical Dysfunction (pp. 3–13). St Louis: Mosby.

Pellerito J.M. (2003). The effects of traditional and computer-aided instruction on promoting independent skin care in adults with paraplegia. Occupational Therapy International, 10, 1–19.

Power, P.W. (2000). A Guide to Vocational Assessment (3rd edn). Austin: ProEd.

Scriven, M. (1991). Evaluation Thesaurus (4th edn). London: Sage.

Söderback, I. (1988). A housework-based assessment of intellectual functions in patients with acquired brain damage: Development and evaluation of an occupational therapy method. Scandinavian Journal of Rehabilitation Medicine, 20, 57–69.

Spenner, K. (1990). Skill: Meanings, methods and measurements. Work and Occupations, 17, 399–421.

Stein, F. (2002). The ergonomic model in occupational therapy. Presentation at the World Federation of Occupational Therapy Congress, Stockholm, Sweden, June.

Stein, F. and Associates (2003) Stress Management Questionnaire: An Instrument for Self-regulating Stress. [Individual Version. CD-Rom] New York: Thomson/Delmar Learning.

Stein, F. and Cutler, S.K. (2000). Clinical Research in Occupational Therapy (4th edn). San Diego: Singular/Thomson Learning.

Stein, F. and Cutler, S. (2001). Psychosocial Occupational Therapy: A Holistic Approach (2nd edn). San Diego: Thomson/Delmar Learning.

Stein, F. and Roose, B. (2000). Pocket Guide to Treatment in Occupational Therapy. San Diego: Singular.

UAW-Ford National Joint Committee on Health and Safety (1996). Ergonomic Action Guide. Detroit, MI: UAW-Ford National Joint Committee on Health and Safety.

Ulin S.S. and Keyserling, W.M. (2004). Case studies of ergonomic interventions in automotive parts distribution operation. Journal of Occupational Rehabilitation, 14, 307–326.

US Department of Labor, Employment and Training Administration (1991a). Dictionary of Occupational Titles (4th edn). Washington, DC: US Government Printing Office. Available at http://www.oalj.dol.gov/libdot.htm

US. Department of Labor, Employment and Training Administration (1991b). The Revised Handbook for Analyzing Jobs. Indianapolis: JIST Works.

Valpar International Corporation (1993). Valpar Component Work Samples. Tucson, AZ: Valpar International Corporation.

Wang, P.P., Bradley, E.M. and Cignac, M.A. (2004). Perceived need for workplace accommodation and labor-force participation in Canadian adults with activity limitations. American Journal of Public Health, 94, 1515–1518.

Watson, D. (2003). Task Analysis, an Individual and Population Approach (2nd edn).Washington, DC: AOTA.

Wheeler, D., Graves, J., Miller, G., O'Connor, P. and MacMillan, M. (1994). Functional assessment for prediction of lifting capacity. Spine, 19, 1021–1026.

World Health Organization (2001). International Classification of Functioning, Disability, and Health [ICF]. Geneva, Switzerland: World Health Organization.

Index